A Guide to Hospital Administration and Planning

Dinesh Bhatia • Prabhat Kumar Chaudhari
Bhupinder Chaudhary
Sushman Sharma • Kunaal Dhingra
Editors

A Guide to Hospital Administration and Planning

Springer

Editors
Dinesh Bhatia
Department of Biomedical Engineering
North Eastern Hill University
Shillong, Meghalaya, India

Prabhat Kumar Chaudhari
Division of Orthodontics
All India Institute of Medical Sciences
New Delhi, Delhi, India

Bhupinder Chaudhary
Department of Hospital Management
H.N.G. University
Patan, Gujarat, India

Sushman Sharma
Department of Hospital Management
H.N.G. University
Patan, Gujarat, India

Kunaal Dhingra
Division of Periodontics, Centre for Dental Education and Research
All India Institute of Medical Sciences, New Delhi
New Delhi, Delhi, India

ISBN 978-981-19-6691-0 ISBN 978-981-19-6692-7 (eBook)
https://doi.org/10.1007/978-981-19-6692-7

This Springer imprint is published by the registered company Springer Nature Singapore Pte Ltd.
The registered company address is: 152 Beach Road, #21-01/04 Gateway East, Singapore 189721, Singapore

Preface

We are happy to write the preface for the book entitled "Hospital Administration and Planning." This book is a compilation of work by experts from different domains working in the healthcare industry, ranging from hospital planning to quality management, and clinical services to disaster management. Since healthcare organization is a very diverse, sensitive, and intricate area, it demands a thorough and flawless planning. The structure should not only be operationally efficient, but also be safe for its occupants and visitors. The book starts with a brief introduction of the healthcare sector at different levels. It also attempts to justify how the changing healthcare landscape has paved the way for establishing a contemporary and ever-evolving specialty of hospital planning and designing, which is dynamic in nature and requires continuous improvements and updates frequently.

This book has been planned in a way wherein clinical and nonclinical departments have been separately classified and their respective standards and guidelines have been incorporated while describing the planning concepts. Critical areas of a hospital such as ICU and CCU have been detailed specifically as the operational requirements and level of different sophistication required.

A chapter on security aspects and disaster management has also been thoroughly envisioned based on the current scenario at global level. Issues and management of hospital-acquired infection have been discussed in different chapters based on its relevance and application in that particular area. Further, the book introduces the concept of green and eco-friendly self-sustainable hospitals. The book also focuses on the planning requirements and statutory considerations as per the "International Patient Safety Guidelines."

We believe that the book would immensely benefit the clinicians, scholars, and researchers working in the field of hospital administration or healthcare management, biomedical engineering, dental studies, paramedical courses, and relevant industries. People working in the field of healthcare, health insurance, policy making, accreditation, and quality management would avail additional knowledge from this book.

The important features of the book include the incorporation of the fundamentals of project management techniques and its implementation in a hospital setup. It provides notes on the planning of facilities with respect to international standards and guidelines suggested by organizations such as the ASHRAE, JCI, WHO, and LEED. The book includes case studies and good practices of healthcare organizations at global level and their methodology. Several illustrations pertaining to the different departments and functional areas, complementing theoretical explanation, have been added to the book to provide better understanding to the audience.

Shillong, Meghalaya, India — Dinesh Bhatia
Patan, Gujarat, India — Bhupinder Chaudhary
New Delhi, Delhi, India — Prabhat Kumar Chaudhari
Patan, Gujarat, India — Sushman Sharma
New Delhi, Delhi, India — Kunaal Dhingra

Acknowledgments

Writing a book involves enormous efforts from all collaborators and contributors. We would like to extend our sincere gratitude to all contributing authors for their painstaking efforts and helping us in incorporating finer details in this book. The book covers diverse topics which would enlighten the readers. We are grateful to our parents and family members for their kind support in allowing us to complete the book in time. We acknowledge the constant support of our employers and the Springer International Publisher for allowing us to complete this challenging task of preparing the assignment in available time. Without their constant support and efforts, it would not have been possible to prepare and improve the quality of the book. We do hope that this book would serve the due purpose for which it was initiated and support people working in the field to enhance their skills and guide budding researchers in the field.

Finally, we thank the Almighty God for his kind blessings, wisdom, and grace to enable us to complete this book. We are thankful to the support of our parents, family members and well-wishers for allowing us sufficient time to complete the book in time. We hope that the readers will be benefitted from the contents present in the book.

Dinesh Bhatia, NEHU, Shillong, Meghalaya, India
Bhupinder Chaudhary, HNGU, Patan, Gujarat, India
Prabhat Kumar Chaudhari, AIIMS, New Delhi, Delhi, India
Sushman Sharma, HNGU, Patan, Gujarat, India
Kunaal Dhingra, AIIMS, New Delhi, Delhi, India

Contents

Chapter 1
Hospital Designing and Planning

Himanshu Bansal, Riya Mittal, and Vijay Kumar

Abbreviations

EPA	Environment Protection Agency
MEP	Mechanical, electrical, and plumbing
NIH	National Institutes of Health
SOP	Standard operating procedure
WHO	World Health Organization
NABH	National Accreditation Board for Hospitals

1.1 Introduction

The word hospital has been derived from the Latin word "hospice"; in fact, the words hospital, hotel, and hostel all are derived from the general Latin root "hospice," which means a place or an establishment where the guest should be received, also known as hospitium or hospitale. The term hospital at different times has been utilized to refer to an institution for the care of the sick and injured people;

H. Bansal (✉)
Amity Institute of Neuropsychology and Neurosciences, Amity University, Noida, India

Ministry of Health and Family Welfare, Civil Hospital Narwana, Jind, Haryana, India

R. Mittal
Ministry of Health and Family Welfare, Civil Hospital Narwana, Jind, Haryana, India

V. Kumar
Department of Audiology and Speech-Language Pathology, Amity University, Gurgaon, Haryana, India
e-mail: vkumar@ggn.amity.edu

D. Bhatia et al. (eds.), *A Guide to Hospital Administration and Planning*,
https://doi.org/10.1007/978-981-19-6692-7_1

providing stay for the pilgrims and the wayfarer was also one of the important functions of the hospital. In its earliest forms, the hospital was usually aimed at poor people's care and the destitute providing the aura of "almshouse." A hospital was no longer an institution where public, i.e., people, went to die. Today, hospital means an institute in which sick or wounded persons are taken care of and treated. As per Stedman's Medical Dictionary, a hospital is defined as "an institution for the care, cure and treatment of the sick and wounded, for the study of diseases and for the training of doctors and nurses." The WHO defines hospital as follows: "A hospital is a combined or an integral part of social and medical organization, function of which should be to provide complete health care to the people in population, both curative and preventive, and whose outpatient services reach out to the family and to its home environment. The hospital is also an institution where training of the health workers and biomedical-research is conducted." The quality and suitability of the hospital environment are key contributors to the patient experience. Early and consistent clinical engagement is an important aspect to enable true alignment of clinical services and facilities. It is necessary that the planning of hospital facilities must respond to changing models of care and is undertaken through an authentic "whole system" approach [1]. Most hospitals are planned and designed for super-specialized medical functions. This purpose might conflict with the need to design the hospital services to evolve and change functions with time [2]. This challenge raises very important questions: Can both our current needs and future demands be met by hospital planning? What is optimal design? Is it a design that fits in a specific function or which supports future change of function [3]? The unprecedented rate of social, technological, and medical change has led to the development of different healthcare architectural approaches to design for a specific medical program while planning for its future change [4, 5]. A more extreme approach by Llewelyn-Davies and Weeks declared that functions change so rapidly that designers should no longer aim for an optimum fit between building and function. The real requirement is to design a building that will allow change of function [6]. Zeidler declared that the concept of "form follows function" does not meet the modern-day requirements of a hospital, and therefore, the true gestalt of a hospital lies in the acceptance of the unpredictability of future needs [7]. Huge hospital building projects provide an ideal opportunity to implement change through the planning and design phases. This will require a planning team approach by doctors, nurses, allied health professionals and administrators, architects, and simulation engineers [8].

1.2 Need of Hospital Planning

An essential service is rendered by the hospital, and hospital planning plays a major role in fulfilling this responsibility and requires certain universally acknowledged principles by providing:

(a) High-quality patient care
(b) Effective community orientation

(c) Orderly planning
(d) Economic viability
(e) A sound architectural plan
(f) Regionalization of hospital service

1.3 Hospital Planning Process

Once the idea to construct a hospital is formulated, a multidisciplinary planning team should be constituted. This is the first step in planning a hospital project. In the very starting, the planning team may consist of:

- Owner/representative of the governing/local body
- Hospital and nursing administrators
- Financial expert
- Architect of hospital
- Health statisticians

At later stage, addition to the planning team is done with:

- Specialist doctors for planning of different areas of hospital
- Hospital consultants
- Engineers
- Landscape architects
- Interior designers of competence

1.3.1 Hospital Planning Team

A suitable qualified and competent planning working staff is required to complete the technical requirements of patients, community, and owners. Participation of professional doctors, specialists, nurses, technical staff, architects, engineers, hospital administrators, and consultants must be involved in a hospital planning team.

1.3.2 Hospital Consultant

A class of professionals known as hospital consultants were firstly emerged in Europe and the USA, which are different from the professional hospital administrators. A hospital consultant is trained like a hospital administrator with proper experience who can profitably do the job of consultant and administrator and provides expert guidance in the areas which cover:

- Local and regional surveys of the medical and health care
- Analysis of demand and need for hospital facilities

- Assessment of the range, type, and extent of services required
- Selection of equipment
- Administrative and institutional relationships

1.3.3 Techniques Adopted by the Planning Team

Techniques adopted by the planning team are the following:

- Each member takes a lead in formulating a proposal, and each proposal is reviewed and modified by the team either in the conferences or through written comments.
- Circulation of questionnaires to medical staff members.
- Need and demands of the population.
- Discussion with other people involved in similar situation.
- Availability of land.
- Means of communication: tele-, rail, road, and air.
- Meteorological data consisting of temperature range, average annual rainfall, humidity, wind velocity, etc.
- Geographical characteristics such as terrain, soil structure, seismic data, subsoil water level, and rivers.
- Demographic pattern: factors such as age, sex, occupational characteristics, and economic and literacy status.
- Mortality and morbidity trends in the population.
- Visit to other hospitals to inspect the units and equipment.
- Existing healthcare facilities' data including use of such patterns.
- Models are constructed to test the room size and arrangements discussed.
- Review of plans in hospital to inspect a specific unit or a piece of equipment.
- Further plans for development of the area including development of industries.

1.3.4 Feasibility Analysis Done by the Hospital Planning Team

Hospital planning team should be aware of the feasibility analysis which is a major component in hospital planning project [9, 10].

Feasibility analysis has the following components:

1. **Data collection**: Demographic data, epidemiological data, geographical data, existing facilities' data, and pattern of the diseases should be recorded.
2. **Need assessment**:

   (a) Types of health, i.e., preventive, rehabilitative, curative, general, or specialized healthcare, should be assessed.
   (b) Types of vulnerable health, i.e., elderly, children, women, and specified disease group.

(c) Financial status and source of earning.
(d) Extent of utilization of present healthcare facilities.
(e) Level of leadership and motivation among people.
(f) Housing and education facility for hospital staff family.

3. **Transport and communication:**

   (a) Better to have close access to railhead or bus stand.
   (b) 24-h public transport and private taxis available.
   (c) Nearby telephone exchange/line with adequate number of pairs.
   (d) Easy access to transmission towers for uninterrupted communication.

4. **Water supply and electricity:**

   (a) Availability of deep table subsoil water.
   (b) Adequate water supply from corporation/Jal Board (400 L/bed/day).
   (c) Good maintained sewerage system (300–400 L/bed/day).
   (d) Easy access to sewerage treatment plant.
   (e) Facility for biomedical waste disposal nearby.
   (f) Electric substation in close vicinity.
   (g) Availability of three-phase electric supply with adequate load (1 kW/bed/day).
   (h) Dedicated electric supply line.
   (i) Standby generator.

5. **Demographic pattern:**

   (a) Type of residents—high, middle, and low class.
   (b) Status of affordability.
   (c) Extent of the people to be covered, i.e., villages and towns.
   (d) People, beliefs, attitude, traditions, practices, and culture.
   (e) Availability of rest houses, lodges, hotels, and dharamshalas.

6. **Environmental study:**

   (a) Area should have clear sunshine, must avoid big buildings, and trees nearby.
   (b) Climate must be moderate.
   (c) No noise nearby or smoke/chemical-emitting industries.
   (d) Fresh airflow.
   (e) Should be away from roads having heavy traffic.

7. **Prioritization of need**
8. **Site selection:**

   (a) Availability of sufficient land depending on the size of the hospital and its future expansion.
   (b) Land required for 25 beds—5 acres, 100 beds—15 acres, 200 beds—25 acres, 500 beds—50 acres, 750 beds—80 acres, 1000 beds—100 acres approximately [11].
   (c) Must have good approaching roads.

(d) Soil condition suitable for construction, not landfill area.
(e) Proper drainage of rainwater.
(f) Subsoil water and mineral level.

Feasibility analysis includes estimation of the level of expertise required, qualitative and quantitative assessment of the possible outcomes, determination of the skill set that is required, and identification of the crucial factors, probable risk, and operational gaps. Feasibility study determines the viability of an idea or a business initiative in the hospital planning process. A feasibility study also contains a detailed analysis report of what is needed to complete the proposed project. The report may include a description of the new product or venture, a market analysis, the technology and labor needed, as well as the sources of financing and capital. Feasibility analysis establishes a base of hospital planning project and hence is the most important phase in hospital planning.

1.4 Size of the Hospital

Two methods can be adopted for determining the size of the hospital [12]:

1. **Bed death ratio:** 0.5 general bed is needed per annual death rate. If we presume 200 deaths per year in a given community, then $0.5 \times 200 = 100$ general beds will be needed for that community.
2. **Bed population ratio** = $\dfrac{A \times S \times 100}{365 \times \text{PO}}$

where ***A*** = no. of inpatient admission, ***S*** = average length of stay, **PO** = percentage occupancy.

If the statistics is not available, then the formula can be used on the assumption from data of other regions.

1.5 Site Selection

Factors necessary to keep in mind for site selection are the following:

(a) **Area and land required:** This depends on the proposed bed strength and the specialized services to be provided. Hospitals should be planned keeping in view the growth of hospital in near future, say 10 years, 25 years, or even up to 50 years. The site should be large enough to enable to expand further.

The usual minimum space occupied by a bed and its accessories is about 100 sq. ft. Minimum area covered in a hospital is about 60–80 square meters per bed.

(b) **Accessibility**: The hospital should be within easy reach of the community. As per the NIH, New Delhi members of the community must be able to reach within 30 min of travel time.

(c) **Environment**: The hospital should have fresh air and sunlight. It should be free from smoke and hazardous industrial emissions.
(d) **Availability of resources**: (1) **Water:** 500 L of water per patient/day is required. Water should be available 24 h. Storage facility for 7 days must be planned in the form of underground water or overhead tank. (2) **Electricity**: Requirement of energy for a hospital with no central air-conditioning and vertical transportation should be 1 kW/bed. In super-specialty hospitals, 7 kW/bed is required for functioning of all the equipment. At present, the trend is at 2 kW/patient/day since the electrical consumption and energy will be required for lighting the area other than the building also. Power supply should be from public utility and at least from two sources with substation in the vicinity of the hospital; it should be continuous, and provisioning of generator should be there. (3) **Waste disposal:** The centralized sewage system should be available near the site selected so that the sewage system of the hospital can be connected to the central sewer. Rate of solid waste should be 1 kg/bed/day, and rate of liquid waste must be 450 mL/bed/day.

1.6 Hospital Architect

The architect has to collect the perception of the complete technical and administrative desires of the hospital. His or her accountability is to translate medical and administrative requirements into architectural and engineering realities, which encompass land site selection, orientation of buildings, supervision of construction, utilities, and electrical and mechanical installation. Architectural creativity is an assignment requiring high inventive approach, an excessively high degree of expert skills, and ingenuity. An architect is of price solely if he or she has experience in medical institution/hospital construction and architecture.

1.7 Preparation of Detailed Architectural Report

Early employment of the hospital architect is the first step towards planning a successful hospital building project. The architect brief (including all the dimensions of the project) is discussed with users and administration and if necessary modified. Then, the architect prepares a detailed report including:

- Architectural drawings/models
- Cost estimates
- Time frame for completion of the project
- Maintenance facilities

1.7.1 Major Departments of a General Hospital

A general hospital is likely to have the following departments:

1. **Administration**
2. **Outpatient department**
3. **Inpatient department**
4. **Hospital services**:
   (a) **Sterilization**
   (b) **Dietary**
   (c) **Laundry**
   (d) **Transport**
   (e) **Stores**
5. **Emergency department**
6. **Engineering services**:
   (a) **Civil engineering: building maintenance, horticulture, water supply, and plumbing**
   (b) **Mechanical engineering: air-conditioning and refrigeration**

1.8 Identifying Equipment Needs

Equipment needs usually generate from the user departments. The need for the new equipment arises from the professional staff to improve the quality of patient care, i.e., both diagnostic and therapeutic services.

The need for equipment falls under three categories:
(a) Acquiring new equipment
(b) Addition of equipment
(c) Replacement of old and obsolete equipment

1.8.1 Acquiring New Equipment

Provision of efficient patient care services of an acceptable standard depends on the right sort of equipment available and maintained in good order. So, careful planning should be done in equipping any health facility whether it be a dispensary in a village or a referral hospital. The following fundamental principles should underline the choice of equipment for all new hospitals:

(a) Reliance on mechanical or electrical should be kept to the absolute minimum.
(b) All equipment should be simple to function.
(c) The equipment chosen should be that which requires locally available spares and maintenance facilities.

The following checkpoints should be applied in the evaluation of the need for new equipment:

(a) Does it suit the socioeconomic environment of the community to which the hospital is providing healthcare?
(b) Type of services provided by the hospital.
(c) Range of services provided by the hospital.

For example, a defibrillator or a ventilator may not be of much use in PHC, whereas an autoclave and routine surgical instruments will serve the purpose.

1.8.2 Addition of Equipment

Expansion of patient care services requires additional equipment. Limiting factors in this aspect are limited resources and limited availability of technical people to maintain the equipment.

Questions coming to mind before going for additional equipment are the following:

(a) Is there increased workload for the existing one?
(b) Is the existing equipment time consuming?
(c) Is it professionally the best method of treatment?
(d) Are there some better alternatives?
(e) Is the extra expenditure justified?

1.8.3 Replacement of Old or Obsolete Equipment

Replacement of old equipment with the new one depends upon the following factors:

(a) **Economic factor/analysis**: In making economic analysis of a potential equipment, capital purchase has to compare the proposed new equipment with the existing old one. The comparison is to determine the measure of profitability.
(b) **Technological and engineering factors**: These factors must be compatible with the buyer's existing equipment, process, and layout. They must also be in accordance with standards established by state and central governments such as occupational safety and environmental protection.

A few major considerations should be kept in mind:

1. **Physical sizes and mounting dimensions**: Will the equipment fit into the existing available space satisfactorily? Can it be tied to existing supporting structures without difficulty?
2. **Flexibility**: Can equipment be moved or relocated easily?
3. **Power requirements**: Can existing power supplies be used?

4. Safety features: Are the safety features comparable with those of existing equipment?
5. **Pollution characteristics**: Does the equipment perform in accordance with the EPA requirements concerning pollution and contamination discharge levels?

1.8.4 Calculation of Requirement of Equipment

Once the need for equipment is over, the next thing is to estimate the requirement of equipment. The estimation should be realistic and should consider the future needs. The estimation of requirement of equipment depends upon:

1. Type of equipment
2. Quantity required
3. Anticipated patient load in future
4. Type and range of services provided by the hospital
5. Expansion plans of the hospital
6. Financial resources

1.8.5 Collection of Information

The next step after assessment of needs and estimation of equipment is to gather the following information:

(a) If there is a purchase department, it keeps a watch on the developments in major equipment industries.
(b) The purchasing department regularly provides information about the new developments of equipment technology to the user department.
(c) The purchasing department's responsibility is to locate the vendors and secure the information required by the user department.
(d) It is the duty of the purchasing department to arrange the display and demonstration of new equipment so that user department can test and compare them.
(e) The purchasing department arranges meeting between potential suppliers and user department.
(f) The purchasing department arranges user's trials.
(g) Arrange visits to other hospitals which are using the proposed equipment already to know more operating and technical details.

1.8.6 Product Evaluation and Specification Audit

The last step is to produce evaluation and specific audit. The product evaluation involves numerous factors:

(a) **Evaluation of professional audibility of equipment**
(b) **Cost comparison and cost-benefit analysis**
(c) **Compatibility with the existing system**
(d) **Existing maintenance capability**
(e) **Utility and facility requirements like water, power, air-conditioning, sewage, and hygiene**

In specification audit, all the technical specifications of proposed equipment should be written as functionally as possible and clearly by the user department. Most of the users hold bias for and against some specific brands, so every effort should be made to prevent this bias in the specifications. The hospital administrator should persuade the user departments to serve the hospital's best interest in unbiased functional specifications.

1.9 Equipping a Hospital

Mechanical and electrical installations and the plant and the equipment component in a modern general hospital have been estimated to cost about 40% of the entire hospital project, out of which about half of it is required for the medical equipment. Universal application of the equipment in a hospital can be classified as:

(a) Physical plant
(b) Hospital furniture and appliances
(c) General-purpose furniture and appliances
(d) Therapeutic and diagnostic equipment

1.9.1 Plants and Equipment Required in the Hospital

(a) Physical plant

- Lifts
- Refrigerators and air-conditioning
- Fixed sterilizers
- Incinerators
- Boilers
- Pumps
- Kitchen equipment
- Mechanical laundry
- Central oxygen, suction
- Generator

(b) Furniture and appliances in a hospital

- Wheelchairs
- Bedside lockers

  - Beds
  - Stretchers
  - Trolleys
  - Dressing drums
  - Operation tables
  - Instrument trolleys
  - Kitchen utensils
  - Bedside lamps
  - Movable screens
  - Handwash stands
  - Bedpans
  - Waste bins
  - Hospital linen

(c) General-purpose furniture appliances

Office machines

- Intercom sets
- Calculators
- Filing systems
- Electronic exchange
- CCTV cameras
- Computers with scanners and printers

Office furniture

- Chairs, tables, sofa sets, resting beds

Crockery and cutlery

(d) Therapeutic and diagnostic equipment

Equipment for general use:

- Surgical instruments
- BP instruments
- Suction machines
- Sterilizers
- Equipment for clinical laboratory
- Rehabilitation department equipment
- Physiotherapy department equipment
- Glassware washers
- Voltage stabilizers
- Refrigerators
- Chemical analyzers
- Microscopes

Equipment for therapeutic and diagnostic procedure:

- Short-wave diathermy machines
- Electric cautery machine
- Defibrillators
- All radiological machines
- Monitoring equipment
- Respirators
- Incubators

1.10 Interiors and Graphics

It was not until recently that the need for interior design was considered important for the better functioning of a hospital. The attitude engaging the services of an interior designer was out of the question in early times, but at the present time after the birth of hospital administrators and hospital consultants, they took the responsibility of design services. Of all the component elements, that form a completed interior of a hospital, the single most important element is space, which can be exhilarating, serene, and cheerful and on the other hand distasteful, depressing, or dreary. The effects of these on the emotional state of patients, patients' families, visitors, and personnel should be considered by a designer. Other components are the ceilings, floors, windows, walls, doors, furniture, accessories, lighting, and fabrics.

1.10.1 Graphic Art and Design

In interior designing, graphic art is gaining its importance. The image of a hospital that a patient and visitors carry with them out of the hospital depends upon the hospital graphics. Elements or components of graphic design are the traits that are applied in a piece of work. Each element of graphic design is combined to create the desired visuals. While the methods may vary, all works of graphic design of a hospital consist of a combination of the following seven elements:

1. **Line**: In graphic design, lines are used for multiple goals such as connecting contents, highlighting a word or a phrase, and creating patterns.
2. **Color**: Color adds vivacity to an art. It impacts the psychology of a viewer profoundly. In graphic design, color is utilized to create visual interest, generate emotions, establish importance, and consolidate branding.
3. **Texture**: Texture adds depth and visual interest. Texture can be applied graphically in the form of a pattern or through the choice of printable surface.

4. **Size**: In graphic design, size is employed to communicate the importance, draw attraction, and create variation.
5. **Shape**: Various shapes are essential for creating visually pleasing and alluring designs. The three essential shape types in graphic design are:
   (a) Geometric (circles, squares, triangles, etc.)
   (b) Natural (leaves, trees, people, etc.)
   (c) Abstract (icons, stylizations, and graphic representations)
6. **Space**: Space is a crucial component of any good graphic design. Space indicates any area around the elements in a design. Space can be used to separate or group information. Space should be used effectively to give rest to the eyes. It also defines the importance and directs the focus to wherever you want it to move.
7. **Value**: Value is everything from the shadiest of black through the brightest of whites. It is used to create depth, contrast, and emphasis.

1.10.2 Types of Graphics

1. **Directional Graphics or the Signage System**: A mass of information must be transmitted visually to the patients, visitors, and personnel to save time and motion. The directional signs must be present both inside and outside of the hospital. Effective signage system (Fig. 1.5) is an art, and hospital administrators should select appropriate terminology supplemented with visual symbols, maps, and directories of floors and rooms. The rooms should be numbered (Fig. 1.2). They should also produce a consistent lettering. Letter style and size are outlined with the design, placement, and color code of the entire hospital.

   Apart from the directional signs (Fig. 1.1), there are other very important signs such as safety signs (Fig. 1.7) that a hospital should be concerned of. Examples are fire emergency, smoking, restricted areas, and safety at workplace. Most of these are warning signs.
2. **The Printed Matter Including Hospital Logo**: This is a part of interior functions such as pamphlets, various forms for laboratory testing, OPD slips, admission cards, and discharge slips. Hospital logo (Figs. 1.3, 1.4, and 1.6) should be thought early so that the interior designer can participate in the total concept of the hospital.

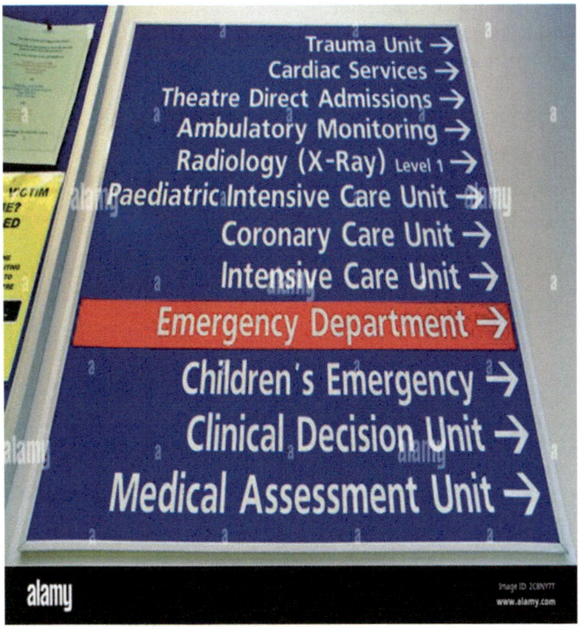

Fig. 1.1 Example of directional graphics (source: www.alamy.com)

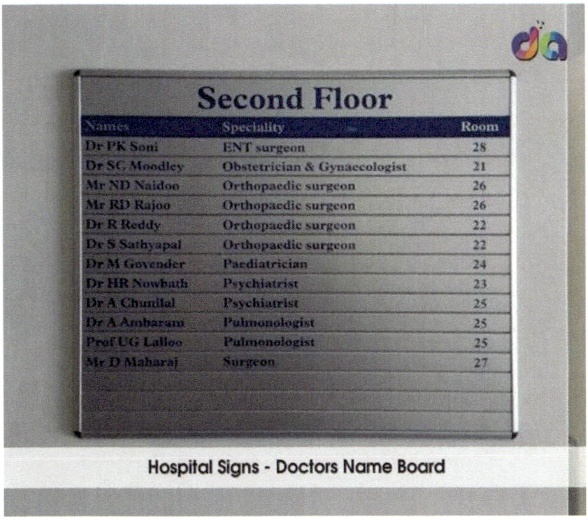

Fig. 1.2 Doctors' nameboard with room number (source: www.city-graphics.co.uk)

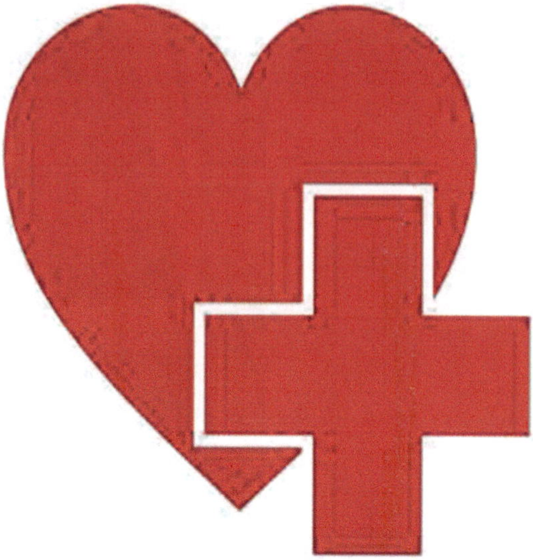

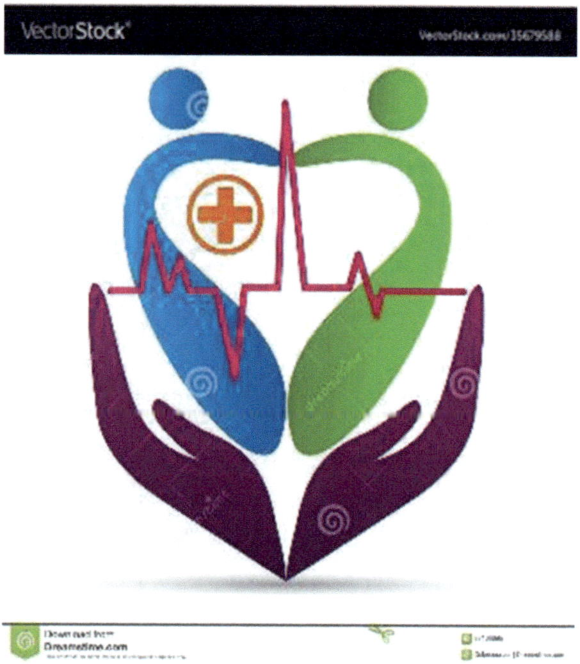

Figs. 1.3–1.4 Examples of hospital logo (source: www.vectorstock.com)

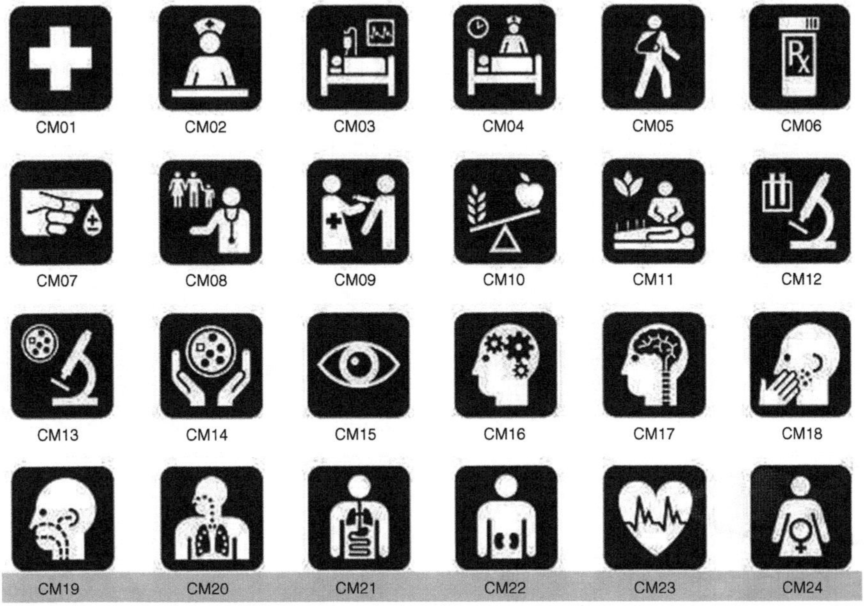

Fig. 1.5 Universal symbols in healthcare (source: www.pinterest.com)

Fig. 1.6 Symbol of health/medical/doctor (source: www.zilliondesigns.com)

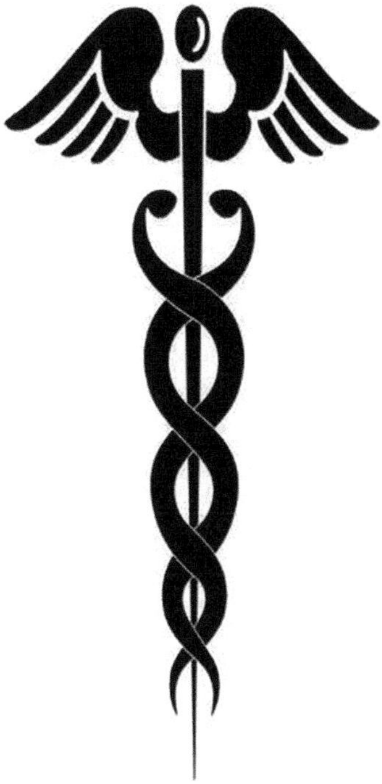

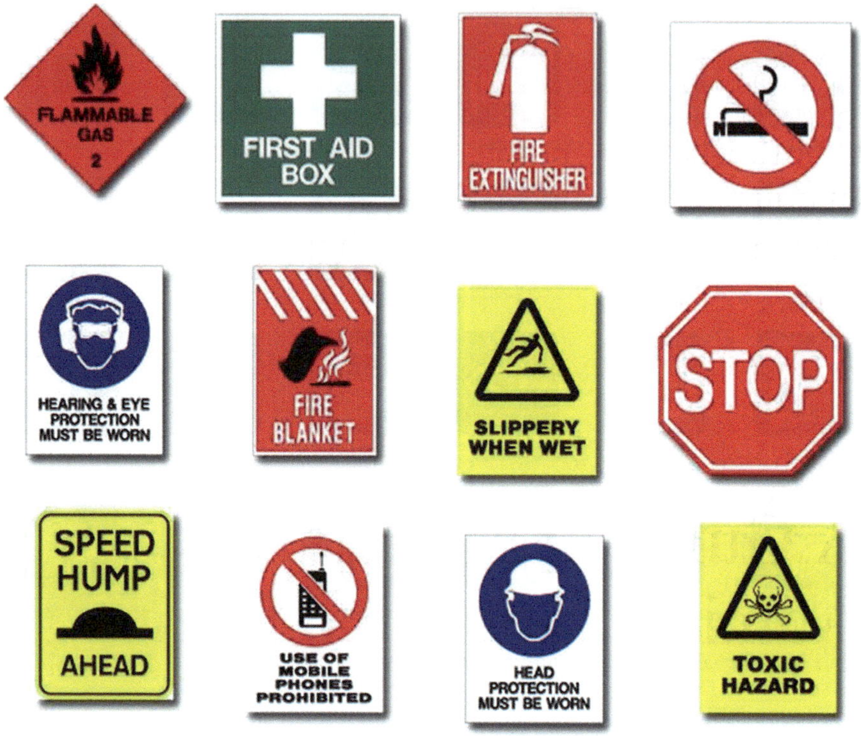

Fig. 1.7 Safety signage/warning signs (source: www.healthfacilityguidelines.com)

1.10.3 Use of Decorative Colors in Hospitals

We have been associated with white color in healthcare since so long. It is clean and sterile. Doctors put on it. So do nurses. But as healthcare plan becomes extra state of the art (i.e., patient centered and supportive of wellness), there is a growing awareness of how necessary it is to fine-tune color palettes. Besides the psychological influence on an affected person (and the pace and probability of their recovery), colors are additionally utilized as a verbal exchange device and signaling device among healthcare staff.

The Cultural Meanings of Colors in a Healthcare Setting

We have made a statement which is that white is related with cleanliness and health. This may additionally be nearly universally authentic in the West and consequently appropriate for a setting that promotes well-being; however, that is not the case everywhere. In China, for example, white symbolizes dying and mourning, no longer the principles you would choose to invoke the place the sick are convalescing.

If we look to older references like Greek and Roman mythology and the Old Testament, the meaning of colors is derived from nature. Yellow was once related with warmness and fertility because of the sun; green color symbolized youth, newness, and hope because of spring; and red color represented strength because it was the shade of blood.

Colors additionally carry psychobiological signals: black could suggest mold, decay, and excreta. "Red is related with blood, mother and baby ties, battle, and hunting. And white coloration is linked with semen, mother's milk, and reproduction."

Psychological Impacts of Colorations in the Healthcare Environment

There are a few broadly held theories on colors' specific effects on patients. Again, however, it is necessary to notice that variations in cultures could alter these effects. Red is believed to be energizing and encourage alertness: It is encouraged for patients with dementia, who want the brain stimulus. It is additionally awesome for memory care offerings in senior homes. On the other hand, red is not encouraged for patients who need a lot of relaxation and sleep, as it can cause anxiety and overstimulation.

Blue, green, and purple, specially in cool muted hues, can be very calming. They are super for health center rooms, wards, waiting areas, and health wellness centers like spa. Perhaps more important, however, is developing stability and contrast with specific colorations and saturations. For example, a room that is predominantly "cool" desires to be balanced with "warm" but some neutral elements like wood. Retirement amenities cannot be predominantly vibrant red, even though a lot of warm, relatively saturated shades against dark and/or neutral backgrounds can supply them a bright, homey environment. In children's hospitals, or even in hospitals that have areas where kids can be active and creative, contrasting colorings can provide that stimulation, or at least a sign that being energetic is encouraged in this area.

A wise use of shade is to preserve most of a patient's room cool or impartial and then use something bold behind the patient's bed. "If someone is coming to visit, they'll stroll in the room and have the sense of something a little extra colourful instead of neutral colour walls. There will be some feel of colour in there, however it's now not something the affected person would be staring at all day," says Jackie Jordan, director of coloration advertising for Sherwin-Williams.

Corridors' partitions ought to reflect light, so honey yellow, gray green, and mild cedar are some of the choices. Colors avoided in patient's rooms are shiny blues, soft purples, lavender tones, and brilliant or strong yellows. Since the affected person stays in the room for 24 h, melon green, dusty rose, rose tone, aqua, pecan grey, and honey yellow are used with a fantastic deal of success. Ceiling of the room is also completed in the same coloration as of side partitions as the affected person is normally in the lying position and sees extra of the ceiling than any other section of the room. Nurseries ought to be decorated with pink or blue color. Pink and blue colors are the traditional shades of the infants. Color in operating rooms, delivery rooms, and workrooms must be restful to the eyes, and as a result an ideal choice is gray-green color.

Colors as a Signage System in Hospitals

Color is additionally a way for hospital workers and individuals to communicate. The International Organization for Standardization (ISO), the Occupational Safety and Health Act (OSHA), and the American National Standards Institute (ANSI) have installed suggestions for markers in hospitals.

Red is a signal for hazard and an indication to stop. It is additionally used to mark safety equipment and apparatus (like fire exits, fireplace extinguishers, stop buttons, and electrical switches).

Green shows safety and the region of first resource equipment like a dispensary, stretchers, and protection deluge showers.

Dangerous parts of machinery or electrical gear that can cut, crush, or injure are marked orange (exposed pulleys, gears, rollers, energy jaws, and more).

Caution and hazards that involve tripping, falling, stumbling, getting caught in between (like building equipment, handrails, and guardrails), and others use yellow.

Purple on yellow signifies radiation dangers like radioactive materials, and containers, burial grounds, and storage areas for radioactive materials.

Black, white, and combinations of black and white are used to direct visitors and for housekeeping (indicating dead ends in aisles, areas and widths of aisles and hallways, etc.).

International and NABH-Accepted Medical Institution Signage Criteria

The National Accreditation Board for Hospitals & Healthcare Providers (NABH) standards for hospitals: This type of standard has been approved by means of the International Society for Quality in Health Care (ISQua). The approval of ISQua authenticates that NABH standards are in consonance with the international benchmarks set by way of ISQua. The hospitals accepted via the NABH will have worldwide recognition. This will provide improvement in clinical tourism. NABH pointers advise that all the signages are in twin languages (sometimes three languages) and use symbols to help in guiding the sufferers around the hospital. Most of the hospitals in India lack an exact signage system and that is why the NABH focuses on enforcing a magnificent signage format as one of the assessment criteria.

Criteria for an excellent signage plan acceptable by the NABH are as follows:

1. Good-quality signboard in terms of materials
2. Readability factor—distance vs. visibility
3. Multilingual—English and one local language acceptable (if you can convince them)

4. Usage of symbols
5. Internal and external wayfinding
6. Services offered
7. Doctors' directory
8. Availability and nonavailability of doctors with days/timings
9. Patients' safety instructions
10. Fire safety instructions
11. Fire exit plans
12. Services for physically challenged
13. Locating lifts and staircases
14. Locating public utility places
15. Patients' rights and responsibilities
16. Service areas
17. No-entry zones

A good wayfinding and a good internal signage system, implemented in a systematic manner, will bring you one step nearer to achieving better client (patient/visitor) satisfaction.

Chromotherapy

Some health practitioners trust in the physical restoration power of light and colors in solving medical health problems. There are, however, virtually many who doubt such medical treatment. Indeed, there exists little authentic scientific research in favor of these beliefs.

A chromotherapist applies particular shades or lights to specific points on the body called "chakras." Different colorations have specific effects. For example, red is the concept to high pulse rate, blood pressure, and respiration rate. Therefore, it is regularly used for circulatory conditions. Blue is believed to bring relaxation and calm. Therefore, blue is used for headaches, pain, cramping, stress, and different conditions.

Though this method can be neither encouraged nor discounted due to a lack of conceivable research, it is a fascinating thought that builds upon the recognized psychological and physiological outcomes of color, imparting one use of integrating the psychology of color in healthcare design.

Color and Health

Color is everywhere, and it influences our moods and feelings greater than we realize. A 2014 article in CodeCondo, "How to Use Color Psychology in Your Web Design Projects," mentioned the feelings often evoked by popular colors. Whereas red conveys power and ardor and increases aggression, blue conveys peace and trustworthiness and conjures up tranquility. Yellow suggests vibrancy and cheerfulness, and orange conveys friendliness and creativity.

There is no scientific research to exhibit that a blue wall in an affected person's room speeds up the healing procedure or that a crimson wall slows recovery. It is noticeably unlikely that coloration has any direct influence on physical health. However, simply as in advertising and retail, coloration in healthcare services can have an effect on mood, which does have an impact on health. The fitness benefits of color are indirect. It is important, then, that designers think about the psychology of color when designing healthcare facilities. The colors they pick out could be extra impactful than they realize.

1.11 Construction

Working, drawing, and specs are prepared by using the architect to furnish to the contractor a precise picture of the work to be done, materials and techniques to be used, and obligations to be assumed for the project. Based on these, contract bidders prepare their proposals and estimates for the construction and put up their tenders when invited to bid competitively. The award of the contractor is made to the lowest bidder and additionally thinking about his or her experience and recognition in the building trade. The architect supervises the construction development to ensure that the work is being carried out as per contract, right high-quality material is used, and all the specifications are followed.

1.12 Commissioning

The medical institution is equipped to be commissioned when its building is ready, all tools have been installed, and the group of workers and manpower has been engaged. The plant, machinery, and therapeutic and diagnostic tools ought to have undergone many check runs before this. The scientific, clinical, medical, and paramedical workforce have to have been recruited and placed a few weeks in advance.

1.12.1 The Commissioning Team

The key individuals of commissioning team who will be linked to the new health facility ought to be the hospital consultant, hospital administrator, senior nurses, chiefs of medical services, personnel manager, material supply officer, and chiefs of all the departments.

1.12.2 Scheduling the Sequence of the Services

Some offerings of the health center/hospital require readiness, while others nonetheless have adequate time. For instance, CSSD requires prolonged trial runs and bacteriological test installation, and calibration of X-ray equipment is a lengthy job. The sequence of opening the departments should be planned carefully.

1.12.3 Categorization of Services [13]

Services are categorized into four groups:

Group 1: Services required immediately

- Telephone
- Domestic services
- Works department
- Linen department

Group 2: Requiring lengthy duration of preparation

- CSSD (for trial runs)
- X-rays/CT/MRI
- OT
- Pharmacy

Group 3: May be partially opened before the admission of patients

- Paramedical service
- OPD

Group 4: Will not be now operational till all the above departments are opened

- Wards

Shake-Down Period

From the time of commissioning of the hospital, some time is taken for functional integration of one-of-a-kind units, services, staff, affected person, and community. This period of duration is known as shake-down period. It is the duration all through which a hospital experiences its teething troubles and till it settles down into a satisfactorily functioning unit and into its normal routine.

References

1. Clark, M., Semple, M. J., Ivins, N., Mahoney, K., & Harding, K. (2017). National audit of pressure ulcers and incontinence-associated dermatitis in hospitals across Wales: a cross-sectional study. *BMJ open, 7*(8), e015616.
2. Kendall, A., Keoleian, G. A., & Lepech, M. D. (2008). Materials design for sustainability through life cycle modeling of engineered cementitious composites. *Materials and Structures, 41*(6), 1117-1131.
3. Pilosof, N. (2015). Planning for change: Evaluation of hospital design strategies. *Summary of the Dissertation Proposal Submitted for the Ph. D. Candidacy Examination, Technion-Israel Institute of Technology, Haifa, Israel.*
4. Pilosof, N. P. (2021). Building for change: Comparative case study of hospital architecture. *HERD: Health Environments Research & Design Journal, 14*(1), 47-60.
5. Preiser, W. F., Hardy, A. E., & Schramm, U. (2018). From linear delivery process to life cycle phases: The validity of the concept of building performance evaluation *Building Performance Evaluation* (pp. 3-18): Springer.
6. James, J. R. (1986). *Considerations concerning the construction of an expert system for control system design.* Rensselaer Polytechnic Institute.
7. Zeidler, E. H. (1974). *Healing the hospital: McMaster health science centre, its conception and evolution*: Zeidler Partnership.
8. Gibson, I. W., & Lease, B. L. (2007). *An approach to hospital planning and design using discrete event simulation.* Paper presented at the 2007 Winter Simulation Conference.
9. Das, S., Yaylacicegi, U., & Menon, N. M. (2010). The effect of information technology investments in healthcare: A longitudinal study of its lag, duration, and economic value. *IEEE transactions on engineering management, 58*(1), 124-140.
10. Mehta, N., & Pandit, A. (2018). Concurrence of big data analytics and healthcare: A systematic review. *International Journal of Medical Informatics, 114*, 57-65.
11. Bowen, S., Dearden, A., Wright, P., Wolstenholme, D., & Cobb, M. (2010). *Participatory healthcare service design and innovation.* Paper presented at the Proceedings of the 11th Biennial Participatory Design Conference.
12. Schuster, M., Neumann, C., Neumann, K., Braun, J., Geldner, G., Martin, J., . . . Group, C. S. (2011). The effect of hospital size and surgical service on case cancellation in elective surgery: results from a prospective multicenter study. *Anesthesia and Analgesia, 113*(3), 578-585.
13. Haupt, M. T., Bekes, C. E., Brilli, R. J., Carl, L. C., Gray, A. W., Jastremski, M. S., . . . Horst, M. (2003). Guidelines on critical care services and personnel: recommendations based on a system of categorization of three levels of care. *Critical Care Medicine, 31*(11), 2677-2683.

Chapter 2
Importance of Hospital Management

Kinjal Jani and Bhupinder Chaudhary

2.1 Healthcare

Healthcare cannot refer merely to medical care, but all the areas of pro-preventive care [1]. It is related to preventive and curative aspects along with the management of illness. It covers the preservation of mental and physical well-being via services presented by the medical, nursing, and associated health professions. In line with the World Health Organization, healthcare encompasses all the services and goods to uphold health, with the inclusion of "preventive, curative, and intervention of palliative care, regardless of individuals or the community" [2].

Healthcare is one of the service sectors that are going through revolutionary change. The nature and framework of healthcare are continuous, as depicted below (Fig. 2.1).

Growing and changing healthcare has built pressure on management to monitor and evaluate the health system and generate efforts to strengthen the response of the health system to overcome the evolving health challenges [4]. Chronic conditions are one of such challenges. Chronic conditions are the twenty-first century's leading public health challenge [5]. It was estimated that by 2020, heart disease, depression, stroke, and cancer would be the bigger contributors to the burden of noncommunicable diseases (NCDs), along with mental disorders contributing to 60% of total mortality in the globe. The number of individuals that need healthcare is quickly growing, and it is estimated to rise at a higher rate in the people of lower socioeconomic class [5]. This has created a need for surveillance, prevention, and control of NCDs. If not handled properly, then it can become the most expensive burden faced by the healthcare industry of the globe [6].

K. Jani (✉)
Department of Hospital Management (DHSI), HNGU, Patan, India

B. Chaudhary
Department of Hospital Management and Hospice Studies, JMI, New Delhi, India

D. Bhatia et al. (eds.), *A Guide to Hospital Administration and Planning*,
https://doi.org/10.1007/978-981-19-6692-7_2

Health care is Changing

Aging Population	Competition for caregivers	Industry Consolidation	Care delivery and payment models	Consumerism	Compliance and security
Chronic conditions	Aging workforce	Growth	Shifting to value-based care	Patient experience	Protected health information
Population health	Shortage of caregivers	Rationalized services and location	Per capita cost	Ratings and ranking	Cyber security
Risk	Clinician satisfaction	Efficiency through scale	Innovation led by technology	Convenience	Government reform
	Work/life balance			Data Portability	Shred responsibility

Fig. 2.1 Healthcare is changing [3]

This has created the need for reorganization of the healthcare system to handle the chronic conditions in an optimum way and eventually resulted in the demand for people-centric care [7]. The nation's ability to strengthen the health system to achieve health goals significantly depends on its personnel. The WHO's "Building Block" or the six core components of analytical framework demand a need for quality health services [8]. The establishment of the high-quality healthcare system comprises the population and their health-related expectations and need, good governance of healthcare and partnership across the various sectors, workforce with skills and in good numbers, platforms for delivery of care, resources and tools, and strengthening of a system from medicine to data. A high-quality health system has four values; they are meant for people, and they are resilient, equitable, and efficient [9]. This global health commission endorses a requirement of system-wide action and health system leaders through which visionary quality of care, strong regulation, a clear strategy of quality, and continuous learning can be achieved [8].

Berman [10] stated reformation of the health sector as a purposeful and sustainable change, to enhance the efficiency, effectiveness, and equity of the health sector. To implement health system reformation in large-scale political sensitivity, strategic thinking and higher order management capacity are in demand.

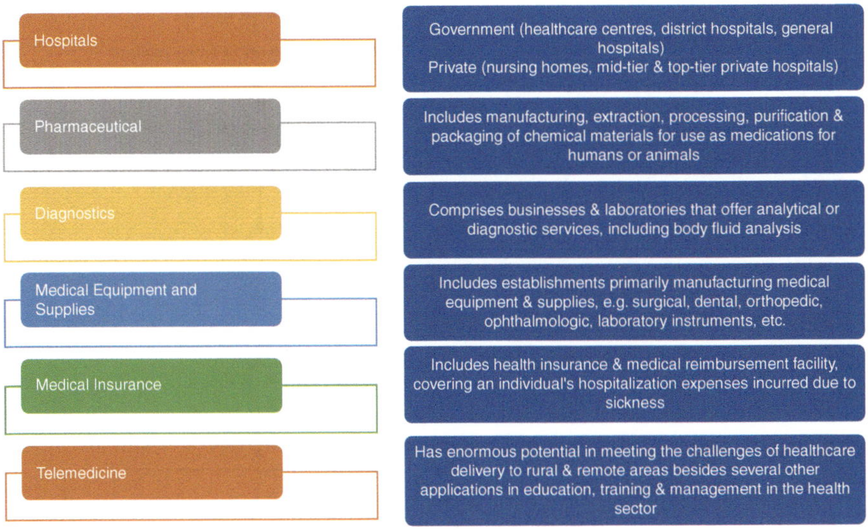

Fig. 2.2 Major segments in India's healthcare sector

2.2 Healthcare Industry

Health is considered as wealth. The health of people holds a social value. In the past, services of healthcare were believed to be philanthropic activities. At that time, the meaning of healthcare was only hospitals. It was beyond imagination to consider the healthcare industry as a commercial industry. But now, the narration of the healthcare industry has changed. It encompasses comprehensive meaning [11]. In the words of the World Health Organization, healthcare holds all the services intended to promote health, i.e., preventive, curative, and rehabilitative related to individuals and/or populations. The provision of organization of such services encompasses a healthcare industry [2]. The healthcare sector is complex with several goals, products, and beneficiaries. This industry encompasses hospitals, medical equipment and devices, health insurance, telemedicine, clinical trials, and medical tourism (Fig. 2.2).

2.3 Classification of Healthcare Industry

2.3.1 Based on Funding and Governance

The healthcare system in India is pluralistic based on funding and governance, public sector, and private sector. Public healthcare is mainly delivered by the government via the national healthcare system. However, private healthcare is delivered via "for-profit" hospitals and freelancer practitioners along with nongovernment providers who are "not for profit" [12].

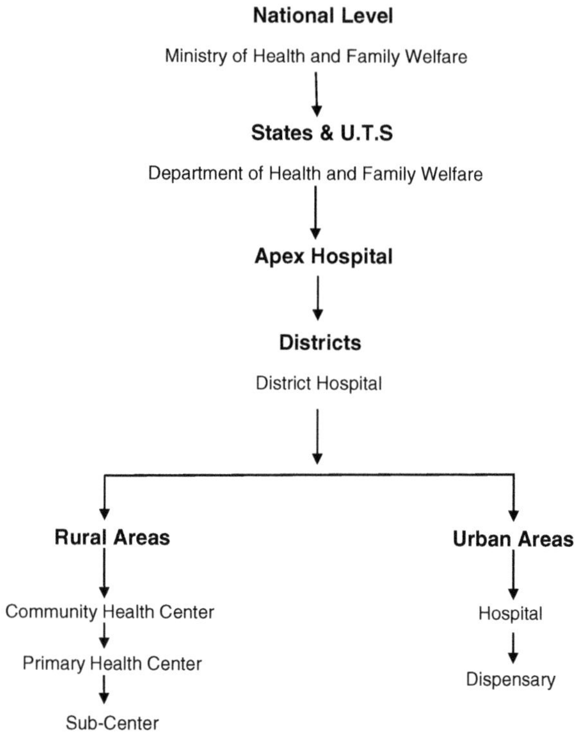

Fig. 2.3 The health system infrastructure in India [2]

Public Sector in Healthcare

The public healthcare industry includes amenities governed by central and state governments. These public health facilities offer free or subvention rates to the families of the lower income group in urban and rural areas (Fig. 2.3).

In India, responsibilities of health-related actions are divided between the central and state governments by the Constitution of India. The national government shoulders the responsibility to conduct medical research and maintain technical education, whereas state government maintains the responsibility for employment, infrastructure, and delivery of services. The states have ample autonomy to manage their health system, while the national government works out financial control over the health system of the state government.

Private Sector in Healthcare

India has been uplifting the investment in the healthcare sector for years. The private sector has played a significant role in all the areas of medical education and related training, diagnosis and medical technologies, pharmaceutical sales and manufacture, hospital construction, and allied ancillary services along with the core focus on medical care. Approximately, 75% of manpower and advanced technologies of medical care, 37% of total beds, and 68% of hospitals in the nation are counted in the private sector [2]. The numbers of solo practitioners and/or nursing homes with bed capacity make the composition of the private sector in India. Moreover, there are corporate bodies, pharmaceutical segment, and numbers of nonresident Indians (NRIs), whose investments in Indian healthcare are also a part of the private sector [13]. In addition, traditional healthcare providers, i.e., Ayurveda and Yoga, are also counted in private sector providers.

Nongovernment hospitals, based on the pattern of ownership [14], are classified as below:

1. Private (personnel)
2. Partnership
3. Private (family) trust
4. Public charitable trust
5. Cooperative society
6. Private limited company
7. Public limited company

2.3.2 *Based on Service Delivery*

Based on the areas of service delivery, the healthcare industry is divided into three core segments:

1. Healthcare providers
2. Healthcare financiers
3. Life sciences [15]

Healthcare Providers

Hospitals and other related medical centers: They perform diagnosis and treatment of illness, research, academic work, and pertaining training. Hospitals are operational with medical equipment and amenities of all kinds together with medical professionals.

Nursing homes and centers of rehabilitative care: In this segment, short-term and long-term care-related services are offered. Short-term services encompass rehabilitative care after undergoing surgery, injury, or illness. Physical therapy, speech-language therapy, or occupational therapy may be included in this segment. Services for sick, disabled, and elderly are included in long-term care.

Ambulatory service providers: Physicians and allied health professionals deliver outpatient health services and/or nonhospital-based care.

Healthcare Financiers

Government agencies and companies of private firms are the healthcare financiers that provide funds and health insurance policies to healthcare services. They pool the medical funds via the contribution of employer and/or individual insurance policies. Healthcare financiers state the accessibility of people for healthcare and cover the type of healthcare.

Life Sciences

This segment encompasses firms of pharmaceutical industries which produce drugs and chemical products required for the healthcare ambit. It also includes manufacturers who produce high-tech equipment for medical care and a biotechnology firm that organizes research work and develops new drugs and new methods of treatment. The rest of the miscellaneous services fall in this ambit which provide services related to diagnosis, treatment, and patient monitoring.

2.3.3 *Classification of Healthcare Based on Nature of Work*

According to available literature, healthcare consists of three kinds of services. Based on their nature of work, there is a distinction among the three services [16]:

- Line services
- Staff services
- Auxiliary services

The line services are responsible to perform direct work for the attainment of organizational goals. The line services encompass outpatient services, inpatient services, and emergency services. The agencies of staff services assist the agency of line services in their respective activities. The staff services include diet, central sterile supply department, laboratory, laundry, nursing, and radiology services. However, the auxiliary services are important too as they are in demand to ensure a nurturing and comfortable work environment where they provide a helping hand to line agencies [17]. It encompasses indoor care records, registration, engineering, transport, stores, and mortuary.

2.4 Value Chain of the Healthcare Industry

A Harvard Business School Professor and Economist, Michel Porter, states that value chain as the chain of end-to-end production begins from input to output as the input of the raw materials to the final services and/or product output. Value chain of

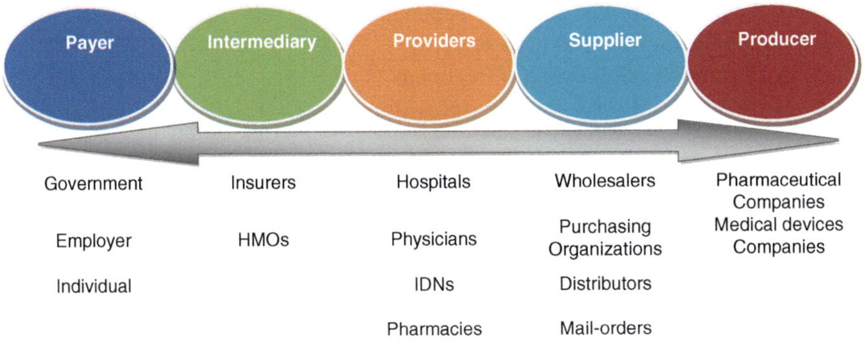

Fig. 2.4 Healthcare value chain [18]

an industry is also narrated as a supply chain [3]. The chain is named a value chain because the value is added by each link to the input [18] (Fig. 2.4).

Nowadays, value and quality are pluralistic convergent concepts of healthcare. In healthcare, the management of the value chain is a bit complex as it involves several stakeholders. Value chain or supply chain is the management of the relationship of upward and downward streams aligned with suppliers and customers to convey superior customer value at a lower cost as a whole.

Currently, hospitals are in the search of new sources to gain competitive advantages and measurement of cost cutting, whenever feasible. It is necessary to take a look into the supply chain management ambit and to identify the feasible area of patient-centric care to improve the quality of care [19]. From the management point of view, resource management, supply management, optimized goods, and service delivery promote an efficient value chain in healthcare.

Hospitals occupy a majority of the healthcare industry, and the terms healthcare management and hospital management are used interchangeably. As the hospital is the point that provides the services to maintain health, it is significant to run at full efficiency, particularly related to the quality of services, affordable pricing, material consumption, turnaround time, and largely outputs. In the current scenario, as every patient invests time, mind, and money into maintaining their well-being, "hospital management" turns into more pivotal to run and set up the best healthcare systems.

Hospital management acknowledges to set a benchmark and to lead to improvement in healthcare delivery. A systematic approach motivates innovations to be developed at every sign of challenges and issues. Hospital management accords in the coordination with medical professionals, pharmacies, paramedical services, nurses, and other nonmedical staff who are related with the hospital industry.

Hospital management helps in the healthcare's structured functioning and makes the easy and smooth delivery of various services. An expanded hospital offers the following:

- To follow better financial decisions by effective planning of fund flow, and to control expenses and better investments
- To maintain patient-doctor confidentiality secure the data

- To eradicate and control errors by benchmarking of process, lean management, and continuous improvement in services
- To make improvised delivery of treatment
- To enhance patient satisfaction by providing better services and innovations at affordable prices
- Through accreditation of organization, to enhance quality ratings and standards
- To maintain record keeping and track digital reports in the scenario of paperless operations
- To build a harmonious relationship with doctors, nurses, paramedical staff, investors, suppliers, vendors, etc.

The various services, i.e., outpatient, inpatient, lab or clinical services, record keeping, imaging services, waste disposal, and store operations, need to be fulfilled with accuracy and close coordination. Hospital management lets these operations happen smoothly and effectively. Moreover, on the economical aspect, it also helps to market and promote the services of the hospital to generate noteworthy sales and revenue. Profit shows its evidence. Thus, hospitals are a complex structure, and they need to be run by an efficient management system.

2.5 Healthcare and National Economy

A healthy society portrays the qualitative well-being of a country as a significant contributor to the growth of the economy. On top of it, the nation's future healthcare needs will be decided by the growth of population and economic aspirations. In the Indian economy, a segment of healthcare has emerged as one of the largest ambits, in the phrases of employment and revenue. In terms of revenue since 2016, it has been on the rise at a Compound Annual Growth Rate (CAGR) of 22%, and in terms of employment, the health sector has been creating an opportunity for employment of 4.7 million individuals directly [20].

- The Indian health market is about to attain $372 billion at a CAGR of 39% by 2022.
- The hospital industry occupies 80% of the total healthcare, and it is expected to account for $132 billion by 2023 and is creating an influx of investment opportunities in the domestic and global market.
- The primary healthcare sector is estimated at $13 billion.
- The contribution of health insurance is 20% to the business of the nonlife insurance, becoming the second largest portfolio.
- The digital health market is expected to reach INR 485.43 billion by 2024.
- The market of telemedicine is expected to reach $5.4 billion by 2025 expanding at a CAGR of 31% [20].
- According to the report of KPMG and FICCI, in 2015, the healthcare sector emerged as the fifth largest employer, employing 4.7 million people directly [21].
- In India, the health sector has potentially produced 2.7 million additional jobs between 2017 and 2022, approximately 500,000 fresh jobs every year.

2.5.1 Investment Opportunities in India

Over the last two decades, India has grown as one of the fastest-developing economies and received hefty FDI inflows that have increased from USD 2.5 billion to USD 50 billion in the year 2019–2020. The nation's comparative cost competitiveness and presence of skilled labor have attracted medical tourism, and the country has emerged as a favored destination for treatment.

In the segment of hospitals, the expansion and relocation of private players to tier 2 and 3 cities provide an attractive investment opportunity. As per the words, available from India's investment grid, 600 investment opportunities are lying in the nation's medical/hospital infrastructure that is worth $32 billion (2.3 lakh crore INR).

In the segment of medical equipment and devices, expansion and development of pathology and diagnostic centers show higher potential to grow. Moreover, medical value travel has bright prospects to attract foreign individuals, and eventually, it also shows new opportunities to invest.

The emergence of advanced health technology, i.e., artificial intelligence, offers several investment avenues. Even the development of facilities of emergency care, medical infrastructure, patient-facing mobile health education, robots, and complete technology-driven optimization open the door for investment opportunities.

2.5.2 Healthcare Drives the GDP Growth

The strong healthcare industry generates GDP growth related to adequate investments and an encouraging environment. It not only drives productivity and employment but also stands as a magnet to bring foreign exchange opportunities along with entrepreneurship and innovation (Fig. 2.5).

Thus, healthcare is a productivity enhancer, employment generator, a driver for entrepreneurship and innovation, and a foreign exchange generator.

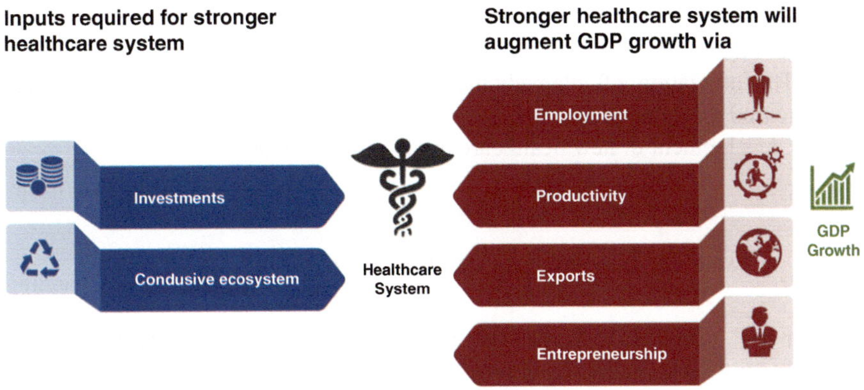

Fig. 2.5 Healthcare drivers for GDP growth [21]

Quality of Care and Economy

In lower income and middle-income nations (LMICs), more than eight million individuals die per year from the treatable illness. In 2015 only, it is estimated that there was $6 trillion economic loss in the USA due to treatable conditions. Poor-quality care can emerge as a bigger barrier in the reduction of mortality in comparison to insufficient access. 60 million people shifted to below poverty line due to high spending on healthcare, which directly affects the national economy [22]. In terms of macroeconomics, the majority of estimates narrate that the NCDs in India account for a higher economic burden that ranges between 5 and 10% GDP, which hampers development. It requires precise management to deal with "chronic emergencies" [23].

2.5.3 *Key Drivers of Healthcare Growth*

1. Epidemiological, demographic, and health transition
   Trends of demography and epidemiology are about to boost the high demand for healthcare, for instance, economic capacity; it is estimated that 8% of individuals of India will earn $12,000 annually and more by 2026 [21, 24]. The life expectancy of India is prone to exceed 70 years by 2022. On the other hand, India is facing a dual burden of disease. There is also a rise in lifestyle disorders.
2. Medical value travel
   MVT is a strong magnetic driver to boost wellness and medical tourism.
3. Enabling policy environment
   Recently released several policies will help to boost the expansion of healthcare. For instance, GDP spending on public healthcare is expected to increase 2.5%, with an announcement from the government to spend $200 billion by 2024 in medical infrastructure, by implementation of Ayushman Bharat.
4. Demand-supply gap
   Currently, India witnesses availability of 1.3 hospital beds/1000 population, skilled worker shortage, 0.65 physicians/1000 people, and 1.3 nurses/1000 individuals.
5. Other factors
   The utilization of telemedicine and technologies in the COVID era has increased the demand for public–private partnerships. Accreditation of hospitals and development of new healthcare models are observed.

2.5.4 *Post-COVID Analysis of Healthcare*

Kapoor et al. [25] state the state-wise estimation of hospitals, hospital beds, intensive care units, and ventilators in post-COVID time. Estimates suggest 25,778 hospitals in the public sector, 43,487 hospitals in the private sector, and 69,265 total hospitals in India. Approximately, 19 lakh hospital beds, 48,000 ventilators, and 95,000 ICU beds are on hand in the nation. The majority of beds and ventilators are strenuous in seven states: 14.8% in Uttar Pradesh, 13.8% in Karnataka, 12.2% in Maharashtra, 8.1% in Tamil Nadu, 5.9% in Telangana, and 5.2% in Kerala. The influx of COVID-19 patients demands a rapid expansion of ongoing capacity or alteration in inpatient care.

In the 15th Finance Commission, the World Bank narrated "fault lines" in the health system of India just after the influx of COVID-19 patients [22]. They found large and persistent gaps between the states. The World Bank's presentation found insufficient focus on main functions of public healthcare, i.e., disease surveillance, contact tracing and testing, weaker service delivery irrespective of improvement in the access, quality of care with high variations, and insufficient attention to the urban health system. On the economical aspect, a team from West Bengal said that India will pay the highest economic cost in Asia related to healthcare, surpassing China [22].

India is one of the worst-hit nations by the impact of COVID-19. As a result of this, the healthcare system has faced alarming collapse, and numbers of entities were in chaotic conditions to manage the second wave. The mismanagement of the supply chain was evident. Scarcity of essential resources, i.e., oxygen supplies, hospital beds, and medicines, forced people to struggle for the endurance of their loved ones [26]. Moreover, healthcare seemed unable to manage and absorb the quick and constant pressure on their functions, particularly in acute care [27]. Licensing, credentialing, reimbursement, and problems related to technology, privacy, security, litigation, and safety are still challenges of healthcare [28, 29].

Thus, COVID-19 has proved to be a reality check for the healthcare industry. It acts as a catalyst of transformation. There is a need for the development of political, legislative, and healthcare management systems (Fig. 2.6).

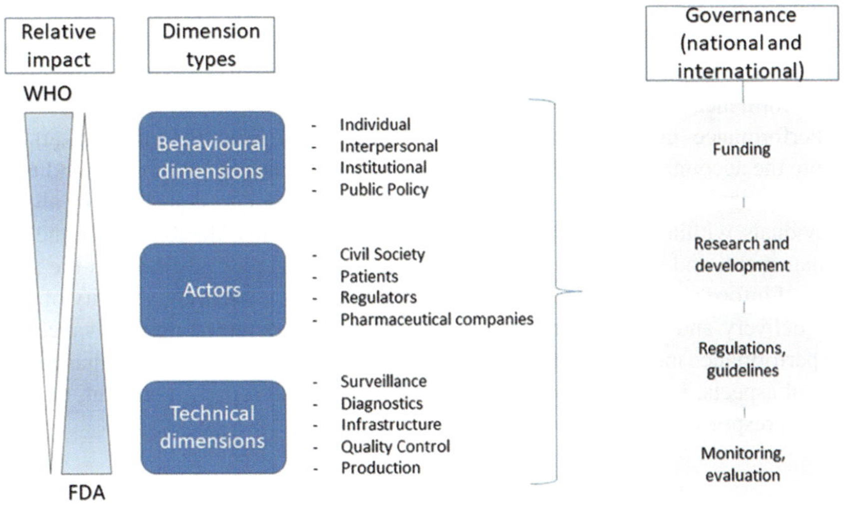

Fig. 2.6 Influencing domain to healthcare in pandemic [27]

Actors affected by other dimensions are shown in the model of the WHO. Coordination of management, technology, and economy are emphasized in the manuscript to deal with the post-COVID era. Eventually, the challenges of the healthcare industry will turn into opportunities. For instance, in 2020, our health technology (health-tec) industry reached a $1.9 billion value, and it is expected to mark $5 billion at a CAGR of 39% by 2023.

2.6 Health System Performance

As the healthcare sector is complex and multilayered, it generates difficulty to unlock its utmost potential and to provide true quality services. Accessibility, quality, and efficiency are the three dimensions of health system performance. These three dimensions together determine the extent to which services are achievable [30].

- Accessibility refers to the degree to which patients are supposed to get the right care as per their needs and when they require it.
- Quality refers to the degree to which the right quality of care is provided in the right way.
- Efficiency explains the degree to which effectiveness and accessibility are optimized related to resources.

Thus, health system performance is concerned with the measurement of these three quantities, their understanding, and focus on the factors that influence the performance. Moreover, it is significant to discover and evaluate the ways to enhance the performance. The expectation of healthcare consumers for the performance of the health system is about to rise over time because access to qualitative care is the ultimate goal of patient safety and satisfaction. To meet these requirements, hospital management can offer noteworthy opportunities to change and to build up the overall performance of healthcare.

Performance measurement extends a major opportunity to policymakers to secure the accountability of healthcare delivery and the health status of individuals. It plays a significant role in the improvement of qualitative decisions taken by all the individuals within the health system, for instance patients, doctors, personnel of management, and government at each unit. Recent foremost advances in the segment of information technology and influx of demand for the accountability of service delivery and particular patient preference have determined rapid advances in the performance measurement of the health system. Health system performance has several aspects, i.e., population health, outcomes of health from treatment, quality of care, responsiveness, productivity, and equity [31].

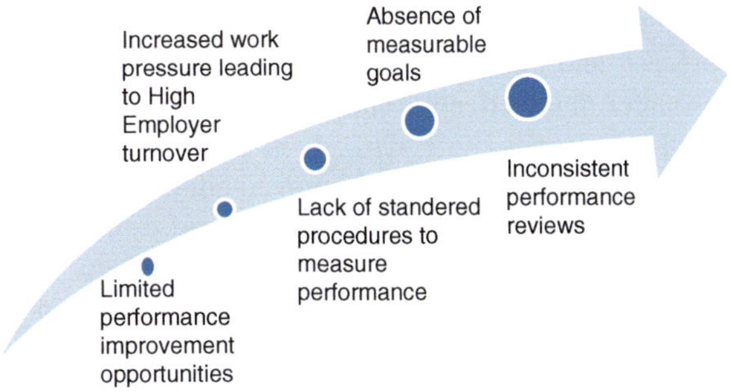

Fig. 2.7 Performance challenges in healthcare

2.6.1 Performance Management Challenges in Healthcare

Along with doctors and nurses, healthcare has support staff that includes personnel from front desk to backside transactional operations. It is indeed a fact that this healthcare sector is considerably workforce intensive [32]. Several performance challenges in the healthcare sector affect the performance of institutions currently or lately, and they are depicted in Fig. 2.7.

To manage such a big task force of employees in healthcare and to take a patient-centric decision are pressing issues in healthcare. To manage an individual's performance, to improve the quality of services, and to build a motivated, productive, and occupied personnel that delivers qualitative healthcare need effective management to streamline all the said outcomes in the conceptual framework.

There is a need for a decisive link between organizational operational aspects and manpower. Growing and changing health challenges have built pressure on the management ambit to monitor and evaluate the service to strengthen the healthcare delivery system.

To set a robust conceptual framework within the system is the first necessity of the performance measurement system. To develop a conceptual framework, hospital management plays a contributory role. For instance, to fulfill patient safety, statistical surveillance, presentation of data of performance measurement, obtaining the feedback from the practitioners and patients, and principles of hospital management are useful. A proper mechanism can be placed to monitor such tendencies.

2.7 Application of Hospital Management Principles to the Healthcare

According to the WHO, management and effective leadership are significant to scale up the quality and quantity of health services and to enhance population health [33]. Henri Fayol (1916) stated the rule book of management. In a simple world, management is getting things done by people. Management is a set of processes to forecast and plan, organize, lead, coordinate, and control the organizational resources in the effective and efficient attainment of specified goals of an organization [34].

Streamlined operations, improved administration, controlling, patient care with priority, strict cost control, and enhanced profitability are the outputs of hospital management [35]. For instance, Tamil Nadu Medical Services Corporation (TNMSC) has administered an admirable logistics management framework for the coordination of the activities, i.e., purchase, storage, and distribution of medicines and drugs in Tamil Nadu [36]. This framework deals with 75 vendors for 600 items of 120 crores per annum. It assures the ready availability of qualitative medicines through the 11,000 government medical institutions that comprise 9000 subcenters, 1500 PHCs, and 250 headquarter hospitals. Several other states, i.e., Rajasthan and Maharashtra, have planned to follow this example.

Hospital material management can help to meet the challenges of cost reduction in healthcare. Healthcare should take a proactive stance to meet up the challenges of technology crosswise industry [37].

Alverson [38] mentioned the significance of inventory management for healthcare to surpass the missed contract compliance, lack of inventory control, workflow interruption, and requirement of manpower.

Three significant concepts of hospital management apply to the healthcare industry: effectiveness, efficiency, and equity.

2.7.1 *Effectiveness*

Effectiveness is a concept of goal measurement that how well a person or an organization is attaining its goals.

In healthcare: If the goal of healthcare is to provide quality services and people are not satisfied and the provision of healthcare is poor, it results in ineffective services.

If a healthcare provider has set an objective to allocate 400 malaria bed nets annually and succeeds in the distribution of only 100 nets, then the service is not effective.

2.7.2 *Efficiency*

Healthcare uses land, labor, and capital as resources. Efficiency measures the goal of healthcare and how well they are achieving the goal using its resources. Efficiency involves the occurrence of the right thing, with the right resources with minimum waste.

In healthcare: If any health center receives a drug, i.e., antimalarial drug or iron folic acid tablets with the remained shelf life of only 1 month, then it will result in wastage of resources. Moreover, staff shortage, cost inflation, and demand of services point out the need for efficiency in healthcare [39].

2.7.3 *Equity*

Equity means providing healthcare to the patient when they need it irrespective of their sociodemographic profile.

In healthcare, inaccessible areas and all the diversified groups of people should be treated with equality. Social and economical barriers need to be eliminated.

In the current era, the health sector is going through several unparalleled challenges in an ambit of a patient-oriented environment. Nowadays, intensive medical care along with personal care is the requirement of health problems [40]. On the other hand, the healthcare industry has been restructured in the ambit of maturation of the industry, increased competition, and increased cost of care. Professional experts and technically skilled individuals are highly in demand who can relate their skills and knowledge along with their expertise. Here, hospital management performs a significant role in organizing the functional setting of hospitals. In the aspect of patient care, hospital management utilizes resources of healthcare, people, and advanced technology to execute organizational goals.

2.7.4 *Patient-Centric Care*

The focus on patients is reflected by the need assessment of the population. This impulse planning of services and information management drive a redesign of internal processes to enhance patient satisfaction in service outcomes [41]. Management helps staff to reach their goals through proper channels of open communication, motivation, and incentive programs.

To summarize: The healthcare industry is extremely interdependent, and merely one ambit cannot achieve efficiency parting behind others. Healthcare providers are beneath the enormous pressure as a result of increased competition, regulation of governments, mounting costs, rising demand for services with higher quality, and patient-centric care. To meet this requirement, hospital management can offer noteworthy opportunities to change and build up the overall performance of healthcare.

References

1. Srinivisan, R. (2020). *HEALTH CARE IN INDIA - VISION 2020. 2507* (February), 1–9.
2. Kakodkar, P., & GS, M. (2010). Health Care System in India. *Questions and Answers in Community Dentistry, March*, 277–277. https://doi.org/10.5005/jp/books/11018_33
3. Rodriguez, H. (2019). *The Modern Healthcare Value Chain is a Care-centric Supply Chain Session Overview Abstract :*
4. Madlabana, C. Z., Mashamba-Thompson, T. P., & Petersen, I. (2020). Performance management methods and practices among nurses in primary health care settings: A systematic scoping review protocol. *Systematic Reviews*, *9*(1), 1–9. https://doi.org/10.1186/s13643-020-01294-w

5. Epping-Jordan, J. A. E., Bengoa, R., & Yach, D. (2003). Chronic conditions - The new health challenge. *South African Medical Journal, 93*(8), 585–590. https://doi.org/10.7196/SAMJ.2279
6. Tinetti, M. E., Naik, A. D., & Dodson, J. A. (2016). Moving From Disease-Centered to Patient Goals–Directed Care for Patients With Multiple Chronic Conditions: Patient Value-Based Care. *JAMA Cardiology*, *1*(1), 9–10. https://doi.org/10.1001/jamacardio.2015.0248
7. Kuluski, K., Peckham, A., Williams, A. P., & Upshur, R. E. G. (2016). What Gets in the Way of Person-Centred Care for People with Multimorbidity? Lessons from Ontario, Canada. *Healthcare Quarterly (Toronto, Ont.)*, *19*(2), 17–23. https://doi.org/10.12927/hcq.2016.24694
8. Topp, S. M. (2017). The Lancet Global Health Commission on High-Quality Health Systems—where's the complexity? *The Lancet Global Health*, *5*(6), e571. https://doi.org/10.1016/S2214-109X(17)30176-6
9. Kruk, M. E., Gage, A. D., Arsenault, C., Jordan, K., Leslie, H. H., Roder-DeWan, S., Adeyi, O., Barker, P., Daelmans, B., Doubova, S. V., English, M., Elorrio, E. G., Guanais, F., Gureje, O., Hirschhorn, L. R., Jiang, L., Kelley, E., Lemango, E. T., Liljestrand, J., … Pate, M. (2018). High-quality health systems in the Sustainable Development Goals era: time for a revolution. *The Lancet Global Health*, *6*(11), e1196–e1252. https://doi.org/10.1016/S2214-109X(18)30386-3
10. Berman, P. A. (1996). Health sector reform: making health development sustainable. *Health Sector Reform in Developing Countries*, *32*, 13–33.
11. Vora, A. A. (2016). Introduction to the healthcare sector. In *Hospital Management from the service sector* (pp. 1–10).
12. Basu, S., Andrews, J., Kishore, S., Panjabi, R., & Stuckler, D. (2012). Comparative performance of private and public healthcare systems in low- and middle-income countries: A systematic review. *PLoS Medicine*, *9*(6), 19. https://doi.org/10.1371/journal.pmed.1001244
13. Sengupta, A. (2005). The private health sector in India Is burgeoning, but at the cost of public health care. *BMJ British Medical Journal*, *331*(7528), 1157–1158. http://www.cehat.org/infocentre/main1.html
14. BM Sakharkar. (2009). *Principles of Hospital Administration and Planning* (second edition (ed.)). Jaypee Brothers Medical Publishers (p) Ltd.
15. PAT Research. (2020). *All About Automotive Industry: Key Segments, Value Chain, Needs and Competitive Advantage in 2021 - Reviews, Features, Pricing, Comparison - PAT RESEARCH: B2B Reviews, Buying Guides & Best Practices*. https://www.predictiveanalyticstoday.com/what-is-automotive-industry-top-software-in-automotive-industry/. https://www.predictive-analyticstoday.com/what-is-healthcare-industry/
16. Marume, D. S. B. M., Jaricha, E., & Chiunye, T. M. (2016). An Understanding of Concepts of Line, Staff, and Auxiliary in Organization. *IOSR Journal of Nursing and Health Science*, 05(04), 43–46. https://doi.org/10.9790/1959-0504034346
17. Brewer, D. J., & Picus, L. O. (2016). Auxiliary Services. *Encyclopedia of Education Economics & Finance*. https://doi.org/10.4135/9781483346595.n26
18. Burns, L. R., Degraaff, R. A, Danzon, P. M., Kimberly, J. R., Kissick, W. L., & Pauly, M. V. (2001). The Wharton School Study of the Health Care Value Chain. *Book, September 2015*, 3–26.
19. Mathew, J., John, J., Kumar, S., & Management, O. (2013). New Trends in Healthcare Supply chain. *2013 POM 24th Annual Conference of the Production and Operations Management*, 1–10.
20. Invest India. (2021). Healthcare Industry in India, Indian Healthcare Sector, Invest... In *the Healthcare industry in India*. https://www.investindia.gov.in/sector/healthcare
21. KPMG-FICCI. (2015). *Healthcare: The neglected GDP driver*. 1–38. https://www.kpmg.com/IN/en/IssuesAndInsights/ArticlesPublications/Documents/Healthcaretheneglected/GDP/driver-2015.pdf
22. Vishnoi, A. (2020). Indian health care underfunded, delivery poor: World Bank Report. *The Economic Times*. https://economictimes.indiatimes.com/

23. Thakur, J., Prinja, S., Garg, C. C., Mendis, S., & Menabde, N. (2011). Social and Economic Implications of Noncommunicable diseases in India. *Indian Journal of Community Medicine: Official Publication of Indian Association of Preventive & Social Medicine*, *36*(Suppl 1), S13-22. https://doi.org/10.4103/0970-0218.94704
24. Sarwal, R., Prasad, U., Madangopal, K., Kalal, S., Kaur, D., Kumar, A., Regy, P., & Sharma, J. (2021). *Investment Opportunities in India's Healthcare Sector.*
25. Kapoor, G., Sriram, A., Joshi, J., Nandi, A., & Laxminarayan, R. (2020). *COVID-19 in India: State-wise estimates of current hospital beds, intensive care unit (ICU) beds, and ventilators. April,* 12. https://play.google.com/store/apps/details?id=apptodate.myFrequency&hl=en&gl=US
26. Agarwal, V. (2021). The Future of Healthcare Post Covid. *The Economic Times.*
27. Jazieh, A. R., & Kozlakidis, Z. (2020). Healthcare Transformation in the Post-Coronavirus Pandemic Era. *Frontiers in Medicine*, *7*(July), 1–6. https://doi.org/10.3389/fmed.2020.00429
28. Alami, H., Gagnon, M. P., Wootton, R., Fortin, J. P., & Zanaboni, P. (2017). Exploring factors associated with the uneven utilization of telemedicine in Norway: a mixed-methods study. *BMC Medical Informatics and Decision Making*, *17*(1), 180. https://doi.org/10.1186/s12911-017-0576-4
29. Donaghy, E., Atherton, H., Hammersley, V., McNeilly, H., Bikker, A., Robbins, L., Campbell, J., & McKinstry, B. (2019). Acceptability, benefits, and challenges of video consulting: a qualitative study in primary care. *The British Journal of General Practice: The Journal of the Royal College of General Practitioners*, *69*(686), e586–e594. https://doi.org/10.3399/bjgp19X704141
30. Mackillop, W. J. (2012). Health Services Research in Radiation Oncology. *Clinical Radiation Oncology: Third Edition*, 203–222. https://doi.org/10.1016/B978-1-4377-1637-5.00011-0
31. Smith, P. C., Mossialos, E., Papanicolas, I., & Leatherman, S. (2010). Performance measurement for health system improvement: experiences, challenges, and prospects. *Performance Measurement for Health System Improvement: Experiences, Challenges and Prospects*, 1–726. https://doi.org/10.1017/CBO9780511711800
32. empxtrack. (2017). *Top 5 Performance Management Challenges in Healthcare Industry.* https://empxtrack.com/blog/performance-management-challenges-in-health-industry/
33. USAID, & WHO. (2007). *Implementing Best Practices Consortium: A guide for Fostering Change to Scale-up Effective Health Services.*
34. Uzuegbu, C., & Nnadozie, C. (2015). Henry Fayol's 14 Principles of Management: Implications for Libraries and Information Centres. *Journal of Information Science Theory and Practice*, *3*, 58–72. https://doi.org/10.1633/JISTaP.2015.3.2.5
35. Sarab, S. (2019). *Hospital Management System.* https://doi.org/10.13140/RG.2.2.35189.19686
36. Narayanan, D. (2010). Tamil Nadu Medical Services Corporation: A Success Story. *Forbs India.*
37. Liu Li, Tao Ran, Gao Danqi, Qi Ting, Gao Yue, D. B. (2021). *Dd_Citation_Export.* https://www.deepdyve.com/lp/springer-journals/was-mauritius-really-successful-in-banning-plastic-carry-bags-after-ZcrsmeLVIc?
38. Alverson, C. (2003). *Beyond purchasing--Managing hospital inventory.* https://www.semanticscholar.org/paper/Beyond-purchasing%2D%2DManaging-hospital-inventory-Alverson
39. Suter, E., Oelke, N. D., Adair, C. E., & Armitage, G. D. (2009). Ten key principles for successful health systems integration. *Healthcare Quarterly (Toronto, Ont.)*, *13 Spec No* (Spec No), 16–23. https://doi.org/10.12927/hcq.2009.21092
40. Kavitha, R. (2012). Health Care Industry in India. *International Journal of Scientific and Research Publications*, *2*(8), 5–8.
41. Roberts, C. C. (1996). Redefining the healthcare paradigm. A proposal for successful provider integration. *Hospital Topics*, *74*(2), 16–20. https://doi.org/10.1080/00185868.1996.11736052

Chapter 3
Hospital Management Challenges

H. K. Mamatha, N. Shalini, Divya Rao, and Arehally M. Mahalakshmi

3.1 Introduction

Healthcare organizations are complex and constantly changing entities. In terms of functions and resources, they are dynamic and diverse. Healthcare services are frequently delivered through systems and organizations that are made up of three distinct levels of care—primary, secondary, and tertiary care. They all share a common purpose of serving the public irrespective of the nature of the organization whether government-owned, private, not-for-profit, independent, or commercial healthcare providers [1]. Employees working in healthcare organizations have deeply ingrained professional values and culture and possess a belief in their contribution to society in terms of value. They also have self-interested motivations related to reward, recognition, and career advancement.

Healthcare systems are also complex environments, as evidenced by the diversity of their structures, cultures, and services. Managing this complexity by fostering teamwork is regarded as an effective and efficient model [2, 3]. Management is the process of creating and maintaining an environment in which people work in groups to achieve specific goals [4].

Any organization's structure is made up of units and functions. These units and functions have positions where job holders are held accountable for results. Relationships exist between these positions that necessitate the exercise of authority and the exchange of information. That is what is commonly referred to as a "chain of command," which begins at the top and defines a hierarchy of positions.

H. K. Mamatha (✉) · N. Shalini · D. Rao
Department of Health System Management Studies, JSS Academy of Higher Education and Research, Mysuru, India
e-mail: pc_mamatha@jssuni.edu.in

A. M. Mahalakshmi
JSS College of Pharmacy, JSS Academy of Higher Education and Research, Mysuru, India

D. Bhatia et al. (eds.), *A Guide to Hospital Administration and Planning*,
https://doi.org/10.1007/978-981-19-6692-7_3

Managers must work with teams comprised of members with diverse backgrounds whether it is professional, organizational, or cultural backgrounds, and managing these diversities can be difficult. Furthermore, in healthcare, it is very difficult for professionals to relate to only one team, hence pressures related to diverse agendas and time management. Managers have to be sensitive and understanding in managing these employees.

3.2 Hospital Management

Management of healthcare organizations necessitates people with strong conceptual, technical, and interpersonal skills. The manager of a hospital is not only at the top level but also at multiple levels depending on the size of the hospital. Management positions exist at three levels: lower, middle, and upper, with delegation and control at each. A hospital's hierarchy is a top-down approach with power and authority concentrated at the top. Management models for organizational structures can be functional, matrix, team based, or line based. Managers are responsible for planning, staffing, directing, and controlling. Decision-making and analytical abilities are critical at all levels of management.

Healthcare organizations are changing their business models to keep up with technological advances. The incorporation of technology into various hospital processes has resulted in a paradigm shift in hospital operations. Human resources must adapt and equip themselves to provide quality care, so training is an ongoing process in a hospital. Managers must identify training needs and provide opportunities for employees to upskill and upgrade their knowledge.

According to Evans [5], healthcare reform is based on three important questions which are as follows:

- Who pays for care (and how much does it cost)?
- Who receives care (what type, when, and from whom)?
- Who is paid how much and for what?

The patient care process can be infinitely adapted or customized to individual patient needs, disease circumstances, and responses to treatment. However, in modern healthcare, processes are more complex, requiring multiple handovers between healthcare professionals, shortened length of stay, and more risks and complexities of new healthcare interventions. This has made the traditional patient care model increasingly unreliable, unsafe, and prone to error and unexplained variation [6]. Care pathways, treatment plans, and clinical guidelines are increasingly being used by healthcare organizations to have a structure and transparency to the healthcare process.

3.3 Challenges in Hospital Management

Living in the twenty-first century has made everyone adapt to the rapid rate of change in every sector of society, and healthcare is no exception in that. In developed nations, the drivers of change are based on outdated traditional methods, cost containment tools, and increasing consumer demands on quality and sophistication in healthcare.

Healthcare has witnessed a significant amount of evolution. The factors that influence more changes in the healthcare system are:

- Health transition—demographic changes, epidemiological changes, emergence of infectious diseases
- Technological advancement—diagnostic, therapeutic, preventive, and robotics and artificially intelligent computer-assisted medical interventions
- Quality management

Any organization's environment comprises the forces and circumstances that encircle and pervade it. An organization's success or failure is entirely dependent on how well it manages the conflicting demands of its environment.

Like any organization, hospital also has two environmental components:

- External
- Internal

The **external environment** can again be categorized as the macro (general) and the micro (operating) environment.

- The general environment consists of several dimensions such as political, legal, economic, sociocultural, technological, and international dimensions. These dimensions might influence its activities and may act as a threat or an opportunity to it.
- The operating environment includes groups and forces which are external to the organization and with whom the organization has direct contact and transactions. These groups are the patients, healthcare professionals, competitors, regulators, suppliers, agencies, unions, and professional associations.

The basic components of the **internal environment** include self, tasks, process and skills, formal design of the organization, organizational culture, individual employees, or people system, together.

The management should develop strategies and structures to meet the demands by assessing the forces in the macro environment and the interactive effects these have on the micro and internal environments.

3.3.1 *Demands for Change*

Demographic

Demographic conditions are a key factor in the business environment wherein healthcare dealers must compete. For the physicians, hospitals, and bed supply in the hospitals, the predictors include the size of the population and demographic changes in terms of age, structure, and income [7].

According to Gröne et al.'s study, [8] demographic trends are constituting challenges to health systems because of the increase in the need for health and social services at the retirement age and further increase after the age of 75.

There is a significant impact of population dynamics on the healthcare labor force shortage. These factors combine to increase the size and proportion of the population in need of care, namely the elderly. This also decreases the availability of physicians and nurses to care for the growing elderly population [9].

Economic

Healthcare costs are a concern for every country. Several factors influence the choice of services by the patients; one important factor is the influence of the general practitioners who recommend the best of the services and help them find such services.

The cost of healthcare in the world has increased drastically over the decades owing to several changes in healthcare delivery. Medical procedure and hospital stay costs have also risen over the last decade and are expected to rise further.

"Part of the reason we spend more on health care each year is the nation's growing and aging population," said Dr. Joseph Dieleman [10], Institute for Health Metrics and Evaluation, University of Washington. Further, he said, "factors associated with health care spending are population growth, population aging, disease prevalence or incidence, service utilization, and service price and intensity."

Technological

Healthcare IT provides insights into new medical technologies as well as updates on new healthcare technologies. The present healthcare sector is dealing with cost issues and at the same time trying to implement new technologies. As a result, healthcare technology is becoming increasingly important. Healthcare technology incorporates tools that integrate technology in every step of the healthcare experience to determine quality and efficiency.

The latest health and technology news can teach us a lot about the prospects of medical care. Healthcare technologies apply skills and knowledge in the form of tools and devices, as well as inventions, to solve healthcare challenges. The primary goal of healthcare technology is to increase productivity and manage staff and operational processes in healthcare.

Trends in Healthcare Technology

Due to rapidly establishing new technological innovations, healthcare trends are not a new phenomenon in the healthcare industry. Customers are becoming more technologically savvy and are continuously seeking convenience.

In the future, several existing and emerging technologies will have a positive impact on the healthcare industry. Artificial intelligence, machine learning, virtual reality, augmented reality, and wearable technology will all become essential tools for healthcare providers and organizations to improve their performance.

Considering the reforms and changes in healthcare, the future trends in healthcare are as follows:

- Growth in telehealth can precisely aid critical care facilities to a great extent.
- Digital health is progressively capturing a considerable position in our lives with several wearable devices, health sensors, and trackers being used, and combining it with the Internet of Things can enable patients to view their data on their devices.
- Improvement in data science and predictive analytics.
- Artificial intelligence will influence trends in healthcare as it has increased the accuracy of diagnosis through automatic assistance in the workforce, optimization of clinical operation, quantitative imaging, etc.
- Cloud computing makes it easy to share medical records, automate backend operations, and even create and maintain telehealth apps.
- The blockchain system will generate identical blocks whenever a linked device is involved in any form of transaction.
- With the introduction of virtual reality and augmented reality, healthcare technologies have improved drastically. Virtual reality assists patients in certain conditions such as cancer, depression, autism, and vision therapy.

Technological advancement in healthcare is a major driver of cost growth. It also provides effective training, cure, and care by using interactive ways.

Quality Management

Quality of healthcare has a big impact on both the providers of healthcare and the patients who receive it. Quality is a continuous process of improving the quality of what we do. It means doing the right thing the first time and doing it better the next time. As in other industries, where quality is customer centric, healthcare should be likewise customer focused to meet customer needs and expectations effectively and efficiently. Quality can be described in terms of eight dimensions: effectiveness, efficiency, interpersonal relationships, safety, technical competency, access, continuity, and amenities. Each of the dimensions of quality should be met at least minimally to meet the definition. Efforts must be made by everyone at every level at various phases of the healthcare delivery system to acquire and maintain quality.

There has been an increasing interest as well as concerns about the quality of services rendered by hospitals as standards of living change. Service quality has become increasingly important for hospitals in their efforts of satisfying and retaining patients.

Patient satisfaction is a valid indicator of measuring service quality [11], where dissatisfaction helps to improve service. Patient satisfaction explains the degree to which expectations of a patient are fulfilled by medical services. Besides, patient satisfaction is a decisive indicator to understand the patient's expectations.

Patient Satisfaction

Satisfaction means the fulfilment or gratification of a desire, need, or appetite.

The extent of patient content with the care they received from their healthcare provider is a measure of patient satisfaction [12].

Factors influencing patient satisfaction are appropriateness, timeliness, respect and concern, safety of the patient, continuity, effectiveness, efficacy, and availability.

Patient Safety

One of the basic principles of the healthcare system is patient safety. Patient safety is a term used to refer to several actions taken by the healthcare system to protect the patients from any harm during treatment, which includes blunders such as infections, injuries, accidents, and medication errors, and to ensure patient safety and quality of services.

According to the WHO statistics, 1 in 10 patients is harmed during hospital care in developed countries, and studies showed that around 4,40,000 patients die owing to the lack of patient care at hospitals. These results suggest that patient safety is very much important as the healthcare system becomes more complex.

Human Resource Development

Despite technological developments, one cannot rule out the significance of manpower in hospitals. Most recent and new technologies cannot substitute the contribution made by specialized manpower in the healthcare industry. Human resource managers in the healthcare industry are responsible for various issues like employee retention, legal matters, and recruitment of staff.

The issues that face healthcare HR professionals today and tomorrow are:

- Recruitment in healthcare
- Wage competition
- Turnover and retention

- Burnout
- Training and development
- Doing more with less
- Compliance with quality standards
- Implementing diversity planning and culturally competent care
- Preparing healthcare workers for new technologies
- Balancing professional and personal lives
- Succession planning

In the research conducted by B. E. Smith, for the annual Healthcare Trends white paper, numerous challenges to healthcare executive teams include the following:

- Leadership compensation and competencies
- Succession planning
- Physician leadership
- Workforce engagement

Each of these trends presents unique opportunities for human resource executives to strengthen their healthcare organization throughout the year.

Leadership and Beyond

Theories about management and leadership keep changing over time. Some people hold strong beliefs about the attributes and behaviors that a natural leader should exhibit. Situational leadership, however, postulates that there is no universal "best" leadership style.

Effective leadership behaviors adjust to the specific situation, particularly the degree of direction or support that a particular employee requires from their supervisor to perform tasks successfully.

Effective healthcare leaders should possess:

- Emotional intelligence
- Technological management
- Adaptive and quick decision-making
- Relationship development
- Powerful communication

Effective healthcare leaders lead organizations through service delivery and help them flourish by improving patient outcomes in an ever-changing environment. The dynamic nature of healthcare delivery requires competent, innovative leaders to drive the organization through human resources, technological and service quality concerns, and improvements. Healthcare leaders should manage complex operational arenas, maintain service consistency, and help the organizations stay abreast of medical advancements.

3.4 Conclusion

Hospital management is confronted with a variety of challenges and problems. These are often caused or aggravated by external factors, which are out of the hospital management's control.

Hospital management needs to tackle these challenges and issues in a systematic and sometimes creative way. There is no guarantee of a final resolution, but mitigating a problem is already an achievement. A manager needs to develop a good understanding of the issues, their underlying causes, and the resources, techniques, and tools available to tackle the challenges.

References

1. Drucker P. Managing the Nonprofit Organisation. London: HarperCollins. 2006.
2. Ingram, H. and Desombre, T. (1999) Teamwork in healthcare: Lessons from the literature and good practice around the world. Journal of Management in Medicine, 13: 15.
3. West, M. and Markievicz, L. (2004) Building Team-based Working – A Practical Guide to Organizational Transformation. Oxford: Blackwell.
4. Adeleke A. Management concepts and applications. Lagos: Concept Publication Limited. 2004.
5. Evans, R.G. (2005) Fellow travelers on a contested path: Power purpose and the evolution of European health care systems. Journal of Health Policy Politics and Law. Special Issue: Legacies and Latitude in European Health Policy, 30(1–2): 277– 93.
6. Walshe K, Boaden R. (eds) Patient Safety: Research into Practice. Maidenhead: Open University Press/McGraw Hill. 2005
7. Pol LG, Tymkiw DR. Demographic change and the supply of physicians, hospitals, and hospital beds: marketing implications. J Hosp Mark. 1990;4(2):71-83. https://doi.org/10.1300/J043v04n02_07.
8. Gröne O, Garcia-Barbero M; WHO European Office for Integrated Health Care Services. Integrated care: a position paper of the WHO European Office for Integrated Health Care Services. Int J Integr Care. 2001;1:e21.
9. Cohen, Steven A. DrPH, MPH. A Review of Demographic and Infrastructural Factors and Potential Solutions to the Physician and Nursing Shortage Predicted to Impact the Growing US Elderly Population. Journal of Public Health Management and Practice July 2009 - Volume 15 - Issue 4 - p 352-362. https://doi.org/10.1097/PHH.0b013e31819d817d
10. Dieleman JL, Squires E, Bui AL, Campbell M, Chapin A, Hamavid H, Horst C, Li Z, Matyasz T, Reynolds A, Sadat N. Factors associated with increases in US health care spending, 1996-2013. Jama. 2017 Nov 7;318(17):1668-78.
11. Natarajappa S, Ravi MD, Chandrashekar BR, Nagesh P. Evaluation of Service Quality in a Tertiary Care Hospital Using A Novel Patient Satisfaction Survey Tool in Mysore City, India–A Pilot Study. EXECUTIVE EDITOR. 2020 Jul;11(7):858.
12. Natarajappa S, Ravi MD, Chandrashekar BR, Nagesh P. Development and validation of a new tool (TerHosQual) for assessing service quality in a tertiary care hospital. Journal of Medical Society. 2020 Jan 1;34(1):17.

Chapter 4
Human Resource Management in Hospitals

H. K. Mamatha, N. Shalini, Divya Rao, and Arehally M. Mahalakshmi

4.1 Introduction

Human resource management (HRM) is managing human resource in an organization. The human resource of an organization is comprised of the capabilities, efforts, and skills of all the people working for that organization. Human resources are regarded as valuable assets and are vital for the growth and development of the organization. Competent and motivated human resources with their dynamism help achieve their goals and build dynamic organization. The quantity and quality of human resources determine largely an organization's performance and productivity, thereby emphasizing the need for effective and efficient management of its people for sustenance and continued growth.

HRM is a multidisciplinary concept and is an integration of many fields such as management, sociology, economics, psychology, and organizational behavior. It is with this integration that human resource management practices and functions affect the performance outcomes of organizations. As HRM involves people and is all about managing people at work, there is no best way to manage. Human beings are complex beings with complex needs, and most often these needs are dynamic and ever changing. Hence, for effective HRM, causes and conditions provided by the organization are essential. In an organization, three basic components—people, purpose, and structure—are important, and the most important among these is the people component.

H. K. Mamatha (✉) · N. Shalini · D. Rao
Department of Health System Management Studies, JSS Academy of Higher Education and Research, Mysuru, India
e-mail: pc_mamatha@jssuni.edu.in

A. M. Mahalakshmi
JSS College of Pharmacy, JSS Academy of Higher Education and Research, Mysuru, India

D. Bhatia et al. (eds.), *A Guide to Hospital Administration and Planning*,
https://doi.org/10.1007/978-981-19-6692-7_4

Human resource management is both a science and an art as it encompasses well-organized knowledge, principles, and techniques and deals with human beings with feelings and emotions. It requires knowledge, skill, and humane approach to deal effectively with people at work to achieve the organizational objectives. This is even more relevant in a hospital as it is a service industry dealing with patients and the service is rendered by humans.

4.1.1 Meaning, Definition, and Objectives

Meaning

Human resource management is constituted by two major terms: (1) **human resource** and (2) **management**. **HR** means people at work, and m**anagement** has drawn its concepts and principles from several disciplines such as psychology, sociology, economics, anthropology, and statistics.

Human resource management (HRM) is the process of several related aspects starting from employing people, providing training, appropriate compensation, developing policies, and strategies to retain them.

Definition

Leon C. Megginson referred to the human resources as "the total knowledge, skills, creative abilities, talents, and aptitudes of an organization's workforce, as well as the values, attitudes, approaches, and beliefs of the individuals involved in the affairs of the organization [1]."

The American Management Association said:

"Human Resource Management is that field of management which has to do with planning, organizing, and controlling various operative functions of procuring, developing, maintaining, and utilizing a work force in order that:

(a) the objectives for which the company is established are attained as efficiently and economically as possible.
(b) the objectives of all levels of personnel are served to the highest degree; and,
(c) the objectives of the community are duly considered and served."

Edwin B. Flippo defined human resource management as "the planning, organizing, directing, and controlling of the procurement, development, resources to the end that individual and societal objectives are accomplished."

Objectives

The primary objective of HRM is to ensure the availability of competent and willing workforce to an organization.

Scott, Clothier, and Spiegel [2] explained the objectives of human resource management as follows:

- To obtain optimum individual development and cordial working relationships between employers and employees and between employees
- To mold human resources to adapt to the requirement unlike other physical resources

These objectives of HRM can be categorized as follows (Fig. 4.1):

1. Societal objectives: To ensure social responsibility of the organization wherein the needs and challenges of the society are given consideration and decrease the influence of such demands on the organization. The organizations should utilize their resources for the benefit of the society in ethical ways, and failure to do so may lead to restrictions.
2. Organizational objectives: To ensure organizational effectiveness by making HRM department assist the organization in achieving its primary objectives. This department should serve the rest of the organization and not as a standalone department.
3. Functional objectives: To maintain the contribution of the department at an appropriate level to the needs of the organization by ensuring that human resources meet the demands of the organization. The value of the department should not be expensive than the cost of the organization.
4. Personal objectives: To assist employees in fulfilling their personal goals and ensuring that these goals enhance the individual's contribution to the organization. It is very important to meet the personal goals of employees to maintain, motivate, and retain employees. If employees are not satisfied, employee turnover may increase in addition to decrease in performance.

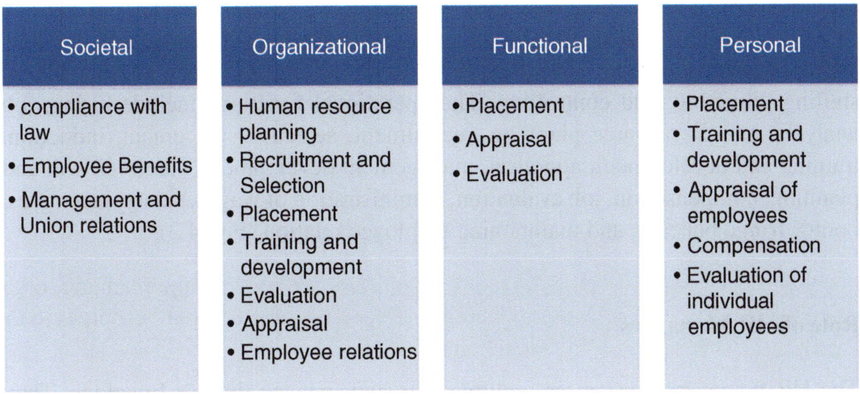

Fig. 4.1 Objectives of HRM

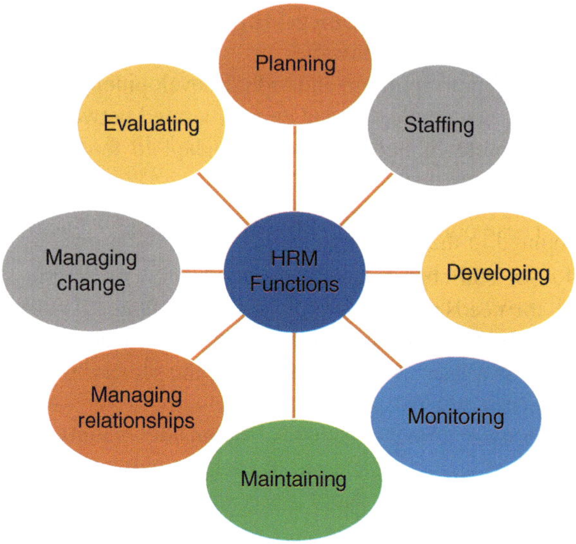

Fig. 4.2 HRM functions

4.1.2 Scope and Functions

The scope of HRM is very vast and includes all major activities in the work life of a worker—from the time of their entry into an organization until they leave the organization. The important activities of HRM include human resource planning, job analysis, job designing, hiring, remuneration, employee motivation and maintenance, and industrial relations.

HRM is a staff function, and the role of human resource manager is to advise line managers across the organization and supply human resources in the right number, right quality, right time, and right cost (Fig. 4.2).

The functions of HR managers can be broadly classified as managerial functions and operational functions. The managerial functions include planning, organizing, staffing, directing, and controlling. The operational functions include hiring, job analysis, human resource planning, recruitment, selection, placement, induction, training and development, appraisal, management development, career growth and planning, compensation, job evaluation, administration of wages, salary, incentives, bonus, fringe benefits, and maintaining employee relation (Fig. 4.3).

Role of HR Managers

The HR managers must wear multiple hats and manage diverse functions. They must have a thorough knowledge of the organization and its intricacies and complexities. The manager's profession can be defined as "playing several roles or planned sets of actions linked to his position" [3]. These may be classified into three folds—informational, interpersonal, and decisional (Fig. 4.4).

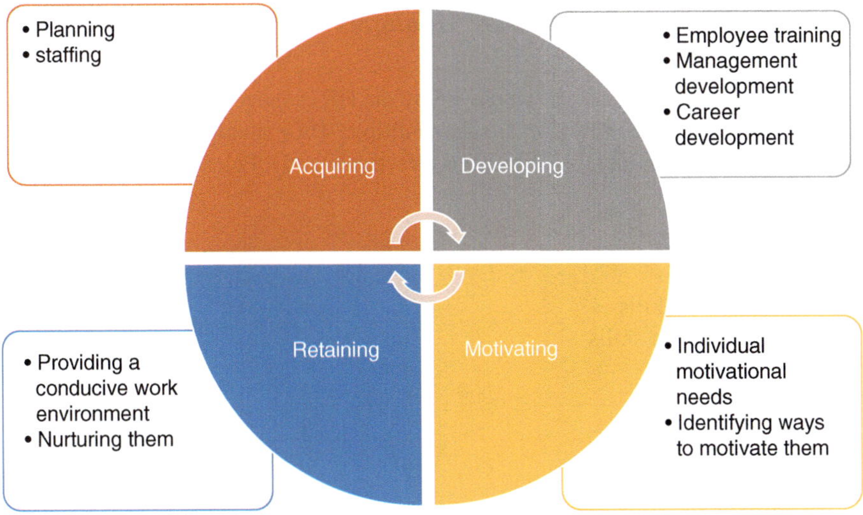

Fig. 4.3 Functions of HRM

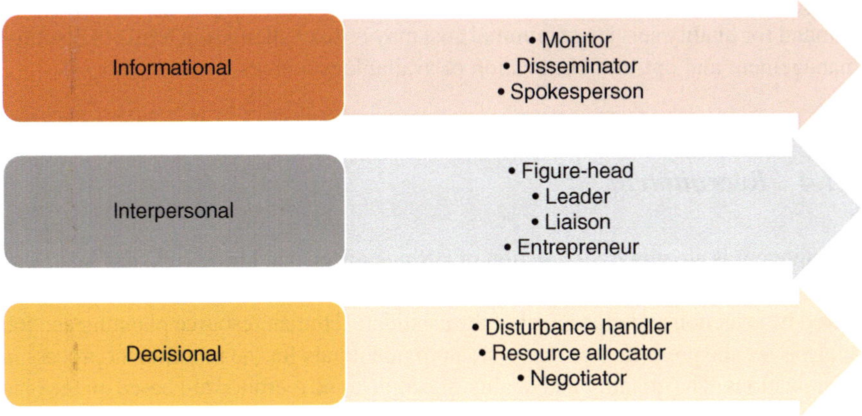

Fig. 4.4 Role of HR managers

Dave Ulrich [4] stated that HR plays four key roles:

1. Strategic partner role—converting strategy into outcomes and building organizations that create value
2. Change agent role—ensuring that change happens and to make it happen faster
3. Employee champion role—talent management of knowledge capital within the organization
4. Administrative role—ensuring that things happen at a pace required to meet the needs

4.1.3 Skills Required for HR Managers

Considering the diverse role to be played by the HR managers, it should be considered that skills required for them are also multiple. They should possess qualities of head and heart to conduct their functions effectively and efficiently. These skills can be considered as:

1. Technical skills
2. Cognitive skills
3. Interpersonal skills
4. Communication skills
5. Empathetic
6. Tolerance
7. Temperament
8. Pleasant
9. Confident
10. People loving
11. Multi-knowledgeable—finance, sales, marketing, operations, etc.

The competencies expected of a HR manager are business mastery, HR mastery, change mastery, and personal credibility [5]. In healthcare organizations, the demand for quality service at minimal cost may pose challenges in terms of resource management and optimum utilization of available resources.

4.1.4 Recruitment

Recruitment is an important function of HR managers, and hiring right candidate can provide an asset to the organization. Recruitment is a step in the process of hiring followed by selection and placement of the candidate. Human resource planning and job analysis are the preliminary steps which provide inputs for the recruitment process in organizations. The quantity and quality of people to be recruited are based on the plan and the need. The supply of right candidate at the right time and right position ensures smooth functioning of the organization without compromising the productivity. Considering the diverse workforce in healthcare organizations/hospitals is particularly important to plan the requirement beforehand for recruitment. Recruitment is "the process of attracting candidates towards a job in an organization." When a vacancy for a job exists, recruitment is initiated. Selection is a "process of hiring right person for a right job at a right time at a right cost." Selection follows recruitment.

Edwin B. Flippo [6] defined recruitment as "the process of searching the candidates for employment and stimulating them to apply for jobs in the organization."

Dale Yoder [7] defined recruitment as "a process to discover the sources of manpower to meet the requirements of the staffing schedule and to employ effective measures for attracting that manpower in adequate numbers to facilitate effective selection of an efficient working force."

The purpose of recruitment is to

1. Assess the present and future requirements of the organization's HRP and job analysis
2. Enhance the pool of job candidates at minimum cost
3. Ensure the success of selection process
4. Determine the composition of workforce to meet the organization's legal and social obligations
5. Identify potential job applicants and appropriate candidates
6. Increase the effectiveness of both organization and individual in terms of short-term and long-term goals
7. Evaluate the effectiveness of recruitment process

Creating a suitable recruitment policy is the first step in the efficient hiring process. According to Dale Yoder, "the recruitment policy is concerned with quantity and qualifications of manpower." The policy gives broad guidelines for the staffing process. Recruitment policy helps ensure recruitment process. Recruitment policy depends upon the organization system. Every organization formulates recruitment policy, which enables to find the best qualified person for each job and retains the best and most promising opportunities for the lifetime, i.e., career growth.

Recruitment process involves planning, strategy development, searching, screening, evaluation, and control. Both direct and indirect methods of recruitment are considered for hiring candidates. Sources of recruitment can be internal or external [8]. Internal recruitment is filling vacant jobs with the employees working in the organization, and external recruitment is recruiting people from external labor market to fulfill the labor requirements. Sources of internal recruitment include the existing employees, former employees, and employee referrals. Sources of external recruitment include employment exchanges, job agencies, advertisements, campus recruitment drives, walk-ins and write-ins, online/internet recruiting, raiding, or poaching.

Recruitment is initiated because of one of the following reasons [2]:

- Vacancies: arising due to expansion and growth of business, diversification, need of more workforce, or employee separation as a result of promotion, transfers, retirement, termination, employee's permanent disability, or death to address shortage of manpower
- Competitive advantage: organizational concerns to achieve more business than formerly
- Expand business: during the recovery period of business cycle
- Market demand: increased demand due to population growth requiring more goods and services to fulfill the requirements of the people
- Increase in standard of living: increased demand for same goods and services and emerging new wants to be fulfilled

4.1.5 Training and Development

Training and development are an ongoing process in an organization. Training is essential for the employees to perform their duties effectively. Training is the process of imparting specific skills.

Development refers to the learning opportunities with the objective of providing help for employees to grow, which need not be skill oriented. Development provides the employees required knowledge and attitudes which will be helpful for them in higher positions.

Edwin Flippo [9] defined training as "the act of increasing the skills of an employee for doing a particular job." It is "a process of learning sequence of programmed behavior."

According to Michael Armstrong [10], "training is systematic development of the knowledge, skills and attitude required by an individual to perform adequately a given task or job."

Reasons for Training

Organizations are dynamic systems and need continuous change in process and techniques. This necessitates dynamic workforce who are continuously upskilling and enhancing their knowledge. This forms the basis for training of employees in organizations.

The training process starts with assessing the training needs of employees. This includes ensuring employees' readiness for training, providing a learning environment, ensuring transfer of training, selecting appropriate training method, and in the end evaluating the training program (Fig. 4.5).

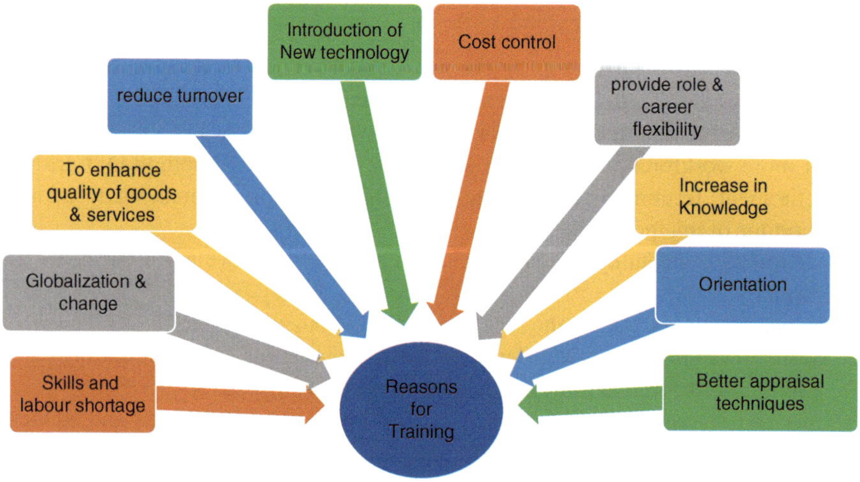

Fig. 4.5 Reasons for training of employees in organizations

On-the-job	Off-the-job	others
• Orientation	• Lecture & special duty	• Computer based training
• Coaching	• Vestibule training	• Internet based training
• Mentoring	• Conference method	• Active learning
• Job-instruction training	• Case study	• Job rotation
• Apprenticeship	• Role play	• Management games
• Internship	• Simulation method	• University related programs
• Job rotation	• Programmed instruction	• Outside seminars
• Committee assignments	• Laboratory training	
	• Virtual organizations and e-learning	
	• Behaviorally experienced training	

Fig. 4.6 Types of training

Types of Training

Training depends on the needs assessment and the method of training. The training methods can be broadly classified as on-the-job training and off-the-job training methods and sometimes a combination of both. The approaches to training are (Fig. 4.6):

- Skill training—explain, relate, respect, encourage, give feedback
- Refresher training
- Cross-functional training
- Team training
- Creativity training—breaking away, generate innovative ideas, delaying judgement (brainstorming)
- Diversity training
- Literacy training
- Orientation training

Depending on the need and objective, the appropriate training method must be selected. The outcome of the training depends on the commitment by both the management and employees in realizing the objectives.

The training in a hospital is provided to employees for the following needs:

- Providing better services to patients
- Minimizing waste
- Filling higher posts
- Promoting safety measures
- Ensuring that employees are taught to efficiently operate new machines which are installed or are likely to be installed soon

At the end of the training, evaluation of training outcomes is done to understand the effectiveness of the training. Benefits of training are both to the employee and to the employer. The evaluation process is explained as "any attempt to obtain information (feedback) on the effects of a training programme and to assess the value of the training in the light of that information" [11].

4.1.6 Performance Appraisal

Once employees join organizations, their appraisal is a critical component. Performance appraisal is the assessment of the performance of an individual with respect to their job and their potential for development in that job. Performance appraisal is a one-time event done annually, and performance management is a continuous, dynamic, and ongoing process.

According to Edwin B. Flippo [6], "performance appraisal is the systematic, periodic and an impartial rating of an employee's excellence in the matters pertaining to his present job and his potential for a better job."

In the words of Dale Yoder, [7]"Performance appraisal refers to all formal procedures used in working organizations to evaluate personalities and contributions and potential of group members." Performance appraisal is a formal program in an organization which not only assesses contribution of the members to the organization, but also aims to recognize the potential of the people.

According to the International Labour Organization, "A regular and continuous evaluation of the quality, quantity and style of the performance along with the assessment of the factors influencing the performance and behavior of an individual is called as performance appraisal."

Performance appraisal is conducted to meet certain objectives, which includes decision about increase in salary, promotion opportunities, identifying needs for training and development, providing employees with feedback, setting targets, and subjecting employees to stress for better performance. An ideal performance evaluation process should not just provide the basis for managing the business of today but also for developing it in the future [12].

Performance appraisal methods are classified as traditional or conventional and modern methods, and the choice of evaluation is based on the need (Fig. 4.7).

They can also be classified as:

(a) Individual evaluation methods: MBO, BARS, critical incident technique
(b) Multiple-person evaluation methods: 360-degree method, ranking method, paired comparison method, and forced distribution method.

Uses of performance appraisal as HRM function areas include:

1. Salary administration
2. Selection program
3. Employee training and development program
4. Decisions about employees' promotion, transfer, and layoffs

Past oriented methods

- Rating scale
- Checklists
- Forced Choice method
- Forced distribution method
- Critical Incidents method
- Behaviorally Anchored Rating Scales (BARS)
- Field Review Methods
- Performance Tests & observations
- Confidential Records
- Essay Method
- Cost Accounting method
- Comparative Evaluation Method (Ranking & Paired Comparison)

Future oriented methods

- Management By Objectives (MBO)
- Psychological Appraisals
- Assessment Centres
- 360 degree feedback
- Online appraisal method, computerized appraisal, electronic performance monitoring (EPM)

Fig. 4.7 Performance appraisal methods

5. Grievance and discipline program
6. Human resource planning

Performance appraisal is often followed by appraisal interview. This interview involves both supervisor and subordinate, wherein the supervisor and subordinate review the appraisal to identify strengths and weaknesses and remedies to overcome the weakness. Appraisal interview is conducted to achieve the following goals:

- Change the behavior of employees who lack performance and who do not fulfill either organizational or individual goals.
- Maintain the behavior of employees whose performance meets the requirements.
- Recognize employees who exhibit excellent performance behaviors and ensure that they continue to do so.

4.1.7 Laws Related to HRM

Labor law is the "body of laws, administrative rulings, and precedents," which encompass the relationship between and among "employers, employees, and labor organizations" pertaining to the issues of public law. The term "labor" *means* "productive work," especially physical work done for wages.

Labor law, also known as employment law, is "the body of laws, administrative rulings, and precedents which address the legal rights of, and restrictions on, working people and their organizations." It includes different aspects covering relationship between trade unions, employers, and employees. Labor law defines the rights and obligations of each of them as workers, members of the union, and employers in the workplace. Scope of labor law includes:

- Industrial relations—Union certification, labor management relations, collective bargaining, and unfair/unethical labor practices.
- Employee safety at workplace.
- Employment standards' minimum wage, working hours, leaves, holidays, unfair dismissals, procedures related to layoff and severance pay.

Labor laws can be broadly classified into two categories

- Collective labor law which is the tripartite relationship between employee, employer, and union.
- Individual labor law which is about employees' rights at work and through the contract for work.

Objectives of labor law are:

- Protection of workers
- Promote cordial industrial relations
- Preserve health and safety of workers
- Protect the interest of women and children
- Establish a legal system

In hospitals, the role of an administrator will be to ensure safety of their own employees from healthcare-associated infections and protect them with preventive measures. Employee safety and benefits are crucial for retention of staff.

The principles of labor legislation are the following:

1. Social justice: Equitable distribution of profit b/w employer and employees. Protection of workers against harmful effects to their health, safety, and morality.
2. Social equality: Flexibility in labor legislation to adjust to the needs of labor society.
3. Social security: Collective action against social risks.
4. Social justice: Provides standards to be set for labor legislation.

There are many labor laws but those which are applicable to HRM are:

(a) Employees' State Insurance Act 1948
(b) Employees' Provident Fund and Miscellaneous Provisions Act 1952
(c) Payment of Gratuity Act 1972
(d) The Minimum Wages Act 1948
(e) The Maternity Benefit Act 1961
(f) The Payment of Bonus Act 1965
(g) The Payment of Wages Act 1936

In addition to the knowledge about these Acts, the HR professionals working in hospitals should also possess knowledge about the Consumer Protection Act 1986, Industrial Disputes Act 1947, Principles of Natural Justice, etc. to conduct their work efficiently and effectively.

4.1.8 Challenges for HRM in Healthcare

Human resource management is one of the most important and complex responsibilities of hospital administration. Human beings being the epicenter of hospitals, it is imperative to have good HR practices. The product of the hospital is service to people provided by its personnel with a variety of skills. The consumers of these services are physically and/or mentally ill and are rendered services within the four walls of the hospital. Individual patients require unique needs, and hence, it must be personalized and customized to meet their requirements. The nature of service required is also variable depending on the patient need, most often under dire circumstances. In a hospital, the situation also varies ranging across birth, suffering, illness, and death. All these unique circumstances necessitate people who have combination of skills and abilities. The service that is rendered may not be by an individual but a team of dedicated members but with a common goal of patient care. Communication, coordination, and teamwork are crucial for delivering quality care.

There are many changes happening in healthcare especially in the VUCA environment, which increases the existing challenges:

- Organizational consolidation
- Declining margins affected by lower reimbursements
- Advancement in technology
- Consumers demanding improvement in clinical performance
- Volatile environmental forces
- Uncertain market forces

Key issues for HR management include:

- Doing more with less due to shortage of workforce
- Comply with quality standards
- Implement diversity planning and provide culturally competent care
- Train healthcare workers for modern technologies
- Achieve balance in professional and personal lives
- Succession planning strategies
- Address any imbalance in practices by management compared to national policy objectives

For example, the aim of health policies is to develop PHC, while the objective of training programs is to train specialized doctors:

- Demand and supply mismatches in manpower
- Disparity in quality: because of gaps between the training programs and the requirements of the nation's health policy
- Unequal distribution of workforce: between regions, areas, professions and categories, health organizations, and specialties
- Paradigm shift in patient expectations from clinical outcome to complete service experience

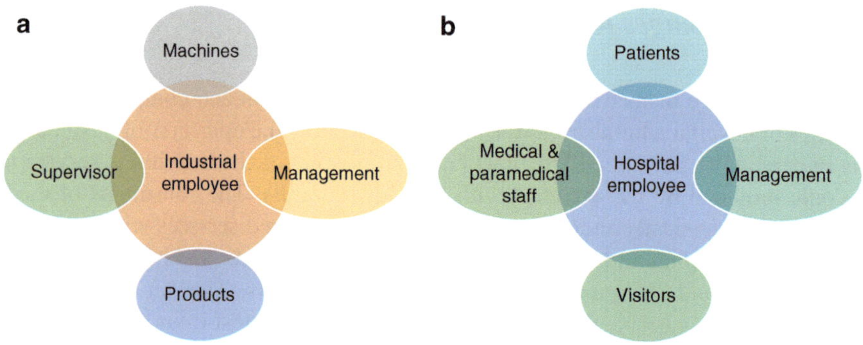

Fig. 4.8 (**a**, **b**) Unique environmental circumstances of employees—industry/hospital

- Demand for promotive and preventive care along with curative and therapeutic services
- Training and retention of workforce
- Developing multi-tasking workforce
- Ensuring accountability by the workforce (Fig. 4.8)

4.1.9 Emerging Trends

Hospitals are also evolving with time and so are its employees. Advancements in technology and its integration in operations have necessitated innovations and reforms across the functions of a hospital. Digitalization of operations, electronic patient record management, and increasing awareness on employees' and patients' rights have all made hospital administration a complex unit. Right from recruitment of employees to providing training and assessment technology plays a crucial role. Employee management through Human Resource Information System (HRIS) and HR auditing ensures reliability and transparency in its functions. Training of workforce to meet the challenges posed by technological advancements is a dynamic and continuous process for HR managers. Employee welfare practices and benefits help in employee retention. Quality of services through accreditations and certifications has been mandatory. Information technology and internet have changed the way hospitals function, with telemedicine and teleconsultation being preferred for routine appointments. Medical tourism is yet another aspect where hospitals with good reputation and quality of services can admit international patients and enhance their branding. All these require dedicated, qualified workforce to meet the challenges and function efficiently. Considering the diverse nature of work and increasing workload, many of the HR functions have been outsourced like payroll management, recruitment, training and audits, and other activities.

Telehealth, remote care, or home care is the next change influencing the management of human resource in hospitals. This necessitates a diverse set of employees who are tech savvy with required digital knowledge and flexibility to adapt to diverse working conditions. Robotics, artificial intelligence, and technological advancements will transform healthcare delivery across disciplines.

References

1. Megginson, Leon C., Personnel and Human Resources Administration, Richard d. Irwin Inc., Homwood, Illinois, 1977, p.4
2. Walter Dill Scott, Robert C. Clothier and William R. Spriegel, Personnel Management: Principles, Practices and Points Of View (New York: McGraw-Hill, 1977), p. 85.
3. Henry Mintzberg (1973) *The Nature of Managerial Work.*
4. Dave Ulrich, "Human Resource Champions" (Boston, MA: Harvard Business School Press, 1997).
5. Yeung. A, Brockbank. W, and Ulrich. D (1994), "Lower Cost, Higher value: Human Resource Function in Transformation, "Human Resource Planning, 17(3).
6. Edwin B Flippo (1984) personnel management, sixth edition-Hill International Edition, Management series.
7. Dale Yoder (1975) - Personnel Management and Industrial Relations, Prentice Hall of India, New Delhi.p.63.
8. Terry L. Leap and Michael D. Crino, Personnel and Human Resource Management (New York: Maxwell Macmillan International Editions, 1990), p. 204
9. Edwin B. Flippo (1984), Personnel Management (New York: McGraw–Hill), p. 200.
10. Michael Armstrong (2001), A Handbook of Human Resource Management Practice, 8th ed. (London: Kogan Page, p. 543.
11. C. Hamblin, Evaluation and Control of Training (Maidenhead: McGraw–Hill, 1974) referred by Michael Armstrong, A Handbook of Human Resource Management Practice, 8th ed. (London: Kogan Page, 2001), pp. 570.
12. Stephen Williams, "Strategy and Objectives" in Frances Neale (ed.) Handbook of Performance Management (Mumbai: Jaico Publishing House, 2002), p. 7.

Further Reading

"Why a Well-honed Performance Management System Is Now Key," Compensation & Benefits for Law Offices, 6 (April 2006): 1–10. (perf. Evln.)

Dave Ulrich and Wayne Brockbank, HR Value Proposition, Harvard Business School Press, 2005, p VIII

Gary Dessler, Human Resource Management (Delhi: Pearson Education, 2005), p. 270.

Chapter 5
Quality Management and Patient Safety in Healthcare Domain

Meena Gupta, Divya Pandey, and Simran Naagar

5.1 Introduction

A healthcare organization (HCO) is a complex association ordinarily attributable to the elusive result of service and a blend of different expert staff. Quality administration in medical care is fundamental and often standardized. However, quality itself is not an actual trait of administration. As such, replacing the term "healthcare" by "medical care services" further characterizes the field as a subject of survey, observation, and improvement. The quality control framework in an HCO is characterized as "appropriate, available, accessible, reasonable, effective, proficient, coordinated, safe, and patient-related" [1]. In addition to medicine and surgery, medical care services also include allied healthcare services, like dentistry, gynecology, radiology, optometry, diagnostic imaging, and physiotherapy.

Quality in healthcare is often synonymous with patient safety. The World Health Organization (WHO) defined patient safety as prevention of errors and blunders, which negatively affect patients of medical care services [2] and to cause no damage to patients [3]. Hazardous healthcare practices are attributed to injury, disability, and even death of innumerable patients globally and consequently occupy scarce organizational resources to deal with the damage. Therefore, patient safety is acknowledged as being fundamental to quality medical care services, and patient safety strategies are being adopted as integral components of HCO across the world [4].

M. Gupta (✉)
Amity Institute of Physiotherapy, Amity University, Noida, Uttar Pradesh, India
e-mail: mgupta9@amity.edu

D. Pandey
Sai Institute of Paramedical and Allied Sciences, Dehradun, Uttarakhand, India

S. Naagar
University of Science and Technology of China, Hefei, Anhui, People's Republic of China

D. Bhatia et al. (eds.), *A Guide to Hospital Administration and Planning*,
https://doi.org/10.1007/978-981-19-6692-7_5

Although patient safety in primary level medical centers has not been as extensively investigated as in hospital settings, primary and outpatient care centers are becoming more popular in such research given the recent research findings [5, 6].

Almost 20–25% of the patients in primary care settings experience harm due to organizational causes, in both developed and developing nations [7]. Such unsafe organizational causes include diagnostic errors, discontinuity in care delivery, hazardous drug practices [8], and poor-quality management. However, the safety of patients and the quality of services delivered can be improved by identifying and rectifying glitches in patient journeys through primary and secondary care.

Both the recurrence and extent of clinical errors in hospital settings attract public health concern worldwide. As such, current research aims to devise thorough strategies for improving and supporting the health outcomes of hospital patients. Hospital accreditation is a commonly employed strategy to enhance healthcare quality and patient safety, which has become fundamental to healthcare frameworks in >90 nations [9]. Developing nations commonly employ hospital accreditation as a strategy to ensure quality and patient safety in its healthcare services. Nonetheless, execution of license guidelines is a tedious task, especially since the research evidence on the advantages of the license is scanty. According to the Joint Commission International (JCI) certification technique, most HCOs transition through certain stages when gaining accreditation [10]. JCI is an international organization, which authorizes healthcare services, institutions, and frameworks outside the USA. JCI had authorized almost 500 medical care associations globally by 2013. To gain JCI accreditation, a hospital is surveyed every third year to evaluate its adherence to JCI's quality and patient safety standards. The surveyors evaluate the healthcare services provisioned and authoritative cycles and aim to promote continuous quality improvement for the organization under study. In India, the National Accreditation Board for Hospitals & Healthcare Providers (NABH) is the highest organization for quality control in hospitals. It is the leading authority for accreditation of hospitals and is responsible for protecting the stakeholders and partners and setting benchmarks for quality, safety, and development of Indian hospitals. The NABH is an autonomous body and is also an institutional member of the International Society for Quality in Healthcare (ISQua). Although inconsistent, evidence supports that the accreditation has a substantial effect on HCO. The evident degree of quality enhancement and value consistency accomplished after the first accreditation survey is almost certainly sustained by HCO. Additionally, repeated surveys decrease variations in quality execution, thereby resulting in long-term quality control, enhanced safety, and high dependability in HCO [11]. Despite the evident business improvement, accreditation can lead to complex organizational dynamics, which makes it difficult to sustain a workforce. While there is theoretical evidence about the advantages of accreditation, observational proof to support it remains inadequate. Greenfield and Braithwaite [12] reported that the experimental proof for justifying accreditation lacks considerably, which is a significant challenge for accreditation institutions, researchers, and policymakers. Considering that accomplishing and maintaining the accreditation status occupy significant organizational resources, it becomes necessary for healthcare organizations to determine if accreditation demonstrates a quantifiable and significant enough difference in the provision of medical care services and the outcomes.

5.2 Quality

Quality of healthcare services can be defined both in strategic and customary terms. It is defined by the American National Standards Institute (ANSI) and American Society for Quality (ASQ) as the integration of characteristics of healthcare or its services, which enables it to fulfill the standard necessities. Quality in itself is a complex and unitless organizational factor, which can be defined along various organizational factors, like patient safety and satisfaction. However, quality in healthcare services is an ambiguous term and includes several technicalities in addition to clinical quality. Content quality is defined in terms of healthcare provider's expectations, whereas delivery quality is defined in terms of consumer expectations and satisfaction [13].

5.3 Quality in Healthcare

Healthcare is a learned profession, wherein the healthcare providers' sole objective is preventive maintenance, rather than total service maintenance. Accordingly, Donabedian suggested employing a tridimensional framework of infrastructure, process, and outcomes for quality assessment in medical services. The infrastructural component is defined by the material and workforce resources to efficiently deliver quality healthcare services. It also includes the ability of both healthcare providers and administrative workforce and the coordination between the two to meet the healthcare requirements of the incoming patient population.

Quality control in medical care as a concept has gradually evolved from solely focusing on the reduction of errors to delivering the ideal patient experiences and satisfaction. Supporting this notion, Philip Crosby advocates that the quality control framework is one centered in prevention and not in appraisal. Considering that a significant proportion of deaths in primary care centers is due to negligence and hospital-acquired infections, it is preventable by establishing quality control frameworks centered in prevention to improvise patient experience. Patient satisfaction is fundamental to quality control frameworks and necessitates patient-centered care and adherence to professional standards. The Institute of Medicine defined patient-centered care as one that is considerate and respectful of patient's preferences and acknowledges it as foundational to all the clinical care decisions. Another component of patient-centered care is shared decision-making, wherein the healthcare professionals assist patients in making most appropriate care-related choices and

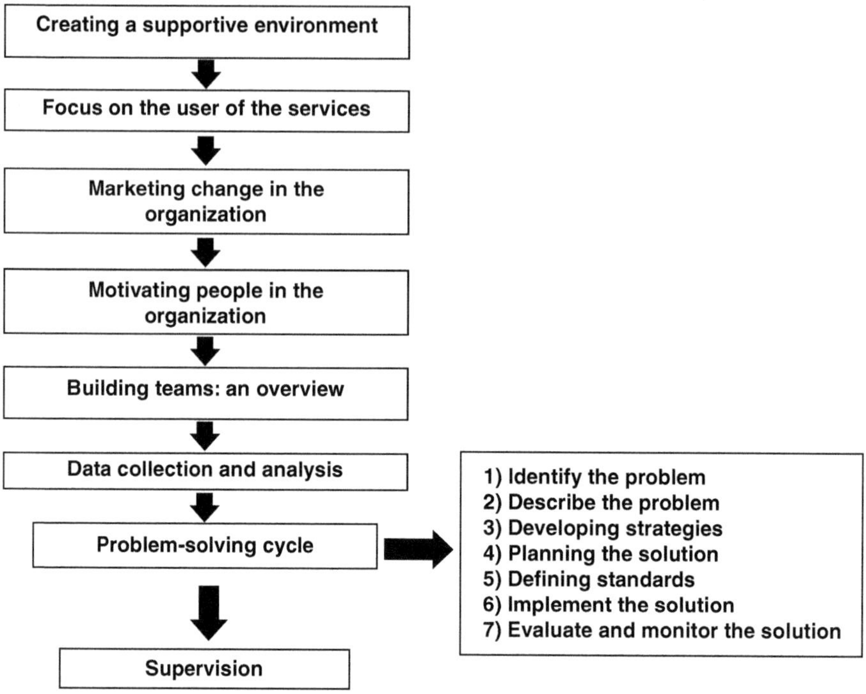

Fig. 5.1 Steps of implementation of quality improvement

decisions. Shared decision-making is also central to patients' inclinations when choosing a healthcare provider [14]. Quality control and management have become most central to the healthcare sector and its services since patient safety and satisfaction are being increasingly recognized as a constituent of quality and administrative outcomes. While the conventional definition of quality control was centered on reducing medical errors, it is now becoming more inclusive of damage prevention, continuous improvement, and result-driven strategies based on the care needs of the patients. Therefore, there is an immediate need to both acknowledge and assimilate that this changes the perspective of quality into organizational frameworks in HCO [15, 16]. Figure 5.1 demonstrates the steps that can be undertaken to achieve quality control and improvement in a HCO.

5.4 Quality Improvement Strategies

Quality control strategies in HCOs aim to establish an administrative framework to ensure the delivery of efficient and effective healthcare service. This can be achieved through the Total Quality Management (TQM), which is defined as an administrative approach centered on human resources and organizational processes to maintain consumer loyalty [17]. It incorporates Content Quality and Delivery Quality. It diminishes the weight of mistakes, guarantees ideal use of foundation and clinical staff, and oversees quality control. It is rooted in both content and delivery quality and aims to reduce service delivery errors, ensure effective utilization of material and human resources, and oversee quality control.

The core elements of TQM are client centeredness, emphasis on quality, scientific approach, cooperation, continuous enhancement, workforce training, and autonomy in the long term [18]. TQM aims to identify and rectify the immediate issues in service delivery but also aims to maintain and continue the developments in the long run. Within the workforce, the nursing professionals and the quality control department are the key executioners of TQM strategies [19, 20]. Together, they aim to ensure quality improvement in service provision, efficient damage control, decreased costs, and elimination of errors before they cause harm. However, evidence on the execution of TQM in developing nations, like India, is limited [21]. Other than TQM, other approaches to quality control and management include the International Organization for Standardization ISO 9000, Zero Defects, Six Sigma, Baldrige, and Toyota Production System/Lean Production. Additionally, the in-house quality maintenance frameworks double-check organizational processes and identification of issues that are likely against the accreditation authority's standards, including documentation and credentialization [22].

In healthcare, TQM is often used synonymously with continuous quality improvement (CQI). CQI is employed as a means to enhance clinical practice [23]. It is an approach, which encourages healthcare providers to persistently inquire: "How are we doing?" "Would we be able to do it better?" And specifically would we be able to do it all the more proficiently? Can we be more effective? Would we be able to do it quicker? Would we be able to do it in an all the more convenient manner? [24]. However, instead of integrating CQI into the organizational culture, the more appropriate way to establish CQI strategies is to evaluate the existing organizational processes and consequently develop frameworks to achieve the idealized future state. Popular CQI strategies include empowering the workforce to actively evaluate the existing service delivery status and formulate strategies to enhance it. Employing an appropriate CQI approach will facilitate the development of an effective strategy based on the existing organizational level and aiming towards the idealized quality and service delivery standards. Accordingly, research evidence reports strong evidence for association between an appropriate CQI strategy and high organizational performance [25]. Therefore, besides improving organizational statistics, employing CQI strategies also facilitate establishing a proactive framework for identification and rectification of errors and organizational improvement.

The steps to drafting an efficient CQI strategy should include [26] the following:

- Identify and employ an appropriate CQI model.
- Install and evaluate performance metrics to periodically assess improvement and outcomes.
- Ensure that all employees understand and acknowledge the established performance metrics.

- Ensure that all the stakeholders, including patients, families, and suppliers, are involved in the CQI framework.
- Establish electronic health records and IT as an evaluation criterion.

Focusing on quality may necessitate changing goals, rules, perspectives, and processes, which can be challenging to do on the organizational level. Consequently, such changes are made gradually over a long time period, rather than overnight. Unlike the private HCOs, quality assurance frameworks can more effectively be established in public sector HCOs considering that they are funded and run by the state, which has significant power and resources.

In terms of healthcare workforce, the healthcare providers undertake medical schooling under expert supervision and the academic curriculum is primarily centered around disease prevention and management. Unfortunately, there is very little consideration on the education of to-be healthcare providers on professional and organizational issues, like patient communication, collaborative care, organizational culture, and behavior. As such, the healthcare professionals only learn about such aspects of care individually, depending on their field of specialty. For instance, a nurse, physiotherapist, and surgeon will have different perspectives on such qualitative aspects of healthcare, which are mostly autonomous and independent of other specialists. Consequently, these differences in professional practice are also significantly reflected on the quality, safety, and satisfaction of healthcare services. Therefore, healthcare provider workforce and their professional practice are essential aspects of quality control and assurance, as advocated by CQI [27].

5.4.1 *Patient Safety*

Guaranteeing patient safety is a significant challenge for healthcare providers and a crucial factor of service delivery for patients in a primary care setting. Considering that the direct healthcare provider-patient communication in a primary care setting is usually scarce, patients should assume a more prominent responsibility in understanding and taking ownership of their illness and well-being. Although resource consuming, it is achievable if the driving forces are identified correctly. Three of such driving forces that impact patient safety in a primary care setting are [28]:

- Behavior of the patient and caregivers
- Role of healthcare professional-patient communication
- Role of healthcare frameworks and the community

Although effective, the above-stated factors also have evident flaws. Intrinsic defects in the healthcare framework may increase the risk of clinical errors, specially like drug and diagnostic errors, which are fundamental to ensure patient safety in service delivery in a primary care setting [29]. Additionally, poor health literacy and ineffective patient education add to the increased risk of clinical errors since patients are unable to fully comprehend their medication, its indication, dosage, use, and potential adverse effects, which can all lead to hazardous clinical errors [30]. Moreover, overseeing test results also adds to the increased risk of missed or misdiagnosis in primary and outpatient care centers. All the above-identified factors lead to significant patient safety and service delivery issues, like [31]:

- Increased mortality
- Increased morbidity (temporary or permanent)
- Treatment delay
- Extra visits to the healthcare providers
- Preventable r-admissions to emergency clinics
- Dissatisfied patients and healthcare providers

5.4.2 *Incident Reporting in Primary Care*

Although incident reporting is perceived as an ideal strategy to evaluate patient safety, it may be ineffective if not undertaken appropriately. An evaluation of local Incident Reporting Procedure (IRP) revealed that it was ineffective in preventing and managing serious clinical errors because the procedure overlooked the emotional and psychological needs of the involved healthcare providers [32]. However, it was also observed that local IRPs empowered healthcare providers to better evaluate incident reports than a centralized rectification framework. Unlike the local IRPs, a centralized system seemed more effective in gathering numerous incident reports and identifying and rectifying repetitive safety issues more successfully. Therefore, it is only justified to combine local and centralized IRPs to achieve more efficiency and better outcomes [33].

Evidence reveals that the most common clinical errors in primary care centers were the communication failure among healthcare providers themselves, followed by errors associated with medicine and misdiagnosis [34]. Analysis of the nature, cause, and outcomes of likely clinical safety incidents at primary care centers revealed that the incidents occurred mostly in out-of-hours primary care centers. While treatment errors were the most common type of safety incidents, there was no harm resulting in 70% of incidents. Additionally, it was revealed that erroneous clinical reasoning was the cause of the majority of the safety incidents, including unavailability of previous patient records, lack of clinical information, and critical cases.

5.4.3 *Transition of Care*

Transition across different segments of the healthcare framework makes patients vulnerable to being subjected to clinical errors. The transition of care refers to the patient entering different phases of healthcare, shifting to different physical locations to receive medical care, or switching from one healthcare provider to another [35]. This includes the transition between home, hospital, primary care centers, and residential care and even consultations with different healthcare providers.

The transition of care becomes even more complex at the primary care level. When patients report at different primary care centers, they may face a new diagnosis or new clinical findings and may be administered a new management plan. Generally, the geriatric patients, who suffer from complex health problems, remain the most vulnerable to the adverse safety and quality incidents since they have to continuously undergo transition of care. As such, managing such service delivery challenges is fundamental to improving patient satisfaction and safety in healthcare services [36].

5.4.4 Current Scenario of Patient Safety in India

Over the recent years, the Indian Government has become more acknowledging and accepting of the quality issues in the Indian healthcare sector and has become considerate to rectifying these quality issues to match the Universal Health Coverage standards. Patient safety is becoming more integral to quality and safe healthcare services, and both the central and the state regulatory authorities are undertaking initiatives to ensure safety in healthcare service delivery [37]. The various patient safety issues in the Indian healthcare system include:

- Poor and fragmented legal and regulatory context for healthcare practice and service delivery.
- Negligence of the Consumer Protection Act and patients' rights.
- Private healthcare sector's low acceptance and adherence to patient safety strategies.
- Lack of consumer awareness and initiative to drive policy changes.
- Poor engagement of public hospitals in the NABH accreditation
- Lack of motivation among healthcare providers in the public healthcare sector to improve patient safety and lack of training frameworks for them.
- Lack of adequate infection control guidelines and frameworks in HCOs.
- Although other infrastructural components, like fire security, device safety, and earthquake resistance, are adequate in Indian HCOs, they are not commonly included in patient safety measures.
- Nonadherence to hospital-acquired infection reporting strategy among majority public and private HCOs.
- Lack of active research in the field of patient safety and its lack of a research-based policy-making framework.
- Lack of funding for patient safety-based research in India.

5.4.5 Strategies for Improving Patient Safety

Patient safety is a complex concept consisting of several organizational and professional factors. Consequently, this necessitates multidimensional strategies to improve patient safety in HCOs [38]. Few of these strategies are as follows:

1. **Engagement of patient and their families:**
   Patient safety in service delivery in HCOs can be improved by employing four evidence-based strategies to increase engagement of the patients and their families in the healthcare service framework.
   (a) Encourage encouragement: This strategy aims to increase readiness among patients and their families to actively engage in their healthcare journey. Patients and caretakers are often unprepared when they visit a primary care center or a healthcare provider. Encouragement strategies will involve giving patients a "Be Prepared" sheet, where they are urged to document their complaints, queries, and health goals. This will enable patients and families to plan their healthcare visits in advance and ensure that they are more prepared to question, enquire, and interact with their healthcare providers. Consequently, the healthcare provider will be able to better address the health issues of the patients. This improves efficiency in healthcare service delivery and outcomes like patient satisfaction.
   (b) Make a medication list together: This strategy will include the patient and their caregivers to bring all their prescriptions to the healthcare provider. The healthcare provider then engages the patient and their caregiver to plan a complete medication list and then the clinician oversees it. This strategy aims to increase the post-consultation engagement of the patient and their caregivers and increase their interest and control over all aspects of their care.
   (c) Actively educate: This strategy requires the healthcare provider to actively educate the patient and their caregivers about all the aspects of their health, so it becomes easier for them to follow and adhere to the plan of care. It is an evidence-based strategy to improve patient safety, commitment, and safety in their healthcare journey.
   (d) Face-to-face handover: This strategy includes a face-to-face patient handover between two healthcare providers, in the presence of the patient and their family. This strategy makes the patient feel actively included in the treatment process and facilitates trust-building between the patient and the healthcare providers [39].

2. **Medication Reconciliation**
   Drug-related errors are the most frequent type of clinical error, and nearly 40% of these drug-related errors occur due to inadequate handover, especially during hospital admission and discharge. Almost 1/5th of these drug-related errors lead to evident patient harm. An evidence-based approach to identify and rectify such

drug-based errors is medical reconciliation, which requires comparing the patient's current medication prescription to all the previous or discontinued drug prescriptions of the patient. This helps the healthcare provider identify similar, synergistic or antagonistic medications that the patient might take or even similar medications with different brand names. Consequently, previous prescriptions may interfere with the current medication, and this may affect the quality of healthcare services delivered to them.

3. **Sharing Information**
   Another strategy to improve patient safety and security in a primary care setting and especially in a transition of care is information-sharing through "yellow" or "release" envelopes. All the information regarding the patient's condition, treatment, management, and care is mentioned in these envelopes, including mentioning the information valuable for handover on the back of the envelope. This is a favorable, dynamic, quick, and cost-efficient method in conveying patient information effectively.

5.5 Conclusion

Medical care services are a more humane and science-based process, instead of just being fundamentally commercial. Skilled healthcare professionals are obliged to guarantee quality and safe healthcare services. Quality improvement in HCOs may require changing organizational perspective, policies, rules, and goals, which can be challenging and can only occur gradually. Additionally, quality and safety assurance in healthcare services is fundamental when trying to accomplish a universal health coverage system and sustainability in healthcare service delivery. As such, it is fundamental from even the policymakers' perspective to target quality and safety of care services in primary and outpatient care centers regardless of the tediousness. This requires HCOs adopting a TQM approach alongside strengthening the medical education and training framework to produce skilled healthcare providers.

References

1. Park K. Health care of the Community. In: Park K., editor. *Park's text book of preventive and social medicine*. 20th ed. Banarsidas Bhanot; Jabalpur: 2009. pp. 780–800
2. World Health Organization. G. Conceptual framework for the international classification for patient safety. *Version 1.1 final technical report January*. 2009;2009
3. Lawati MHA, Dennis S, Short SD, Abdulhadi NN. Patient safety and safety culture in primary health care: A systematic review. *BMC Fam Pract*. 2018;19:104.
4. González-Formoso C, Martín-Miguel MV, Fernández-Domínguez MJ, Rial A, Lago-Deibe FI, Ramil-Hermida L, et al. Adverse events analysis as an educational tool to improve patient safety culture in primary care: A randomized trial. *BMC Fam Pract*. 2011;12:50.
5. Tabrizchi N, Sedaghat M. The first study of patient safety culture in Iranian primary health centers. *Acta Med Iran*. 2012;50:505–10

6. Webair HH, Al-assani SS, Al-haddad RH, Al-Shaeeb WH, Bin Selm MA, Alyamani AS. Assessment of patient safety culture in primary care setting, Al-Mukala, Yemen. *BMC Fam Pract*. 2015;16:136.
7. Michel P, Brami J, Chanelière M, Kret M, Mosnier A, Dupie I, et al. Patient safety incidents are common in primary care: A national prospective active incident reporting survey. *PLoS One*. 2017;12:e0165455.
8. Bucknall TK, Hutchinson AM, Botti M, McTier L, Rawson H, Hewitt NA, et al. Engaging patients and families in communication across transitions of care: An integrative review protocol. *J Adv Nurs*. 2016;72:1689–700
9. JCI. JCI-Accredited Organizations. https://www.jointcommissioninternational.org/about-jci/jci-accredited-organizations/ (Accessed May 2018)
10. Joint Commission international. *Joint Commission International Accreditation: Getting Started*. 2nd edition: Oakbrook Terrace, IL: Joint Commission Resources, 2010
11. Subashnie Devkaran et al. Impact of repeated hospital accreditation surveys on quality and reliability, an 8-year interrupted time series analysis, BMJ Open. 2019; 9(2): e024514.
12. Developing the evidence base for accreditation of healthcare organisations: a call for transparency and innovation. *Greenfield D, Braithwaite J Qual Saf Health Care. 2009 Jun; 18(3):162-3.*
13. Mandeep, Chitkara N., Goel S. Study to evaluate change of attitude toward acceptance of NABH guidelines: an intra-institutional experience. *J Nat Accred Board Hosp Healthcare Providers*. 2014;1:52–55
14. Ungureanu Marius-Ionuţ, Mocean Floarea. What do patients take into account when they choose their dentist? Implications for quality improvement. *Patient Preference Adherence*. 2015;9:1715–1720.
15. Rathee M. Quest for quality: pivotal paradigm for healthcare transformation. *J IDA North West Delhi Branch*. 2016;3(2):55–56
16. Rana B.K., Behera N.S., Nair S.B. QCI - medical laboratory program journey of quality in public medical laboratories": an experience though program evaluation. J Nat Accred Board Hosp Healthcare Providers. 2014;1:7–11.
17. Sadikoglu E., Olcay H. The effects of total quality management practices on performance and the reasons of and the barriers to TQM practices in Turkey. *Adv Decis Sci*. 2014:17
18. Agarwal A., Aeran H., Uniyal S., Nautiyal A. Quality assurance in dentistry: a need in Indian scenario. *Int J Oral Health Dentistry*. 2015;1(4):172–176.
19. Lee P.M., Khong P., Ghista D.N., Mohammad MosadeghRad A. The impact of organizational culture on the successful implementation of total quality management. *TQM Mag*. 2006;18(6):606–625.
20. Al-Shdaifat Emad A. Implementation of total quality management in hospitals. *J Taibah Univ Med Sci*. 2015;10(4):461e466.
21. Murti A., Deshpande A., Srivastava N. Service quality, customer (Patient) satisfaction and behavioural intention in health care services: exploring the Indian perspective. *J Health Manage*. 2013;15(1):29–44
22. Chassin MR. Quality of Care–part 3: Improving the quality of care. N Engl J Med. 1996:1060–3.
23. Wallin L, Bostrom AM, Wikblad K, et al. Sustainability in changing clinical practice promotes evidence-based nursing care. J Adv Nurs. 2003;41(5):509–18.
24. Edwards PJ, et al. Maximizing your investment in EHR: Utilizing EHRs to inform continuous quality improvement. JHIM 2008;22(1):32-7.
25. Shortell SM, Gillies R Siddique J, et al. Improving chronic illness care: A longitudinal cohort analysis of large physician organizations. Med Care 2009;47(9):932–9.
26. Wagner EH, Coleman K, Reid RJ, Phillips K, Abrams MK, Sugarman JR. The changes involved in patientcentered medical home transformation. Prim Care. 2012 Jun;39(2):241-59
27. Subhash S Dodwad, Quality management in healthcare year 2013 volume 57 issue 3, Indian journal of public health
28. Refocusing the lens: patient safety in ambulatory chronic disease care.Sarkar U, Wachter RM, Schroeder SA, Schillinger D Jt Comm J Qual Patient Saf. 2009 Jul; 35(7):377-83, 341.

29. Agency for health care and safety, Ambulatory Care Safety [homepage on the internet] [Last accessed on 2019 Sept 23]. Available from: www.psnet.ahrq.gov/primers/primer/16/patient-safety-in-ambulatory-care
30. To err is human: patient misinterpretations of prescription drug label instructions. Wolf MS, Davis TC, Shrank W, Rapp DN, Bass PF, Connor UM, Clayman M, Parker RM Patient Educ Couns. 2007 Aug; 67(3):293-300.
31. Russell LM, Doggett J, Dawda P, Wells R. Patient Safety – Handover of Care between Primary and Acute Care Policy Review and Analysis. Canberra: National Lead Clinicians Group, Australian Government Department of Health and Ageing; 2013.
32. Zwart DLM, de Bont AA. Introducing incident reporting in primary care: A translation from safety science into medical practice. *Health Risk Soc.* 2013;15:265–78.
33. Measuring perceptions of safety climate in primary care: a cross-sectional study.*de Wet C, Johnson P, Mash R, McConnachie A, Bowie P J Eval Clin Pract. 2012 Feb; 18(1):135-42*
34. Paese F, Sasso GT. Patient safety culture in primary health care [Portuguese] *Text Context Nurs Florianóolis.* 2013;22:302–10.
35. T*echnical series on safer primary care [homepage on the internet]* [Last accessed on 2019 Sept 23]. Available from: https://www.who.int/patientsafety/topics/primary-care/technical_series/en.
36. Improving transitions of care. *The vision of the national transitions of care coalition.* Washington DC: National Transitions of Care Coalition; 2008.
37. *National Patient Safety Implementation Framework, (2018-2025) India [homepage on the internet]* [Last accessed on 2019 Sept 25]. Available from: national patient safety implementation_for web.pdf
38. *Guid to Improving Patient Safety in Primary Care Settings by Engaging Patients and Families [homepage on the internet]* [Last accessed on 2019 Sept 26]
39. The collaborative communication model for patient handover at the interface between high-acuity and low-acuity care.Toccafondi G, Albolino S, Tartaglia R, Guidi S, Molisso A, Venneri F, Peris A, Pieralli F, Magnelli E, Librenti M, Morelli M, Barach PBMJ Qual Saf. 2012 Dec; 21 Suppl 1():i58-66.

Chapter 6
Dental Office Layout and Design

**Lata Goyal, Amrit Preet, Arshad Eranhikkal,
Prabhat Kumar Chaudhari, and Kunaal Dhingra**

6.1 Introduction

The key steps for smooth functioning and efficient patient care delivery are planning and designing of a dental office [1]. Workplace design supports the procedures and various activities carried out in that area; it leads to better patient flow, ease of movement, and better time management. It also helps to create an identity in the competitive era. The architectural design of a complete dental office with its interiors including clinical, reception and even sterilization areas will convey a message to every visitor so as to make judgments about dentists' practice, capabilities and expertise based on what they see around [2]. Dusty and dark offices communicate lack of maintenance while neat, well-organized and equipped offices enhance ideal patient experience. Architectural and ergonomics design can help decrease workplace-related stress and promote an atmosphere of teamwork and collaboration.

L. Goyal
Division of Periodontics, Department of Dentistry, All India Institute of Medical Sciences, Bathinda, Bathinda, India

A. Preet (✉)
Department of Dentistry, B.R. Ambedkar Institute of Medical Sciences, Mohali, India

A. Eranhikkal
Department of Dentistry, All India Institute of Medical Sciences, Bathinda, Bathinda, India

P. K. Chaudhari
Division of Orthodontics and Dentofacial Deformities, Centre for Dental Education and Research, All India Institute of Medical Sciences, New Delhi, New Delhi, India

K. Dhingra
Division of Periodontics, Centre for Dental Education and Research, All India Institute of Medical Sciences, New Delhi, New Delhi, India

D. Bhatia et al. (eds.), *A Guide to Hospital Administration and Planning*,
https://doi.org/10.1007/978-981-19-6692-7_6

Meticulous planning of the dental office is required to strike an operative balance between comfort of the patient, regulatory specifications, clinical efficiency, integrating advance technology and ergonomic design. As there are multiple activities and services involved in rendering care to the dental patient, its design involves consideration regarding collaboration between designer, electrical, civil, plumbing equipment manager and dentist.

6.2 Dental Office

6.2.1 Administrative/Reception Areas

Administrative areas are the spaces meant for the management of financial and other clerical works. Various operations like management of insurance claims and receiving of payable amounts are done here. Patient records are also kept in this area. Nowadays, dental firms are running speciality-oriented clinics as compared to general and interdisciplinary dental practice. So, it has many dental clinics depending upon the different speciality services being provided.

Parking Areas

The design and location of parking area should be taken into account at the beginning of the site planning so that the forefront and entrance to the dental office are not obscured by unsightly parking areas. Distance from the parking area to the main entrance should not be very long. It should include parking for patients, staff, differently abled users, accompanying persons, medical transport and service vehicles. The parking spaces must have designated areas for disabled users and should be accessible for all of them who require assistive devices to move around. The minimum parking requirements are typically determined by the occupancy group (doctors including all staff members) and floor area of your office building (main determinant is the number of dental chairs).

Other key points of adequate parking include easy way finding and exit; clear signing; separate parking for staff and visitors; designated areas for two wheelers and four wheelers; and security against unauthorized parking, vandalism and theft.

Entrance

The main entrance is the place of arrival and departure of the patients and visitors. It further function as an enquiry and information point, security check and waiting area. This area does make the first impression on the visitor about dental settings in a particular dental clinic. So, its planning must include these qualitative effects like warmth, welcoming, considerate, helping, reassuring, efficient, comfortable and clean. These qualitative effects include combinations of appropriate infrastructural lighting, right and warm colour combinations, proper and spacious settings, appropriate displays and most importantly affectionate and considerate human behaviour as this is the first point of contact [3]. Qualitative requirements of this area include ramps and stairs with proper inclination and step width, width of the entrance door, flooring with tactile tiles and other indicators for direction, taking into account all types of visitors including persons with disabilities both sensory and physical, paediatric patients and old-age patients.

Another important consideration is separate entrances for patients and for dentist and the staff. It may be from the back.

Reception

The reception area is immediately inside the lobby after crossing the entrance. It should have a reception desk for enquiry, information and concierge services. It will be the first stop for patient reorientation and the last place to pause before departing. It should be immediately inside the entrance, slightly located back from patient circulation route, clearly signed and should have sufficient space at the reception front for queuing up without obstructing the passage [4]. Signposting to all key destinations should be located beyond the desk.

Desk design: The desk should be visually prominent within the entrance area and designed with good-quality materials. It should be accessible and convenient for patients and accompanying persons, at the same time safe and user friendly for the staff working there. Ideally, a low-level desk in the open main space creates a welcoming quality and provides better patient or visitor and staff contact.

The desk design details will be according to the number of staff members behind it and their functions other than enquiries by visitors. Additional functions may include patient registration, information distribution in the form of leaflets, coordination between different clinics and laboratories, entrance and waiting area supervision, general patient assistance and facilities for persons with disabilities. As the scope of functions in this area increases, provisions should be made for computers, printer and scanners, cabinets for storage requirements, internet router installations, internet and communication connections to other services, security alarm controls and central fire controls, staff security and protection, location suitable for entrance supervision, etc.

Concourse Area

Concourse is the public space in a dental clinic connecting the main entrance to different clinics with other services, laboratories or X-ray room. It ought to be appropriately sized to accommodate communication and circulation for patients, other visitors and equipment. It should preferably be naturally lit.

Main Waiting

The main waiting area should be immediately after the reception desk within its sight. The need for main waiting area space is usually small as after enquiry and registration patients move directly to departmental entrance waiting areas. Therefore, the main waiting area should be planned for small seating groups, with special arrangements for kids and persons with disabilities. Stands or corners for information leaflets and videos are recommended. It is essential to have small waiting areas in front of each dental room with good-quality seating and fabrics. There should be separate washrooms for males and females with infrastructural facilities for persons with disabilities in the main waiting area only.

Waiting areas include seating and walking spaces for the patients. This space also includes entrance doors and access to reception area and operatory area. A minimum of 120 square feet is required for six patients. Waiting area should be utilized for patients arriving early than their appointment time and for emergency patients who are planning to wait until doctor's appointment. Waiting area should be equipped with television and different types of reading magazines. For paediatric patients, a separate area should be maintained inside the waiting room. This area should be equipped with toys and other playing materials. This helps the child to reduce the stress and anxiety before entering the operatory.

Public Area

It includes reception, waiting area, private office/consult, toilets for patients and refreshment area. These areas should preferably be around the entrance only. Toilets for the patients should be close to the waiting area.

6.2.2 The Dental Operatory and Accessory Clinical Area

Dental operatory is the treatment/working area with specially equipped dental treatment delivery systems to perform dental procedures along with all associated tasks by the dentist and his/her team. It is the place where a dentist does all the dental treatments. Various types of instruments and tools for doing dental procedures are kept in a single room. Dental operatory can be found in hospitals, schools, government offices and other health-related establishments. Often, though not always, low-cost treatments are performed. It includes dental treatment room, sterilization, radiographic room, dressing room, clinical photography room, refreshment room, private room for staff and service room.

Dental Operatory

Dental treatment rooms include clinical area with additional clinical spaces like X-ray room, sterilization room, photography area and documentation area. The dental treatment area is the most vital part of a dental set-up as it will determine dentists' treatment efficacy, productivity and ergonomic well-being, and it is the single major decisive factor and determinant of patient experience. Dental room design should be modified according to speciality practices. Various speciality clinics like oral and maxillofacial surgery operatory, implant, periodontics, endodontic, orthodontic, paediatric or multi-speciality set-up can be made.

This includes the operatory areas where the treatment of the patient is done. The dental operatory consists of the dental chair, work surfaces, light unit and some area for storage of consumables. The dental chair should have either inbuilt ultrasonic scaler, curing light and intraoral camera or separate units attached to it. The advanced type of dental chairs have digital radiography units attached to it. The operatory should be very spacious enough for accommodating all equipment, and wheelchair access should be available to the operatory. Depending on the budget and scope, there can be more number of dental operatories inside a service room. Hand-washing stations should be provided inside each operatory or can be shared by two or three operatories.

The optimum size of an operatory usually recommended is 10 × 11 ft. It should not be less than 9 × 8 ft. Equal amount of spacing should be given on both sides of the chair if the operatory is used by both left- and right-handed dentists. According to the Americans with Disabilities Act (ADA) wheelchair accessibility requirements, the entrance of an operatory should have a width of 32 inches. This will help in easy entry of wheelchair patients and their transfer from wheelchair to the dental chair. The sterilization areas may be constructed centrally to all the operatories. This helps in easy transfer of instruments from the sterilization area to the dental operatories. If placement of windows is possible, clinics should be designed in such a manner that operatories are equipped with windows. This provides natural light to both the dentist and patient. Claustrophobic patients will be more relieved in such operatories. Moreover, natural light aids in accurate selection of shades and choice of asthetic procedures.

Dental treatment room planning in modern day has prerequisites, which include investment in technology for better patient experience, better efficiency and better patient perception with minimalist design, which allows more modern open designs with no unsightly wires, cables, cords and foot controls [5]. The operatory space should be flexible at the time of the first set-up so that it can easily accommodate the new equipment with the advent of new and advanced technology.

X-Ray Room

X-ray rooms should be having protection barriers on walls and entrance door. Signage should be properly displayed. Rooms should be having an internal camera system and also technical control.

Sterilization Area

Sterilization room have autoclaves and other sterilization equipments. The sterilization area is one of the most important support areas in a dental office. Due to the widespread increase in different types of life-threatening diseases, sterilization is one of the key factors to be maintained. There are more chances that contaminated instruments can cause the spread of infections from one person to another. Due to this, dental offices should have dedicated sterilizing areas meant for cleaning, packaging and storage of instruments.

In order to promote efficiency of sterilization and to comply with standards, the Centers for Disease Control (CDC), sterilization area should be having such a design which incorporates collection of contaminated instruments for their storage after sterilization process. Initially, there should be an intake area for unloading the trays. Sharp instruments should be placed in sharp containers. Colour-coded foot-tap trash storage should be present for disposal of different types of infected and non-infected wastes.

Changing Rooms and Washrooms

These areas should be part of the clinical area. There should be a provision for separate changing room for staff and doctors. Similarly, separate washrooms should be there for staff and doctors with restrooms to have lunch or refreshment.

System Room for Technological Equipment

This room is called the "heart and lung" of the dental clinic as it includes high-quality vacuum and dental compressed air piping equipment. These potential equipment can be located in a dedicated dental plant room or within the dental surgery. Recently, designing experts have been suggesting different rooms for these instruments for a hassle-free, efficient experience of the patient with future expansion scope for business and staff growth. Power backup system can also be stationed in this room preferably with acoustic insulation system.

Laboratory

Every dental office should have a laboratory area. It is the place where study models and initial impressions are poured up. Fabrication of custom trays and repair of dentures are also done in this area. Laboratory should have a minimum size of 5×7 ft with a small sink along the wall. Basic instruments required inside laboratory include cast trimmer, finishing and polishing instruments and burner. Materials like wax sheets, different types of stainless steel wires, screws, sandpapers, emery papers, finishing and polishing burs, and self-cure acrylic materials should be present in dental laboratory. Fire and safety precautions should be strictly followed in laboratory as there are more chances of accidents to happen.

Storage Area

Ready-made/manufactured cabinets and custom-made cabinets are the two types of cabinets available. Manufactured cabinets are readily available in the market under standard cabinetry designs. They are aseptically designed for easy cleaning and long life. There is ease of installation and can be easily shifted from one place to another. The disadvantage is that sometimes they may not fit properly and cost may be higher than custom made. Custom-made cabinets are less expensive, and unlimited colour choices will be available. Moreover, there will not be wastage of any space, and the dentist can be actively involved in the design process.

6.3 Design Considerations

With all the prerequisites in mind, the dental room layout can be configured following these ideas:

6.3.1 Layout

Open Entry

It is an open cove with many patient dental chairs without partition in-between in the room. It can accommodate more dental chairs, so it is highly cost friendly, but patient privacy is usually compromised in this type of setting.

Single Entry

The dental bay is open from one side only with single entrance into the room, and the dental chairs are separated by walls. Walls are usually translucent, but exceptions can be there. The advantage of this kind of set-up includes patient privacy, more dental chairs' placement in limited office space and high economical benefits. However, restricted staff movements during treatment should be managed by proper planning.

Dual Entry

This dental bay resembles single-entry operatory with dual entrances allowing staff entry from either side of the dental room. As in single entry, the treatment area is divided by partitions to separate clinical area and also at the same time maintain reasonable patient privacy. This design requires more space and wider room design as compared to other settings as it permits a second entry.

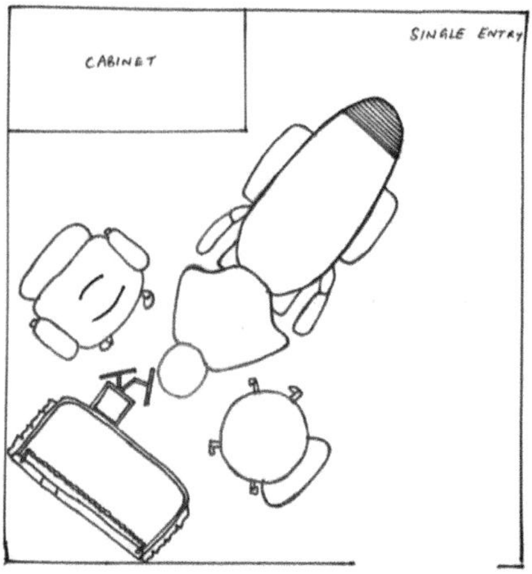

Single Entry

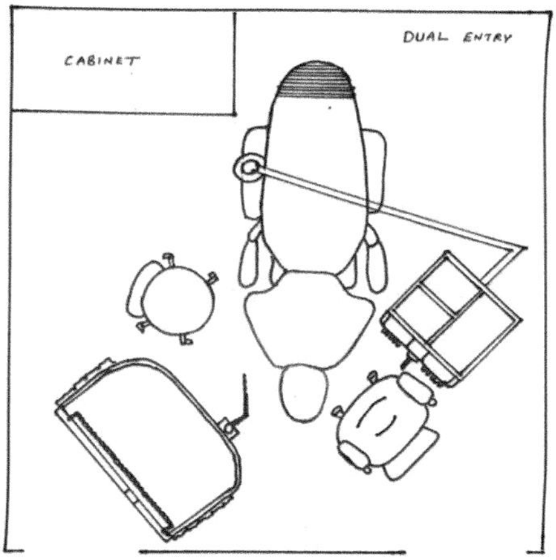

Dual entry type

6.3.2 *Size*

It depends on the room layout, equipment and instrument placement, and delivery while doing patient work, type and site of delivery system such as front, rear, side and over-the-patient systems. During the initial set-up, it may have minimum number of dental chairs installed, but provision should be kept for further expansion. The dental rooms nowadays accommodate portable digital radiography for images to be taken intraoperatively or certain wall-mounted radiographic machines with display screen.

Room should also accommodate equipment like dental room assistant carts, operating microscopes, dental lasers and computers.

6.3.3 *Acoustic System Design*

In a dental office, different types of instruments like high-speed air rotors, low-speed straight and contra-angle hand piece, high-vacuum suction machine, scaling and root planning ultrasonic instruments, vibrators, model trimmers, lathe for polishing the dentures, and cutting and vibrating instruments are used [6]. They produce continuous sounds of different frequencies, which causes auditory effects of noise on health. It is important to decrease the amount of exposure to these sounds for the staff and for better patient experience. Dental operatory should be having soundproof walls and ceilings. Barriers and shields should be considered to absorb or filter the noise. Low-speed devices and low-volume suctions tend to produce less noise and should be preferred. Ultrasonic frequencies can also damage hearing due to the generation of subharmonics, and thus hearing should be protected against these frequencies.

6.3.4 Delivery System Style and Location

The delivery system style selection depends upon the practice to be followed: endodontic, periodontal, orthodontic, oral surgery, prosthetics, oral radiology and diagnosis, oral pathology or pedodontics. There can be multiple delivery locations/styles used within a treatment area. This is named as per clock diagram according to the location of the operator in relation to patient, instrument delivery positioning and assistant positioning. Within the set standard, the clock diagram depicts a patient's head at the midnight or 12 o'clock position and patient's feet kept at 6 o'clock position. Instrument delivery systems are basically of three types: side delivery, over the patient or from back or rear end for efficient workflow settings to be customized.

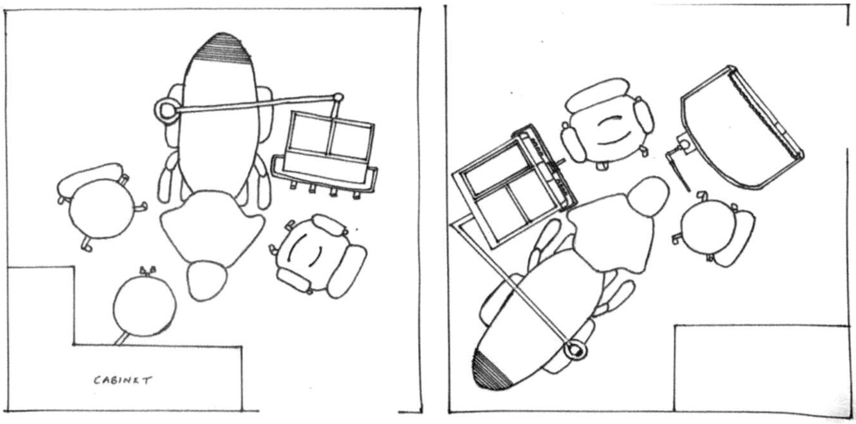

A. Front End Delivery. B. Rear End Delivery

6.3.5 X-Ray Systems

Two types of X-ray systems are used in dental offices:

1. Intraoral X-ray machine
2. Panoramic X-ray machine

Intraoral X-Ray Machine

The intraoral X-ray machine can supply radiation for both digital and traditional film systems. Traditionally, fixed type of X-ray machines were used in dental offices. Nowadays, portable types of machines are available. Intraoral periapical radiographs, bitewing radiographs and occlusal radiographs can be done with this machine. X-ray machine can be installed between the operatories so that two operatories can use the same machine and also be cost effective. If the traditional film system is used, darkroom should be made for processing of the radiographs. Darkroom should have a minimum size of 4 × 6 ft, containing processing tanks for developer and fixing solutions. Safe lighting can be done in darkroom, and the colour of the bulb is preferably red.

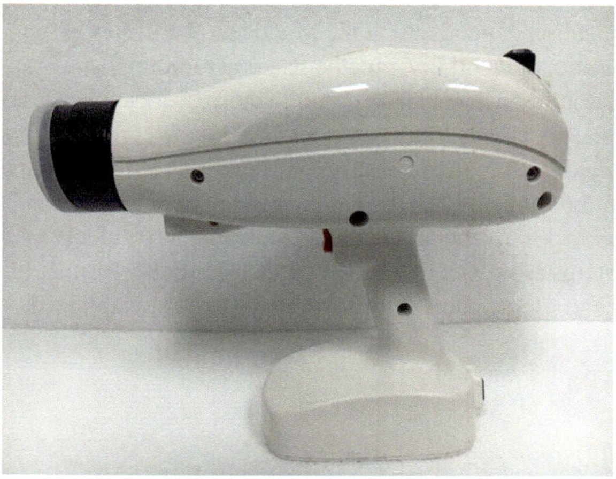

Portable X ray machine

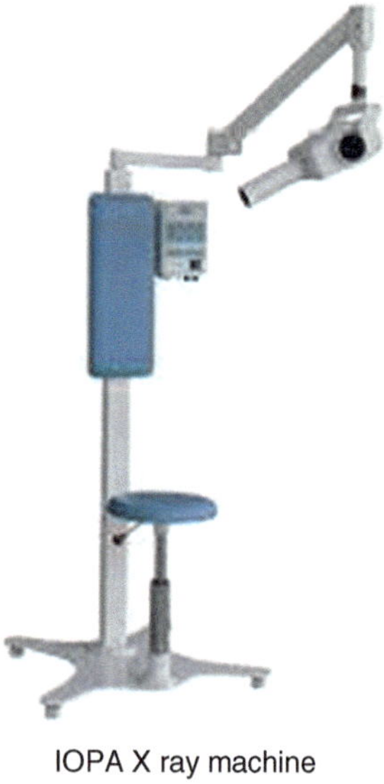

IOPA X ray machine

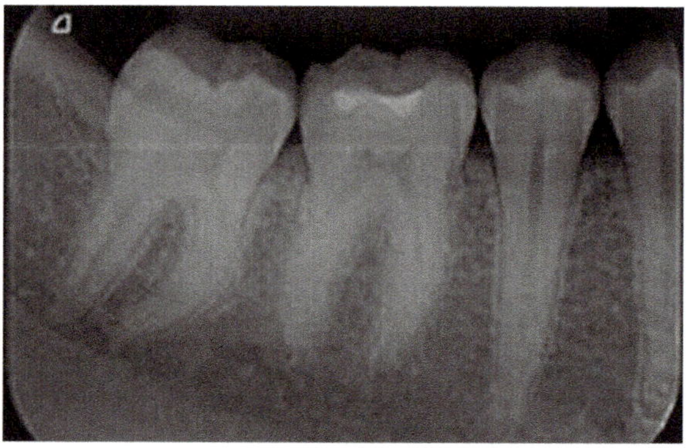

IOPA Radiograph

Panoramic X-Ray Machine

Panoramic radiography is a type of extraoral radiographic technique which is widely used in dentistry. It provides only 2D information about oral and other maxillofacial structures. It is an essential and valuable diagnostic tool, which can provide a one-time image of all teeth, maxilla and mandible, paranasal sinus, temporomandibular joints, inferior alveolar nerve and palate. Through proper positioning of patient and applying standardization techniques, good quality of panoramic images can be obtained. This type of images are less expensive than computerized tomography (CT) images.

For the fixation of panoramic X-ray machine, "5 × 5" ft of clear floor space is required. It is efficient and user friendly to locate the panoramic X-ray machine space near the clinical area.

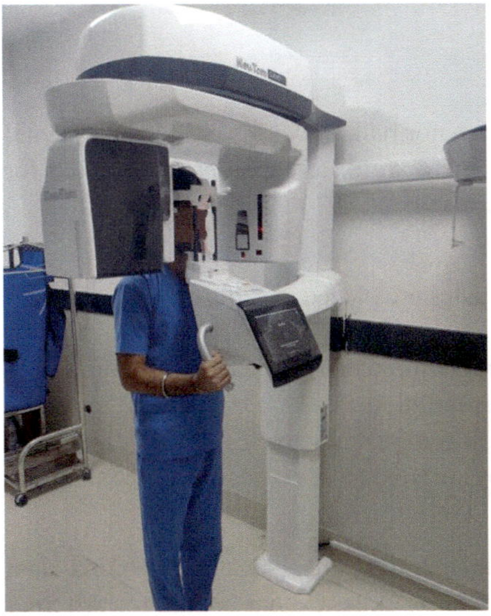

Panoramic X ray machine

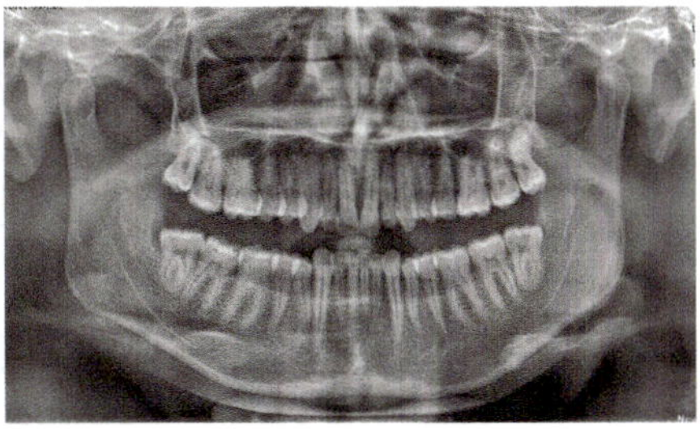

Panoramic X ray

6.3.6 Data Collection

Dental records may include treatment planning notes, radiographs, diagnostic study models, investigations, clinical photographs, prescribed medication and progress of patient and medical history. This information is very essential and should be maintained in an easily accessible manner. Electronic or digital records maintained by computer-assisted methods are of high quality and are very beneficial for patients in terms of safety [6]. Another advantage of storing digital records is that less space is required for storage than paper records [7–9]. Moreover, photographs of casts can also be stored in some cases [8].

6.3.7 *Waste Management System*

Different types of wastes are generated inside a dental office including general wastes, chemical wastes, infectious wastes and sharp wastes. Proper segregation and disposal of waste are required in order to prevent the spread of infections. Two types of wastes are generally produced in a dental clinic which include:

1. Hazardous wastes
2. Non-hazardous wastes

Hazardous waste	Non-hazardous waste
Infectious waste Pathological waste Sharps Chemical waste Cytotoxic waste Radioactive waste	Disposable paper towels Paper mixing pads Disposable covers of operating surfaces

Non-hazardous wastes also constitute a major bulk of wastes produced in dental offices but should be managed properly. There are different steps to be taken for waste management. These include the following:

1. Waste survey: identify different types of wastes.
2. Waste segregation: different types of wastes are placed in different colour-coded containers.
3. Waste accumulation and storage: accumulation means keeping waste for shorter duration and storage is meant for longer duration.
4. Waste transport: transport of materials in designated vehicles.
5. Waste treatment: treatment of waste by different techniques like decontamination or disinfection.

The most essential part of waste management is the segregation of biomedical waste. For this, colour coding of the container is done. Colour coding for different types of waste categories is listed below as per biomedical waste management rules 2018 by the Central Pollution Control Board (Table 6.1).

General Waste Management

This includes all types of wastes produced in a dental office other than biomedical waste. These wastes are not in contact with any infectious, chemical or biological secretions. Moreover, waste sharps are also not included in this group. General office wastes can be reduced by using materials with minimum packaging. Moreover, plastic containers and cardboards, if clean, can be sent for recycling. The clothing materials used in dentistry should be sent to laundry in red laundry bags labelled as biohazard. Otherwise, disposable aprons or uniforms should be used.

Table 6.1 Color coding of biomedical waste

Option	Waste category	Treatment and disposal	Colour coding
1	Human anatomical waste, extracted tooth, cotton contaminated with blood, alginate impression material	Incineration/deep burial	Yellow-coloured non-chlorinated plastic bags
2	Infected plastic waste, disposable suction tips, gloves, syringes, broken dentures	Incineration/autoclave	Red-coloured non-chlorinated plastic bags
3	Waste sharps—needles, scalpels, blades that may cause puncture and cuts—both used and unused	Disinfection/autoclaving/ microwaving and mutilation/shredding	White-coloured translucent puncture-proof, leak-proof containers
4	Glassware and metallic body implants	Disinfection/autoclaving/ microwaving and mutilation/shredding	Blue-coloured puncture-proof, tamper-proof containers

Infectious to Potentially Infectious Waste

This includes any materials contaminated with blood or any other secretions. Gauze pieces and cotton rolls infected with blood should be segregated in yellow-coloured bags and should be discarded properly. Wastes like suction tips and gloves must also be placed in leak-proof red bags and labelled appropriately. Once the waste is collected, licensed biomedical waste management team should be informed for proper waste disposal.

Mercury-Containing Wastes

Mercury is a natural metallic element which is a bio-accumulative toxin. It can cause potential risk to human health. A major constituent of dental amalgam fillings is mercury, and thus a large amount of mercury waste is produced in dental clinics. So proper management of mercury wastes is very important in a dental clinic. Amalgam-containing traps should not be rinsed in the sink. Moreover, any mercury-containing materials like broken amalgam restorations, extracted teeth having amalgam and filters containing amalgam should not be mixed with normal solid waste. Instead, it should be segregated and stored in an airtight container designated as "scrap dental amalgam". Apart from this, staff should be properly trained for minimal usage and disposal of mercury without wastage, and precapsulated dental amalgam should be preferred than bulk elemental mercury.

After the segregation of wastes, the next area is meant for cleaning of the debris from the instruments and trays. Ultrasonic cleaners and undercounter instrument washer system can be used for efficient removal of debris from the contaminated instruments. A sink is required for the rinsing of contaminated instruments and for handwashing purpose. Sterilization areas can be equipped with suction devices to remove water from the surface of instruments and for emptying of the instruments at a faster rate.

After cleaning and drying of instruments, there is a need of packaging of instruments. Wrapping of the cleaned instruments and cassettes is done in the area. Proper bagging of instruments is required for ready access to different types of instruments. Actual sterilization space should be separated from cleaning and processing area so that splattering of wastes will not happen over cleaned instruments. A space for cold sterilization should also be present for sterilizing instruments which cannot tolerate heat and for disinfecting trays and lids. Autoclaves should be installed for proper sterilization of instruments with in-built vacuum for cleaning of water reservoirs.

The last step is the storage of sterilized items. Storage can be done in different types of cabinets and drawers. Instruments can be divided according to the order of use and type of procedures. This type of organization process is effective for storage of surgical, endodontic and prosthodontic procedures.

X-Ray Processing Wastes

Even though most of the dental clinics now use digital radiography techniques, there are some centres that still use conventional radiographic techniques. Different types of chemicals like developer, fixer and cleaning agents are used during the process, and each of them requires special techniques for proper management. The fixer and developer solutions should not be mixed. Waste developer solution can be poured to the normal drain if the pH of the developer solution does not exceed pH standard of the local sanitation agency. In most cases, developer is caustic in nature, which recommends a separate disposal of the developer rather than draining to sewage. The fixer solution will be having silver, which is valuable and should be recycled. Two techniques are generally used of which one is onsite treatment. Onsite treatment and disposal involve the usage of silver recovery units or electrolytic units. If onsite treatment is not possible, offsite treatment can be done. In such cases, the used fixer should be collected and stored in a plastic container labelled as "Silver-containing Used Fixer—To Be Recycled" and sent for recycling.

6.3.8 Internal Network for Water, Osmotic, Suction, Electricity Systems

Internal network and storage within the delivery cart give a neat appearance to the operatory. A single tube should be placed for the passage of compressed air, electrical wires, computer cables and other wires. This allows for a neat arrangement and should be routed to either an in-wall or an in-floor junction box. Another aspect to be considered during clinic design is the placement of the foot control. The foot control tubing can be kept under the floor through a conduit from the junction box to the patient dental chair. This helps in creating easy access to the foot control without tubing running across the floor [10].

6.4 Summary

Planning and designing of dental clinic are one of the important steps, which should be done with utmost care and precision. A dental clinic should be designed in such a way that smooth functioning of the clinic and proper patient management will be possible. Dental office should be designed not only according to recent technologies, but also anticipating future advancements. The architectural design and structural framework should be pleasing to the patients. In this post-COVID period, patients are more concerned about the hygiene, sterilization and infection control. At any cost, proper waste management and sterilization protocols should be followed. The clinical environment should be maintained in such a manner that a positive attitude can be induced in patients regarding the treatment. Architectural and ergonomic design can help decrease workplace-related stress and can promote an atmosphere of teamwork for the dentists and supporting staff. So, it is very important to plan and design dental office to meet the clinical and functional demands.

References

1. Unthank M. Dental office planning. *J Am Dent Assoc* 1999;130:1579-82.
2. Infection control recommendations for the dental office and the dental laboratory. ADA Council on Scientific Affairs and ADA Council on Dental Practice. *J Am Dent Assoc 1996;127:672-80.*
3. Hamula W, Bucher B. Creating your next office. *J Clin Orthod* 2000;**34**(12):723–30.
4. Jain et al. Strategic planning of a dental clinic in India. *International Dental Journal of Student's Research* 2019;6(4):74-6
5. De Bruyne MA, Van Renterghem B, Baird A, Palmans T, Danneels L, Dolphens M. Influence of different stool types on muscle activity and lumbar posture among dentists during a simulated dental screening task. *Appl Ergon* 2016;**56**:220–6.
6. T.K.L. Schleyer, Why integration is key for dental office technology, *Journal of the American Dental Association* 2004*;* **135:** 4–9
7. Haeger RS. Establishing an all-digital office. *J Clin Orthod* 2005;**39**(2):81–95
8. Hamula W, Hamula DW. Orthodontic office design: the paperless practice. *J Clin Orthod* 1998;**32**(1):35–43
9. Keim RG. The paperless office. *J Clin Orthod* 2005;**39**:61–2.
10. Varghese J, Doshi V. Orthodontic office design: principles and practice. *Semin Orthod* 2016;**22**:289–96.

Chapter 7
Hospital Information System

Divya Rao, Venkatesh, H. K. Mamatha, and N. Shalini

Objectives

This unit on HIS fulfils the following objectives:

1. Understanding the basic structure, layout, and design of hospital information system (HIS)
2. Functioning of hospital information system (HIS)
3. Decision-making and support
4. International coding of disease

7.1 Introduction

Healthcare is a crucial component of our society; healthcare professionals must carry out their duties properly and efficiently. Hundreds or thousands of patients enter medical facilities every day expecting the administration to handle the work. And to do that, the staff must integrate and manage the clinical, operational, and financial data that is changing along with the practice.

All of this data was initially organized manually in the absence of a system, which was not only time consuming but also fell short of expectations for efficiency. As a result, to increase efficiency, the majority of professionally managed clinics

D. Rao (✉) · H. K. Mamatha · N. Shalini
Department of Health System Management Studies, JSS Academy of Higher Education and Research, Mysuru, India
e-mail: divyaraobj.dhsms@jssuni.edu.in

Venkatesh
Padmashree College of Hospital Administration, Bangalore, India

D. Bhatia et al. (eds.), *A Guide to Hospital Administration and Planning*,
https://doi.org/10.1007/978-981-19-6692-7_7

and hospitals today rely on hospital information systems (HIS) to manage all of their administrative and medical data.

In the era of intense competition, the healthcare sector is seeing a greater emphasis on patient care quality and successful clinical outcomes. Therefore, in order to keep up with the changing market, hospitals and other healthcare providers must streamline procedures and models while cutting operational expenses.

The administrative, financial, and clinical aspects of hospitals and healthcare facilities are managed by modern hospital information systems (HIS), which are extensive, integrated, and specialized information systems. They are regarded as one of the most crucial hubs on which the provision of healthcare within hospitals and various types of medical facilities depends [1]. These systems' play a very critical role in maintaining patient data and information, including vital information about the patient and other comprehensive medical data, as well as in documenting all medical services provided to the patient, including examinations, diagnoses, treatments, follow-up reports, and crucial medical decisions, makes their significance clear [2].

7.2 Information

According to Wikipedia:

"Information can be recorded as signs, or transmitted as signals. Information is any kind of event that affects the state of a dynamic system that can interpret the information".

Conceptually, information is the message (utterance or expression) that is being conveyed. Hence, in a general sense, information is "knowledge communicated or received, concerning a particular fact or circumstance". Information cannot be predicted and resolves uncertainty [3].

7.2.1 Information vs. Data

Information	Data
Raw facts that are organized, structured, and interpreted and created into a useful message are information	Raw facts which are unstructured, unprocessed facts and figures and collected plainly
Interpreted data: they are created from processed, organized, and arranged data in a specific environment	Groups of non-random symbols that depict objects, actions, and numbers in text, graphics, and voice

According to Davis and Olson [4]:

"Information is data processed to give meaningful content and which is real and has perceived value in the current action or in the future action or for decision making process by the recipients".

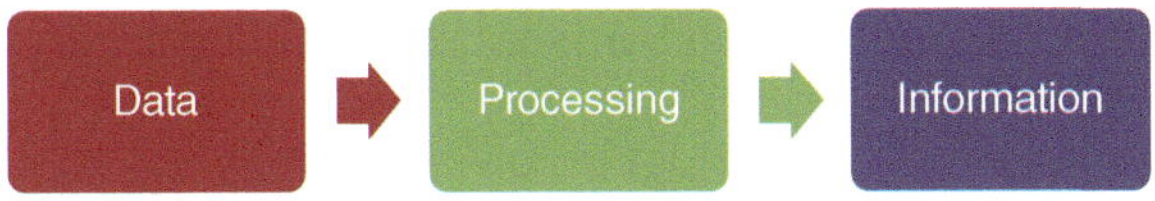

Professor Ray R. Larson of the School of Information at the University of California, Berkeley, provides an *Information Hierarchy*, which is

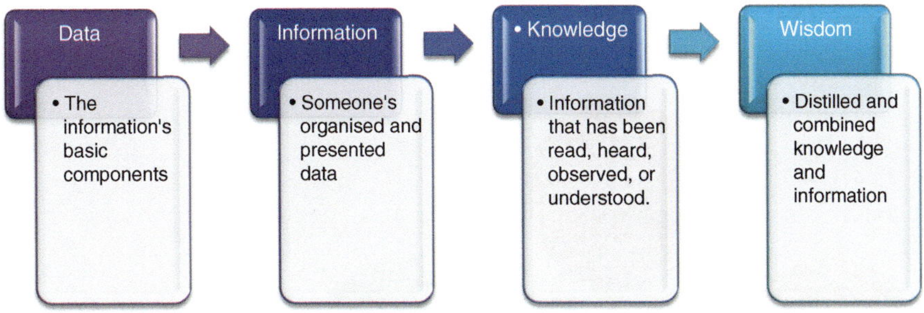

Information Continuum as explained by Scott Andrews' [5]

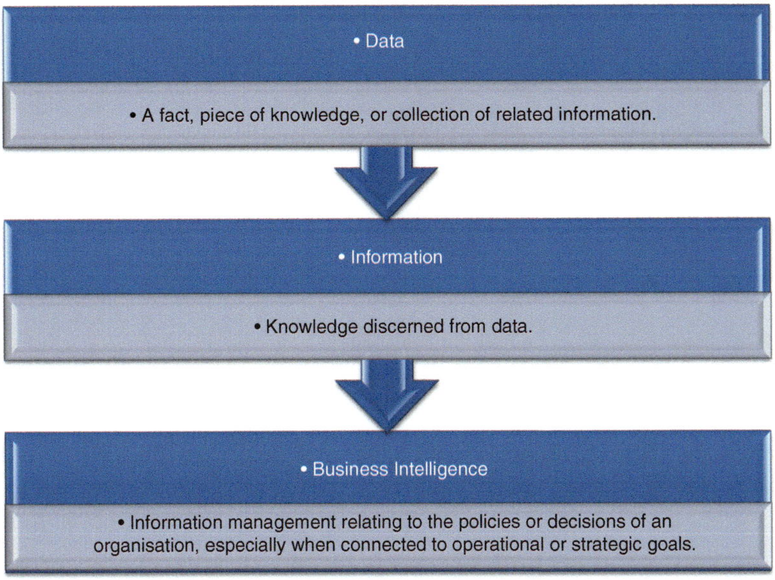

7.3 Management Information System (MIS)

"The study of people, technology, organisations, and their relationships is known as management information systems (MIS). MIS specialists assist businesses in getting the most out of their investments in people, technology, and operational procedures. MIS is a people-centric approach with a focus on providing services using technology".

Management information systems can be utilized by any level of management, and executives who are in charge of business typically make decisions about which management information system (MIS) to adopt and business's entire technology strategy, including assessing how a new technology might benefit the firm. They make decisions on the new MIS's implementation.

The MIS is a product of contribution of functional features from various fields, which depicts its nature and scope [6].

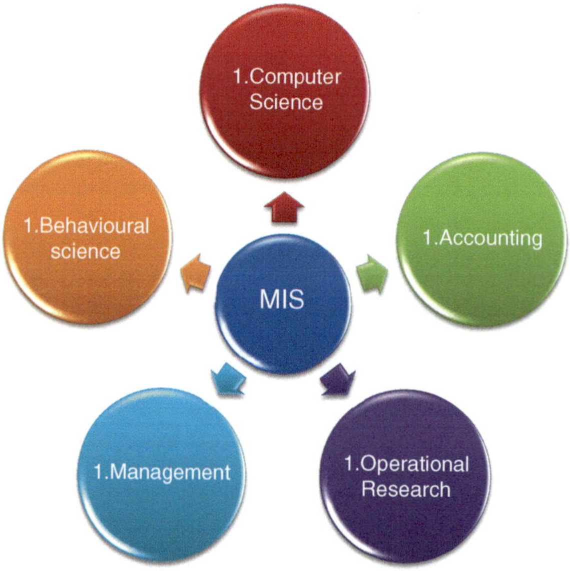

7.3.1 Types of MIS [7]

Hossein states that there are different forms of information systems that help middle and operational level managers prepare reports, extract data, and make decisions.

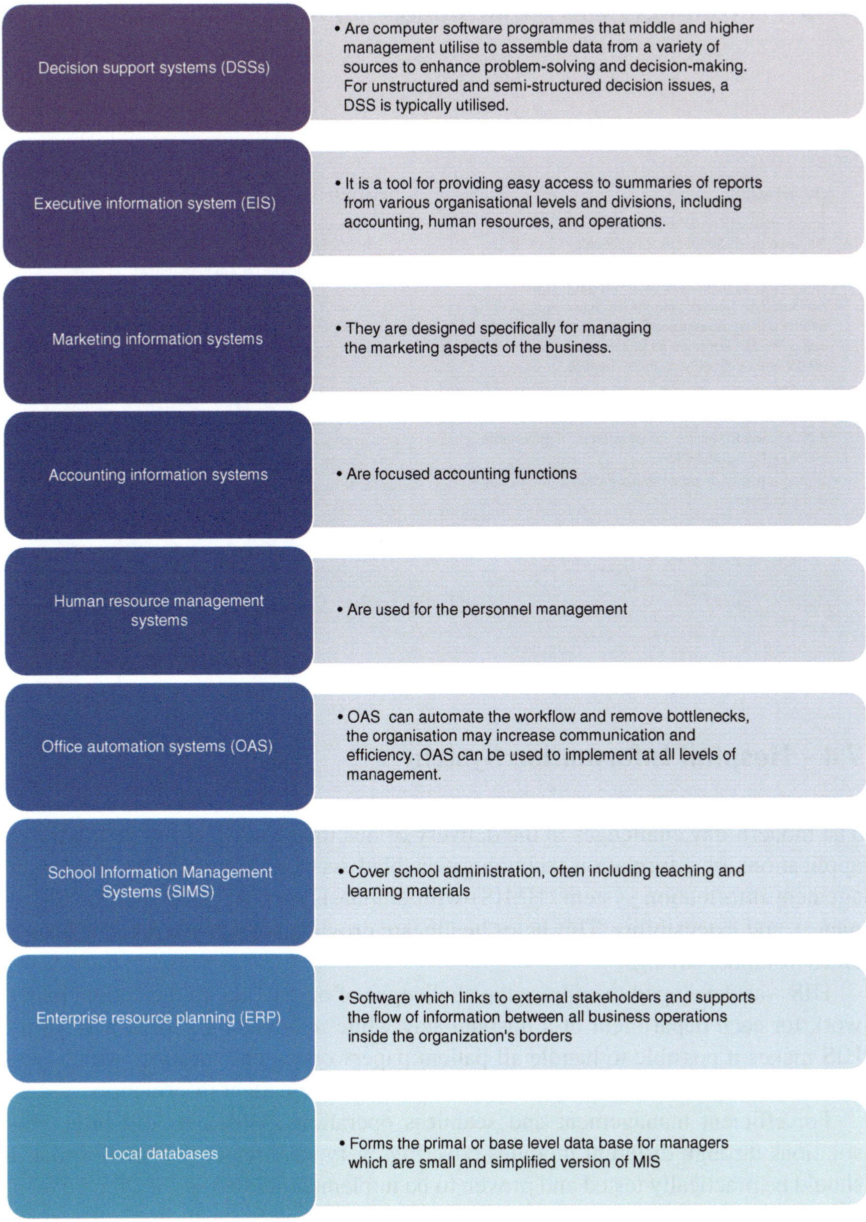
Decision support systems (DSSs)
• Are computer software programmes that middle and higher management utilise to assemble data from a variety of sources to enhance problem-solving and decision-making. For unstructured and semi-structured decision issues, a DSS is typically utilised.
Executive information system (EIS)
• It is a tool for providing easy access to summaries of reports from various organisational levels and divisions, including accounting, human resources, and operations.
Marketing information systems
• They are designed specifically for managing the marketing aspects of the business.
Accounting information systems
• Are focused accounting functions
Human resource management systems
• Are used for the personnel management
Office automation systems (OAS)
• OAS can automate the workflow and remove bottlenecks, the organisation may increase communication and efficiency. OAS can be used to implement at all levels of management.
School Information Management Systems (SIMS)
• Cover school administration, often including teaching and learning materials
Enterprise resource planning (ERP)
• Software which links to external stakeholders and supports the flow of information between all business operations inside the organization's borders
Local databases
• Forms the primal or base level data base for managers which are small and simplified version of MIS

7.3.2 Advantages and Disadvantages of MIS [7]

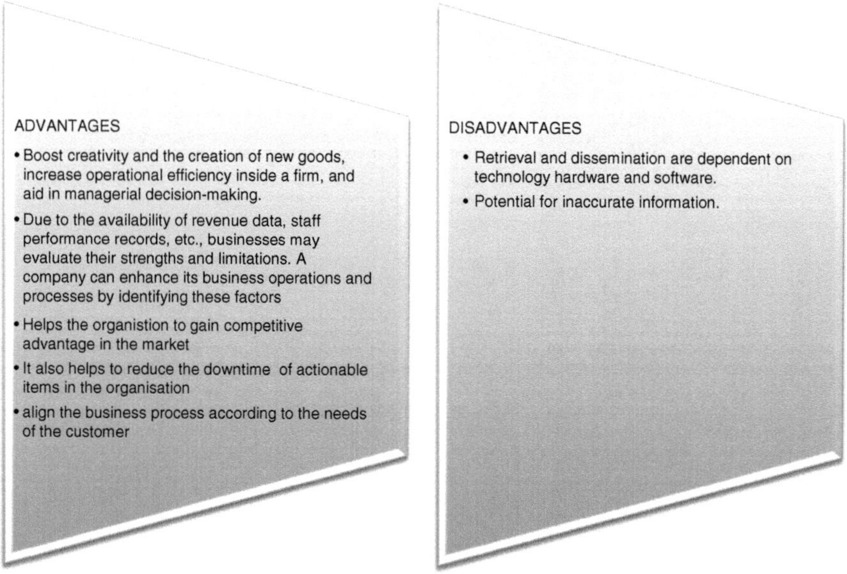

7.4 Hospital Information System

The modern-day challenges in the delivery of healthcare services are addressed by applications of information technology-enabled services known as hospital management information system (HMIS) with emphasis on cost-effectiveness, convenience, and extensibility. This helps healthcare providers to achieve revenue growth and substantial savings.

HIS was developed to address the challenges of organizing all the patient paperwork for each department of a hospital stay while maintaining patient anonymity. HIS makes it possible to handle all patient paperwork in one location, which frees up staff members from having to organize and analyse patient information.

For efficient management and seamless operations, HMIS should offer 360° solutions through different modules covering every requirement of the hospital. It should be practically tested and proven to be implementable across healthcare facilities, and the HMIS provider should have enough experience in implementation. The solution should be highly scalable to fulfil most of the requirements of various kinds of healthcare facilities and providers when they grow and scale up in terms of business and introduction of newer facilities.

Any HMIS should be designed keeping in mind the needs of the customer and should be easy to learn and use. The needs of the hospitals should be met by tailoring the functions within the modules.

7.4.1 *Development* [8]

Since its introduction in 1960, hospital information system has evolved and kept pace with technological advancements while improving healthcare facilities. In the modern world, patient needs are met by starting the management of healthcare in the hands of patients through their mobile phones.

7.4.2 *Definition*

The general meaning of management information system (MIS) is a structured and systematic arrangement and presentation of facts (information) that is generally required and helps the management of an organization in taking effective and better decisions for the organization. The MIS derives data from several units of the organization or from other sources linked to it.

The term "Hospital Information Systems (HIS) refers to the component of health informatics that places focus largely on the administrative, financial, and clinical needs of hospitals. These systems augment the ability of healthcare professionals to coordinate care by providing a patient's health information and visit history at the place and time that it is required" [9].

7.4.3 *Objectives of HIS*

The main goal of any organization is to manage itself in an improved manner by utilizing the potential of the HIS and gain competitive advantage.

Following are the basic objectives of the HIS [10]

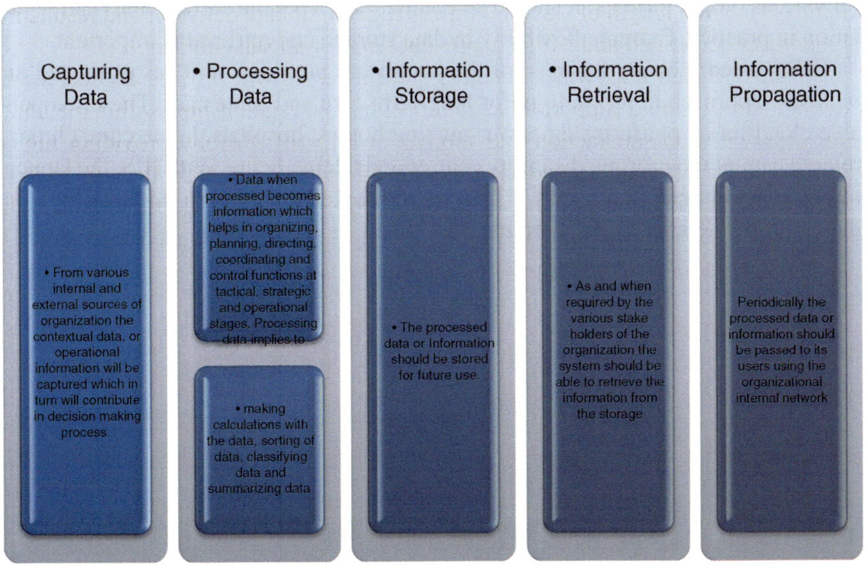

Characteristics of HIS [11]

The HIS exhibits the following characteristics:

It is designed for a long-term planning providing a holistic view of the dynamics and the structure of the hospital by comprehensively interconnecting sub-systems of the organization.

The hospital manager's needs, such as strategic, operational, and tactical information, should be met; it should also report any exceptional situations which are detrimental to the users and hospital.

Decision makers or users should be able to make estimates and forecasts, generating advanced information which provides a competitive advantage.

All sub-systems within the hospital should be linked between each other and provide an integrated view, which helps the decision maker to take the right decision.

The redundancy and duplicity of data will be avoided by allowing easy and clear flow of information through various sub-systems, simplifying the operations with as much practicability as possible.

Although the HIS is an integrated system linking all sub-systems, it should also be able to function as a stand-alone sub-system without interfering with other sub-systems, thus providing autonomy between each sub-system and vice versa.

The backbone of any HIS is its database without which the HIS cannot fulfil the needs of the hospital management and the users.

With the advancement in the computer hardware and software configurations, the HIS should be capable of processing data accurately and with high speed.

Since the hospital generates large amounts of raw data, both related and unrelated in nature, from various internal and external sources related to the organization related to the various activities, this data should be collected, organized, and updated for processing meaningful information.

As there will be constant activities being exhibited in a hospital, the HIS should provide real-time information of these activities without delay and provide support for various output formats. It should be compatible as per the current rules and regulation in practice. Extreme flexibility in data storage and retrieval is important

HIS is used globally by most of the healthcare providers and has promoted an inclusive approach in technology for long-term care and acute care. The interoperable cloud-based platforms empower nursing homes, hospitals, home care, clinics, remote patient monitoring, disability centres and telemedicine. With HIS, the launch of any new service is possible for healthcare providers with least possible time on the cloud with comprehensive access.

Functioning of HIS

The hospital information system functions online and uses the intranet to access the relevant hospital network. Information about the medications needed to treat pertinent ailments is stored on database servers. Additionally, it monitors patient financial information and makes online appointments for doctors.

7.4.4 Features or Modules of HIS [12]

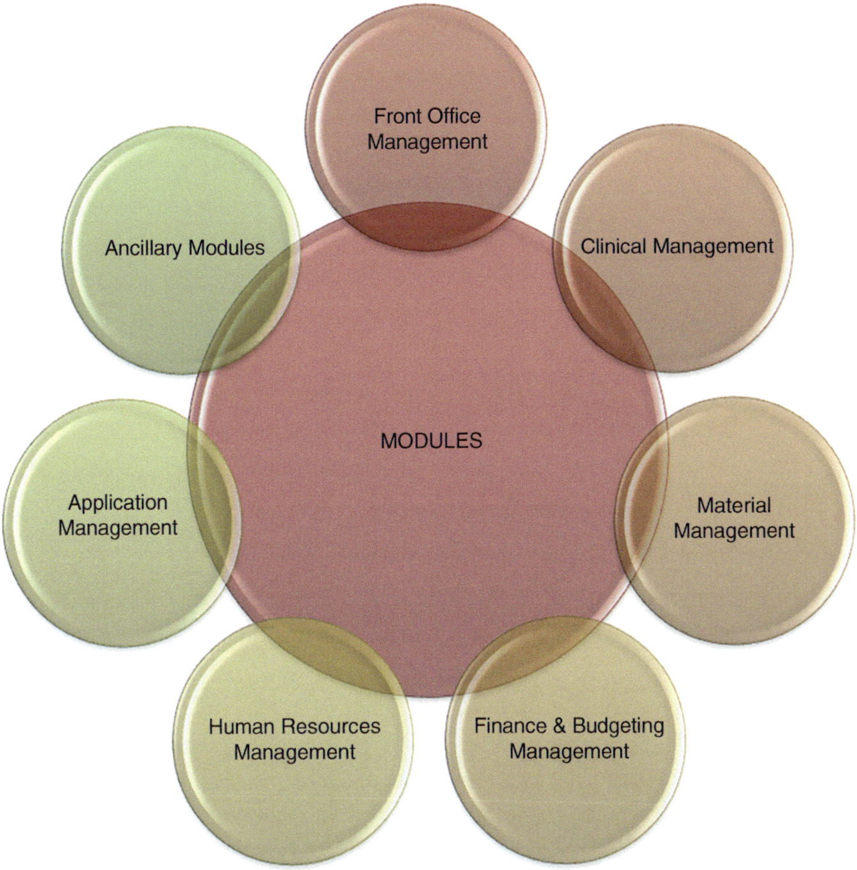

Features/Outlook of the Modules

The modules could possess features like:

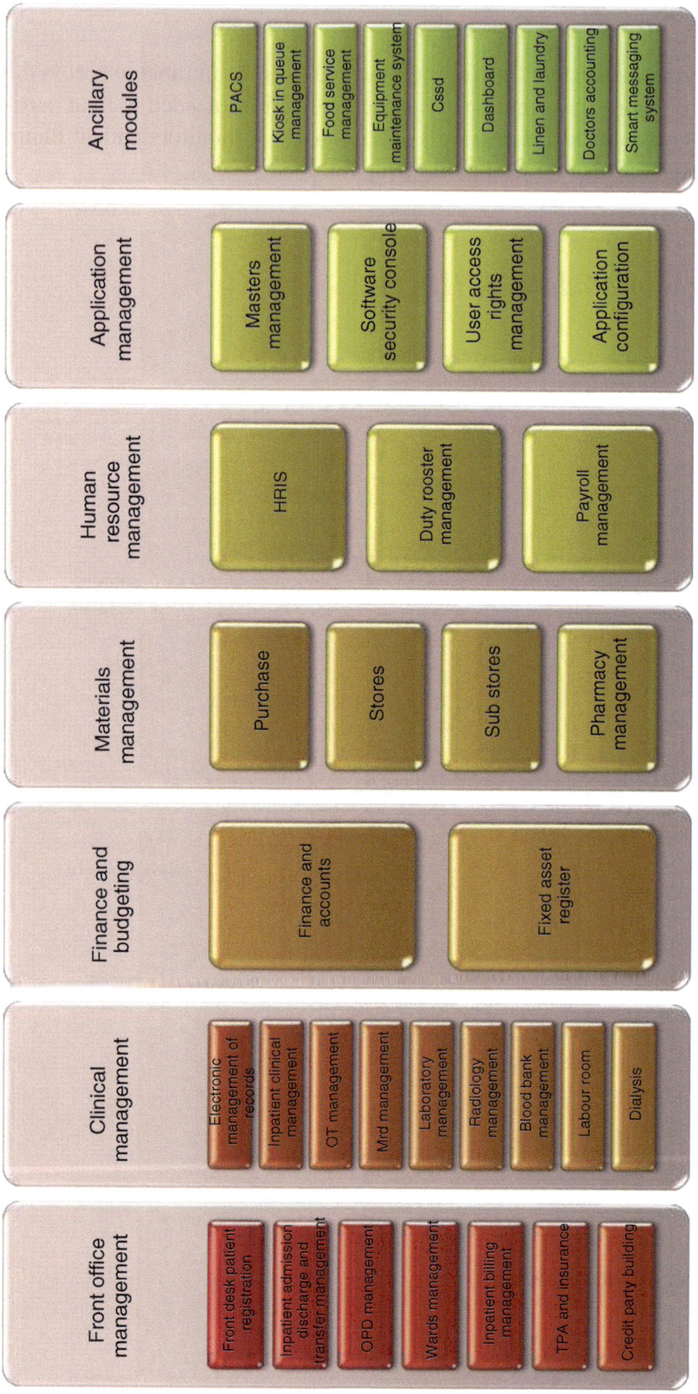
Front office management
Front desk patient registration
Inpatient admission discharge and transfer management
OPD management
Wards management
Inpatient billing management
TPA and insurance
Credit party building
Clinical management
Electronic management of records
Inpatient clinical management
OT management
Mrd management
Laboratory management
Radiology management
Blood bank management
Labour room
Dialysis
Finance and budgeting
Finance and accounts
Fixed asset register
Materials management
Purchase
Stores
Sub stores
Pharmacy management
Human resource management
HRIS
Duty rooster management
Payroll management
Application management
Masters management
Software security console
User access rights management
Application configuration
Ancillary modules
PACS
Kiosk in queue management
Food service management
Equipment maintenance system
Cssd
Dashboard
Linen and laundry
Doctors accounting
Smart messaging system

Example of HMS Workflow with Associated Activities

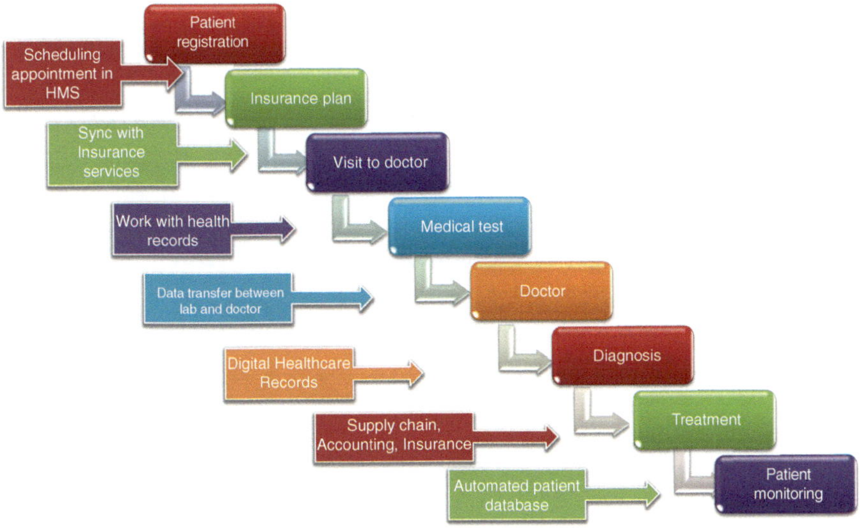

Functioning of HIS

See Fig. 7.1.

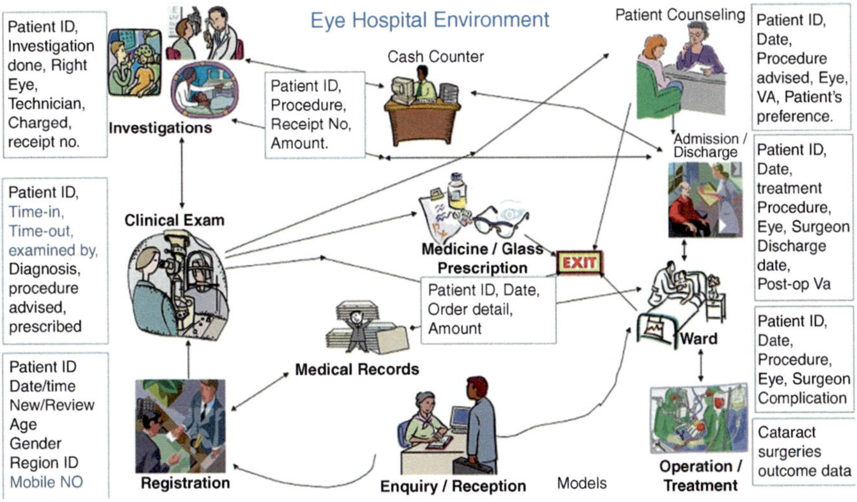

Fig. 7.1 Eye hospital functions and key data generated [13]

Benefits of HIS [14]

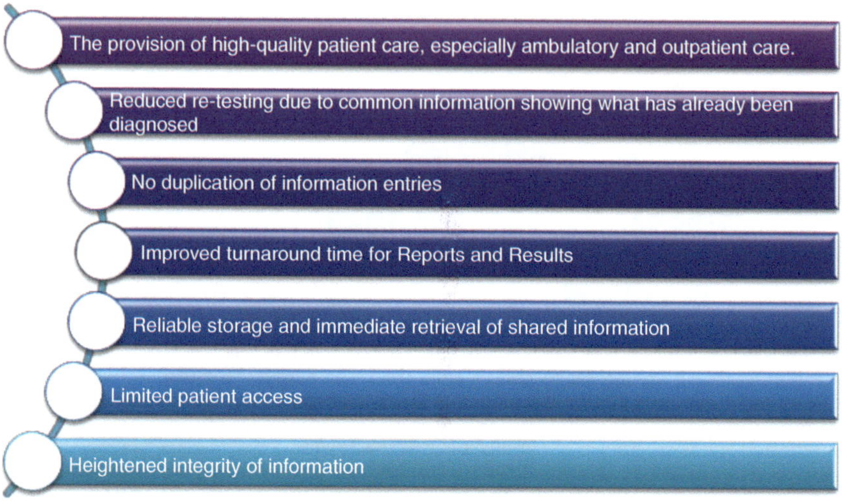

7.5 Decision Support System (DSS)

7.5.1 Introduction

The HMIS acquires data and processes the data to form a useful information which is used by the organization for taking better decisions, which involves the user discretion and interpretation ability based on the individual's capability and requirement [15]. Furthermore, when the same information is presented by the system/program itself which can support determinations, judgments, and course of action in the hospital or business, it is termed as decision support system. The DSS is a computerized program which shifts through and analyses large amounts of data, compiling comprehensive information which can help to solve problems and can be used in decision-making [16].

7.5.2 Definition

"A decision support system (DSS) is a computer programme application that helps businesses make better decisions. Large volumes of data are analysed, and the best solutions are then presented to an organisation. To give users information beyond the typical reports and summaries, decision support systems combine data and knowledge from several fields and sources. This is meant to assist people in making defensible decisions" [17].

The hospital information system incorporates a clinical decision support system (CDSS), which analyses large data within electronic health records to provide prompt reminders to help doctors and clinicians in implementing evidence-based clinical guidelines at the point of care [18].

CDSS helps to improve the delivery of healthcare and enhance physician decisions with goal-oriented clinical acumen supported by a software program, which aids in clinical decision-making known as clinical decision support system or CDSS. The traditional CDSS consists of a software program, which helps clinicians to take decisions based on the information available pertaining to a particular patient such as patient-specific assessments, disease history of the patient, earlier medications used, laboratory investigations, and other inputs.

CDSS can be used to provide care in multiple ways: for example, by reminding providers to screen for certain (cardiovascular) diseases' risk factors, highlighting/flagging cases of high blood pressures or hyperlipidaemia, providing info on treatment protocols, prompting questions on medication adherence, and offering customized recommendations for health behaviour changes.

Thus, the CDSS software presents with certain recommendations to the clinician for arriving at a decision. Nowadays, the CDSS are used at the point of care, where the clinicians use his/her knowledge and discretion along with the suggestions presented by the system (CDSS). The advantage of today's CDSS is the availability of software program that can process large volumes of data and interpret meaningfully, which will help clinician to arrive at a best possible option of treatment. Otherwise, normally these large volumes of data cannot be processed and interpreted by human capabilities. Quality of care in screening, testing, and treating patients can be increased significantly. However, there is lack of evidence to suggest that CDSS directly affects health outcome.

7.5.3 Evolution [19]

Evolution of DSS started early in the 1950s and 1960s from the research conducted at the Carnegie Institute of Technology, but came into practical usage in the form of executive information system (EIS), group decision support system, organizational decision support system, and clinical decision support system in the early 1980s, i.e. when all the organizations worldwide were focusing on data-driven decision-making and the decision science or decision intelligence started gaining prominence [19]. Decision scientists emerged as the new professionals who can unlock the potential features of decision science systems. By combining together applied data science, managerial science, social science, and design science and focusing on selecting between options, thus reducing the effort required to make higher quality decisions, the DSS started delivering its output.

The computer-based CDSS emerged during the early 1980s with limited developments and poor system integration; back then, it was time consuming and was only limited to academic activities. There were many unanswered questions such as the use of computers in medicine, physician independency, and responsibility of wrong decision when computers used for decision-making were not clear, as ethical and legal framework for usage of computers in medicine was not specified. With the advancement in the field of IT, there are lot of Web applications available which can integrate with electronic health records (EHR) and computerized provider order entry (CPOE). Also, the accessibility of CDSS through desktop, tablet, smartphone, and wearable health devices which may or may not produce outputs directly on the devices or be linked into EHR databases has popularized the usage of CDSS.

7.5.4 Functioning

A clinical decision support system works by combining the raw data with document and personal knowledge, associated with business models to help users make decisions. The data sources used by a clinical decision support system are from various sources, input data captured at various points in the electronic medical records (EMRs), and projections from marketing departments and finance departments such as revenue projections, sales projections, data warehouses, and more.

7.5.5 Components

There are generally three components in DSS [20]:

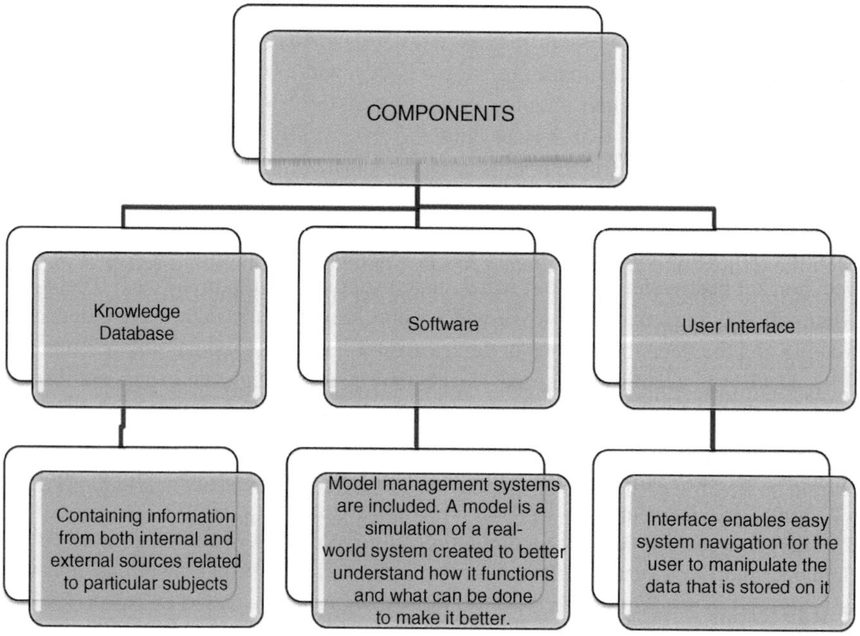

7.5.6 Types of DSS [21]

Data-Driven DSS

A computer programme that bases “its judgments on information from either internal or external databases” is known as a data-driven DSS. A data-driven DSS typically uses data mining techniques to identify trends and patterns, which allow it to foretell future events. Data-driven DSS are frequently used by businesses to support decision-making on inventories, sales, and other business activities and are utilised to aid in decision-making in the public sector.

Model-Driven DSS

Model-driven decision support systems are “tailored in accordance with a preset set of user needs to help analyse various situations that satisfy these requirements. These systems are built on an underlying decision model”. A model-driven DSS might help with scheduling or creating financial statements.

Communication-Driven and Group DSS

Using a number of communication channels, such as voice chat, instant messaging, or email, a communication-driven and group decision support system enables multiple people to work on the same task at once. The purpose of this kind of DSS is to boost user-system collaboration while also enhancing the system’s overall efficacy and efficiency.

Knowledge-Driven DSS

“The information that powers this kind of decision support system is stored in a knowledge base that a knowledge management system continuously updates and maintains”. Users of a knowledge-driven DSS receive information that is in line with the business procedures and expertise of the firm.

Document-Driven DSS

“An information management system that employs documents to retrieve data is known as a document-driven DSS”. Users can conduct searches on websites and databases or for particular search phrases using document-driven DSS. A document-driven DSS might access documents like policies and procedures, meeting minutes, and company records.

7.5.7 Types of CDSS [22, 23]

Knowledge based: It requires a data source, and a particular rule is created and the system retrieves data and examines or evaluates it with the rule to generate an output or action. The rules are based on the literature, practice, or patient-directed evidence [16].

Non-knowledge based: It does not need a rule to be created to evaluate the data, but still the data is required and the decision is arrived at with the application of artificial intelligence (AI), machine learning (ML), or statistical pattern recognition [17]. Non-knowledge-based CDSS is rapidly growing but with a lot of challenges, and understanding the logic that AI uses to generate recommendations is a puzzle in itself, combined with problems of data availability; these types are yet to have widespread implementation. Both types of CDSS have common components with a few subtle differences (Fig. 7.2).

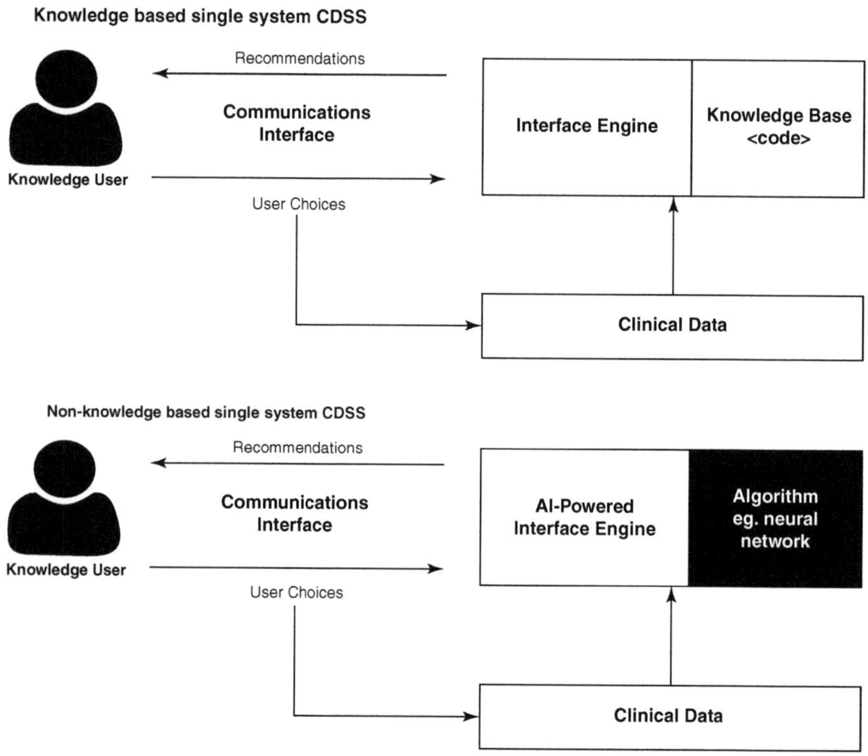

Fig. 7.2 Diagram of key interactions in knowledge-based and non-knowledge-based CDSS. [Image Courtesy: npj Digital Medicine (*npj Digit. Med.*) ISSN 2398-6352 (online)] [16]

7.5.8 *Features* [16]

They are composed of the following:

1. Base: The data provided, the algorithm used to model the decision (non-knowledge based), and the rules that are coded into the system (knowledge based).
2. Inference engine: The inference engine uses the programmed or AI-determined rules and data structures to process the clinical data of the patient and provide an outcome or action that is displayed to the user (e.g. physician).
3. Communication mechanism: The front-end interface of a website, app, or EHR that the user uses to interact with the system [18].

7.5.9 *Implementation* [24]

For implementing CDSS, there are several considerations, such as the following:

1. **Areas of usage:** Although healthcare providers are using CDSS in various ways, very few studies are available about the usage as the systems used may be different. CDSS is used primarily for outpatient care and hence lacks the evidence supporting and justifying the implementation of CDSS.
2. **Policy and law-related guidelines**: The vendors should fully disclose the sources used to build the knowledge base for their CDSS since they interpret and translate the guidelines into algorithms used by the HMIS-CDSS systems, i.e. software along with its limitations and drawbacks. In order to account for changes in evidence and guidelines, the providers must ensure that CDSS is updated regularly, for changes in clinical evidence and guidelines. The HMIS having CDSS feature should track complete and up-to-date information about a patient's medical histories and hypersensitivity and allergic details. If not, the CDSS would not be able to offer comprehensive output and the providers would be burdened and avoid the CDSS guidance, which would become a barrier for successful implementation and outcome, and hence it should be mandatory to have repeat trainings about CDSS implementation and guidelines.
3. **Implementation:** In order to implement the CDSS, various guidelines available from different sources must be used as it requires vast and unique inputs specific to certain diseases and conditions so that the CDSS would work better. By combining the processing of data with inferential models, deductive logics, and predictive algorithms that enable not only the search for relationships among data but also existing trends, causes, and consequences, the incorporation of the "intelligent" characteristic to the "decision support system" seeks to address this challenge. To create a decision system with low uncertainty and exceptional

accuracy, it is crucial to properly combine and complement all these statistical, inferential, and predictive methods.

7.5.10 Functions and Advantages of CDSS

Patient Safety

This helps in reducing medication errors, drug–drug interaction errors [19], dosing and prescribing errors, contraindication warnings, and more [25]. These are done through drug safety software, which are designed with safeguard features for dosing, identifying duplication of treatment patterns and drug–drug interactions; CPOE systems use this software.

Clinical Management

Traditional clinical guidelines and care pathways have demonstrated difficulty in implementing and practice due to very low adherence by the clinicians [26]. If these guidelines can be formulated as a rule and encoded into CDSS, it can serve in a variety of forms, such as standardized order sets for a customized case, alerts to a specific protocol for a specific patient, and reminders for testing. CDSS can also help in managing patients who are on observation protocols on research/treatment. Follow-up for referrals and ensuring preventative care is possible [27].

Cost Reduction

By reducing test duplication, prescribing cheaper drug alternatives [28], and suggesting lower cost treatment, thus reducing insurance denials and decreasing length of stay for inpatients by timely clinical interventions, CDSS can help in cost reduction and help providers to offer cost-effective healthcare.

Administrative Tasks

CDSS helps in quick patient triage by providing support to physicians in arriving at quick decisions in selecting the most suitable diagnostic coding and ordering of tests and procedures through specifically designed algorithms. As per a study, CDSS was conceived to address the inaccuracy of ICD-9 emergency department (ED) admission coding (ICD is International Statistical Classification of Diseases, standardized codes used to represent diseases and diagnosis) [29]. CDSS helps in improving the quality of clinical documentation. An obstetrics CDSS protocol can adopt an enhanced alerting system, which helps in improving the documentation of indications for labour induction and estimated foetal weight as compared to control parameters of the organization [30]. Proper documentation helps in effective implementation of clinical protocols.

It is not very popular due to negative perceptions of the physicians and their biases; inaccuracy due to lack of data availability and system integration has prompted for a manual entry of data [31].

Diagnostics support has a huge potential, especially in countries with resource shortage in terms of established clinical experts, where there are also desires for systems that can supplement specialist diagnostics [32]. Electronic reference-based systems offer probable diagnosis on the basis of patients' clinical presentations of signs and symptoms [33].

DDSS in Radiology and Imaging

Diagnostic radiology and imaging use knowledge-based CDSS for image ordering; radiologists use this to select the most appropriate test to run; and the DDSS system sends reminders of best practice guidelines and gives alerts on contraindications to contrast [34]. It was also known to reduce the number of investigations which were not necessary by assessing the signs, symptoms, and clinical queries prior to image ordering (POC). Moreover, if an image was denied, an alternative was suggested by the system.

There is a great emphasis on non-knowledge-based clinical decision support systems for enhanced imaging and precision. With large amount of data and image acquisition, interpreting manually is difficult and limited. With the advanced pixel recognition and image classification algorithms such as deep learning (DL), several companies are at the forefront of developing solutions for tumour detection, medical imaging interpretation, and diagnosis. IBM Watson has developed "Eyes of Watson", which can combine image recognition of a brain scan with text recognition of case descriptions to provide comprehensive decision support system called as "cognitive assistant" [35].

The Google-invented deep convolutional neural network can detect diabetic retinopathy with high sensitivity and specificity from a data set of 130,000 retinal images. The system algorithms' performance was on par with the US board-certified ophthalmologists.

CDSS in Laboratory and Pathology

CDSS is used extensively in laboratory testing and interpretation. Reminders are set for abnormal lab results in EHR systems. Artificial intelligence is used to enhance accuracy where multiple tests are combined (serum markers, imaging, and gene tests); the CDSS is used in the interpretation where test's reference ranges are highly personalized and are age, sex, and disease subtype specific [36]. CDSS is used in tumour grading and estimating recurrence with 93% accuracy in urinary bladder tumours and brain tumour classification and grading. It is also used in arterial blood gas interpretation, protein electrophoresis reports, computerized ECG analysis, and blood cell counting [37].

With the invention of personal health record (PHR) decision support system useful to patients, the CDSS functionality is integrated, similar to EMRs, with the patient as the end user or manager of the data, which is a great move towards patient-centric care, and the CDS-supported PHRs aid in the implementation of shared decision-making between patient and provider; this will help in removing the barrier and help in patients' participation in their care.

Several PHRs are available, which can be fully integrated into the institutional EHR. This helps the patients in deciding the level of care they need and then help them seek treatment [38].

The data collected by the PHRs is limitless such as allergies to insurance coverage to prescription and medications. Also, data from other wearable devices can be integrated to PHRs to create an actionable insight for providers.

Challenges of Clinical Decision Support System [16]

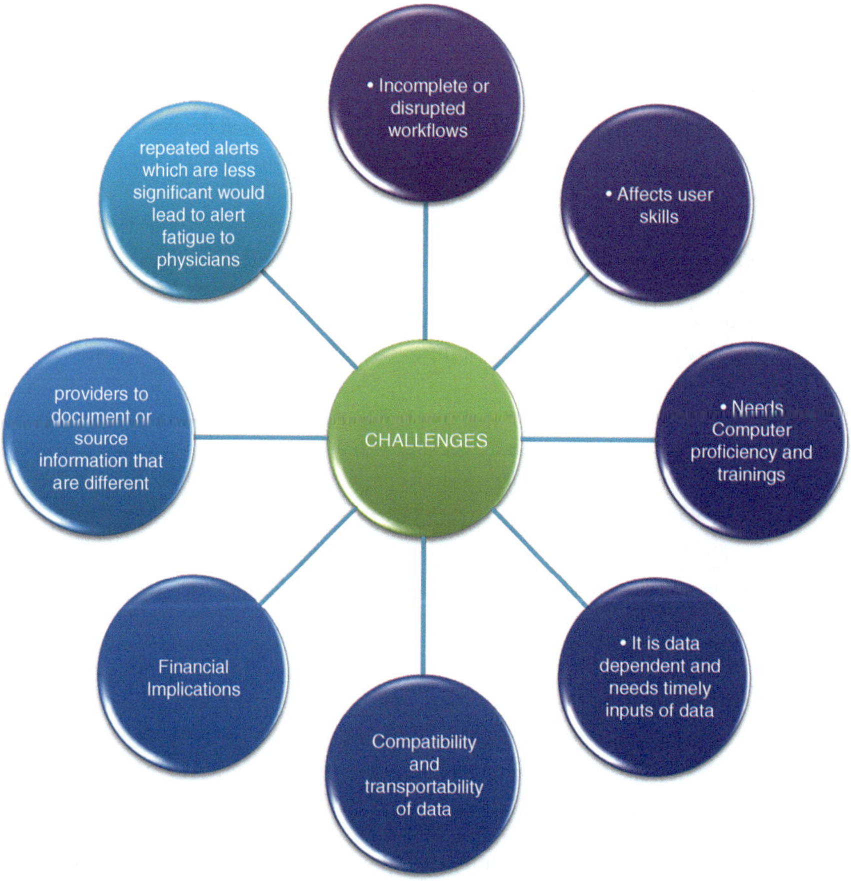

Drawbacks of CDSS [39]

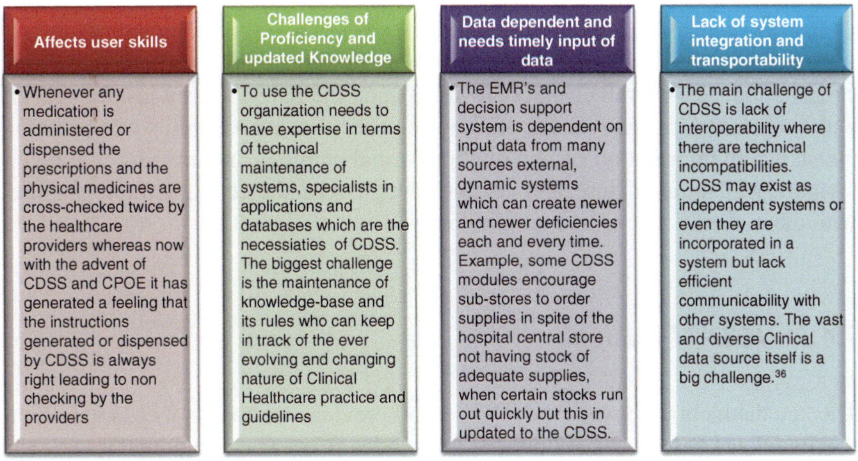

7.6 International Classification of Diseases (ICD)

Diseases have to be analysed in terms of prevention, treatment, and allocation of resources. To understand this, a measurement system has to be followed. Measurement must be accurate to enable cogent summarization of massive amounts of data as well as reliable comparisons between locations and over time. For this measurement, a classification of diseases and related issues is necessary [40].

The International Classification of Diseases (ICD) has been the primary basis for comparable statistics on causes of death and non-fatal diseases for more than a century and was adopted by the International Statistical Institute in 1900 in Paris [41, 42]. This was followed with the updating in every decade, till the task was handed over to the WHO in 1946. It started with the ICD1 to the various versions that have come into vogue after that. The ICD-9 was adopted in 1985, and after an interval of 17 years, the ICD-10 was adopted in 1992 [43].

The WHO started working on the ICD-11 in 2007 with the involvement of experts from over 90 countries. The ICD-11 was adopted in May 2019 (27 years after the ICD-10) by the World Health Assembly, to be effective for use from January 2022.

The ICD is used widely and diversely all over the world. The use of data coded according to the ICD supports a majority of what is understood about the scope, causes, and effects of human disease globally.

Since the inception of the ICD-10, medicine has developed significantly, and our understanding of many diseases has also evolved significantly. The adjustments required to consider these developments were beyond what could be accomplished by merely revising the tenth edition. The advent of the digital age, as an extrinsic element today, influences practically all aspects of life and is another justification for conducting a significant overhaul of the ICD [40].

Inadequacies of the ICD-10 were addressed in the 11th revision, which was approved by the 72nd World Health Assembly in May 2019 after much debate and consultation. The overall changes are significant; the ICD-11 is not just the ICD-10 with a few extra categories. The ICD-11, on the other hand, is a distinct and more potent health information system built on formal ontology, intended for use in contemporary IT infrastructure, and flexible enough to be altered in the future and used with other classifications and terminologies.

7.6.1 ICD-11 Design

The key distinction between the ICD-11 and previous editions is its adaptability to the digital age based on a computable knowledge framework. Although the ICD-11 can be utilized in paper-based systems, the framework's features and capabilities are expected to make electronic use appealing to the majority of users.

7.6.2 Framework of the ICD-11 [40]

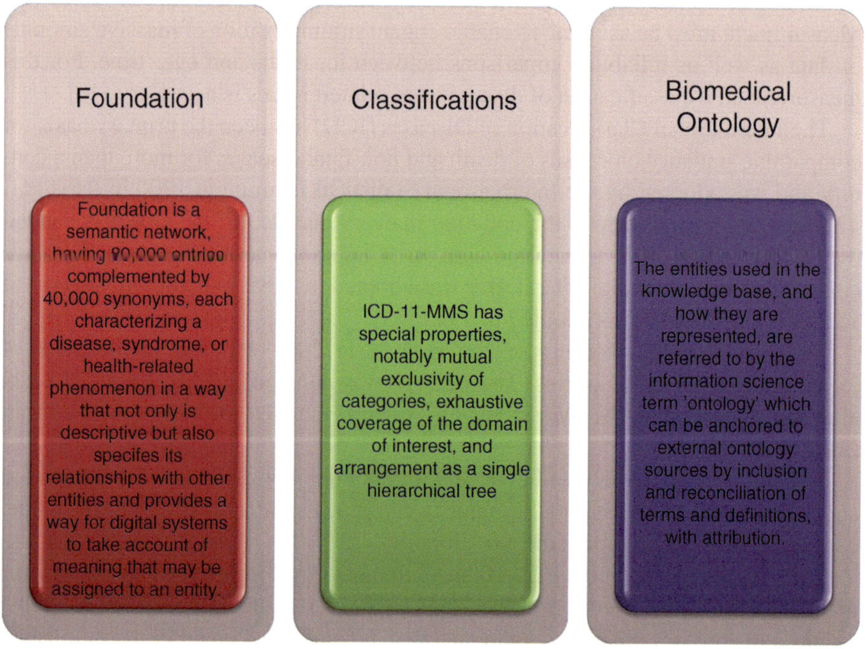

ICD-11 had 28 chapters, 6 more than ICD-10. ICD-10 has around 10,607 codes and ICD-11 has 14,662 codes.Three new chapters, among the first 25 chapters, are [40]:

Chapter 4 Diseases of the immune system

Chapter 7 Sleep-wake disorders

Chapter 17 Conditions related to sexual health

The other 22 chapters are almost similar to the chapters of the ICD-10 [40].

ICD-10 chapter		Corresponding ICD-11 chapter
I	Certain infectious and parasitic diseases	1
II	Neoplasms	2
III	Diseases of the blood and blood-forming organs and certain disorders involving the immune mechanism	3 and 4
IV	Endocrine, nutritional, and metabolic diseases	5
V	Mental and behavioral disorders	6
VI	Diseases of the nervous system	8
VII	Diseases of the eye and adnexa	9
VIII	Diseases of the ear and mastoid process	10
IX	Diseases of the circulatory system	11
X	Diseases of the respiratory system	12
XI	Diseases of the digestive system	13
XII	Diseases of the skin and subcutaneous tissue	14
XIII	Diseases of the musculoskeletal system and connective tissue	15
XIV	Diseases of the genitourinary system	16
XV	Pregnancy, childbirth, and the puerperium	18
XVI	Certain conditions originating in the perinatal period	19
XVII	Congenital malformations, deformities, and chromosomal abnormalities	20
XVIII	Symptoms, signs, and abnormal clinical and laboratory findings, not elsewhere classified	21
XIX	Injury, poisoning, and certain other consequences of external causes	22
XX	External causes of morbidity and mortality	23
XXI	Factors influencing health status and contact with health services	24
XXII	Codes for special purposes	25

New chapters and sections in the ICD-11-MMS [40]

Title	Reason for addition
Chapter 3: Diseases of the blood or blood-forming organs	These two chapters were split from a single chapter in the ICD-10, recognizing differences in aetiology, manifestations, and care
Chapter 4: Diseases of the immune system	
Chapter 7: Sleep-wake disorders	This topic has become more prominent since the tenth revision. The chapter mostly includes new concepts with some concepts moved from other chapters in the ICD-10
Chapter 17: Conditions related to sexual health	This topic has become more prominent since the tenth revision. The chapter mostly includes concepts moved from other chapters in the ICD-10, combined with some new concepts
Chapter 26: Traditional medicine conditions	This entirely new supplementary chapter in the ICD-11 enables coding in terms of traditional medicine concepts, where required
Extension codes section	Codes in this section can be combined with a stem code to provide additional information
Functioning section	Some national modifications of the ICD-10 added sections to allow patient functioning to be recorded. The ICD-11 provides a supplementary section for functioning assessment, aligned with the WHO International Classification of Functioning

7.6.3 Coding Tool as an Index

The ICD-10 and older editions advise using the index book to locate the correct code for diseases. The ICD-11 offers users a new method for locating and choosing categories. The WHO developed a Web-based coding tool that takes advantage of partial word matching, word-order independence, synonym management, hierarchy traversal, and other digital capabilities. The tool can return the completed cluster when a search word corresponds to a cluster rather than a single stem code [43, 44].

Benefits of ICD-11 [40]

Global Reach, Accessibility, and Standardization

The ICD-10 is utilized extensively in several nations, but not at all in certain others. The ICD-11-MMS's digital and Web-based design will remove several obstacles to the ICD's more widespread implementation. It will be simple for someone with online access to have virtually equal access to the same version of the ICD-11-MMS, thanks to the improved language support, the coding tool, the API on which it is built, and the expected apps that will tap the potential of the API.

Health Metrics

ICD-coded data have served as the foundation for both international and national statistics on cause-specific death for many years. More recently, assessments of the global and local burden of disease and injury have relied heavily on mortality data as well as ICD-coded morbidity data.

The ICD-11-MMS has been created to offer statistical continuity for main causes as well as numerous specific causes, and these measures frequently deal with rather broad types of causes (e.g. tuberculosis, suicide).

Integrated Support for Hospital Case Data

Patient records that have been admitted to the hospital as well as several other kinds of healthcare data have long been coded using the ICD. Many users felt that the WHO-published version of the ICD-10 lacked enough specificity for clinical applications as well as for a related goal of enabling activity-based billing and payment systems. To achieve these goals, a few WHO member nations created "clinical modifications" of the ICD. While there are some similarities across the various clinical modifications, there are also many differences that make them an inadequate basis for cross-national comparisons.

Capability to Operate Within Health Information Systems

The ICD-11-MMS is a "native citizen" of the age of networked, cooperative health information systems, thanks to its digital foundation. For administrative or research purposes, it is becoming more common to merge data from several sources, which increases the value of already existing data. When the combined sources contain information on mortality and morbidity, for instance, classification of the data in both sources in accordance with the ICD-11-MMS will assist analysis and interpretation.

ICD-11-MMS Support for Activity-Based Funding Systems

Codified diagnosis data are utilized in activity-based systems, which are frequently used to manage and distribute payments for hospital care. It is reasonable to anticipate that the ICD-11-MMS will serve as a solid foundation for activity-based systems given the parallels between the ICD-10 and ICD-11-MMS and the new revision's enormous expressive potential.

Quantitative Derived Measures

Case mix cost weights are well-known quantitative measurements that are primarily obtained from ICD-coded data. Other ICD-based quantitative measures have come into existence, such as those that assess the likelihood of surviving to discharge and the occurrence of post-injury persistent disability. It is anticipated that the ICD-11-MMS's significant expressive capability, particularly with regard to features of case severity, will facilitate more effective quantitative measures across a larger range of issues.

Governance, maintenance, and updates: It is believed that getting the ICD-11-MMS ready for use in various contexts will highlight omissions and other areas that could use improvement that was not seen during pre-release testing. Naturally, as long as the ICD-11-MMS is in use, new information regarding diseases will also call for modifications. ICD-11 updates will be made in an open and transparent manner. This updating approach, along with the adaptable ICD-11 framework, may prevent the need for another significant modification for a while.

Since the introduction of the ICD-10, information systems have evolved more than they did in the preceding century. Health information has not yet fully adapted to the era of globally networked and nearly real-time data systems, which have altered many other parts of life. The ICD-11 has been created to make that shift possible right now, from its foundation, information framework, and API to a range of tools for users.

The ICD-11 can be accessed at icd.who.int.

7.7 Conclusion

One of the health information systems that have seen extensive use is the hospital information system (HIS). The quality of these systems is a source of concern. Therefore, it is essential to regularly assess HISs. The implementation of HIS also needs a significant financial commitment. To meet administrative needs and enhance healthcare efficacy and efficiency at a reasonable cost, hospitals have established health information systems that deliver timely and accurate information. The primary requirements for hospital information systems are accurate data storage, dependable utilization, quick access to data, secure data storage, and decreased usage costs. According to Damen [45], the goal of the hospital information system is to elevate "managing" to a level of system insight, system knowledge, and system problem resolution from one of fragmentary patchy information, intuitive guesswork, and isolated problem-solving. The information system in an organization must be user friendly, and regular training of the employed system will help the employees to use the available software and help in delivering quality care to the patients.

References

1. Ismail NI , Abdullah NH, Shamsudin A, and Ariffin NAN, Implementation Differences of Hospital Information System (HIS) in Malaysian Public Hospitals., International Journal of Social Science and Humanity, Vol. 3, No. 2, March 2013,115
2. Clifford, G.D. Shortliffe Edward H, Cimino James J "Biomedical Informatics; Computer Applications in Health Care and Biomedicine". BioMed Eng OnLine **5**, 61 (2006). https://doi.org/10.1186/1475-925X-5-61
3. https://www.dictionary.com/browse/information
4. Davis/Olson: Management Information System, 1985, http://www.perflensburg.se/Privatsida/cp-web/INFODAOL.HTM
5. https://www.esraa.edu.iq/modules/lect/lect/98590123852570080.pdf
6. Hossein Ahmadi, Mehrbakhsh Nilashi, Alireza Almaee, Mohammad Soltani, et al, Multi-level Model for the Adoption of Hospital Information System: A Case on Malaysia, JOURNAL OF SOFT COMPUTING AND DECISION SUPPORT SYSTEMS, Vol 3 No 1 (2016)
7. Mehdi Babaei, Jafar Beikzad, Management information system, challenges and solutions, European Online Journal of Natural and Social Sciences 2013; vol.2, No. 3(s), pp. 374-381, ISSN 1805-3602
8. Morris F. Collen, Randolph A. Miller, The Early History of Hospital Information Systems for Inpatient Care in the United States, The History of Medical Informatics in the United States, January 2015, https://doi.org/10.1007/978-1-4471-6732-7_6
9. https://medicalequipment.moreptt.com/info/129436
10. News Letter, European Union of General Practitioners, Objectives for Health Care Information Systems and Electronic Health Records in Primary Care,11/03/2004
11. James A O'Brein, George M Marakas, Ramesh Behl, Management Information Systems, Ninth Edition, Chapter 1, Section II, pg 31, Tata McGraw Hill Education Private Limited, New Delhi
12. Shaw C (2003). How can hospital performance be measured and monitored? Copenhagen, WHO Regional Office for Europe (Health Evidence Network report.
13. https://www.iapb.org/news/effective-utilization-of-hospital-management-information-system-hmis/
14. Ashmita Gupta, Ashutosh Niranajan, Hospital Management and Control System, European Journal of Molecular & Clinical Medicine, Volume 07, Issue 06, 2020, pg1079–1085, ISSN 2515-8260
15. Osheroff, J. et al. Improving Outcomes with Clinical Decision Support: An Implementer's Guide. (HIMSS Publishing, 2012).
16. Sutton, R.T., Pincock, D., Baumgart, D.C. *et al.* An overview of clinical decision support systems: benefits, risks, and strategies for success. *npj Digit Med.* **3,** 17 (2020). https://doi.org/10.1038/s41746-020-0221-y
17. Vonbach, P., Dubied, A., Krähenbühl, S. & Beer, J. H. Prevalence of drug-drug interactions at hospital entry and during hospital stay of patients in internal medicine. Eur. J. Intern. Med. 19, 413–420 (2008).
18. Koutkias, V. & Bouaud, J. Contributions from the 2017 Literature on Clinical Decision Support. Yearb. Med. Inf. 27, 122–128 (2018).
19. Cornu, P., Phansalkar, S., Seger, D. L., Cho, I. & Pontefract, S. International Journal of Medical Informatics High-priority and low-priority drug–drug interactions in different international electronic health record systems: a comparative study. Int. J. Med. Inf. 111, 165–171 (2018).
20. D. J. Power, A Brief History of Decision Support Systems, Editor, DSSResources.COM, https://dssresources.com/history/dsshistory.html
21. Dan Power, Types of decision support systems (DSS), https://www.gdrc.org/decision/dss-types.html
22. Berner, E. S. (Ed.). Clinical Decision Support Systems (Springer, New York, NY, 2007).

23. Osheroff, J., Pifer, E., Teigh, J., Sittig, D. & Jenders, R. Improving Outcomes with Clinical Decision Support: An Implementer's Guide. (HIMS, 2005).
24. Iacopo Cricelli, Genomedics Srl, Ettore Maconi, Health Search, Italian College of General Practitioners and Primary Care and Francesco Lapi, Clinical Decision Support System (CDSS) in primary care: from pragmatic use to the best approach to assess their benefit/risk profile in clinical practice, March 2022, Current Medical Research and Opinion 38(5):1-8, https://doi.org/10.1080/03007995.2022.2052513
25. Jia, P., Zhang, L., Chen, J., Zhao, P. & Zhang, M. The effects of clinical decision support systems on medication safety: an overview. PLoS ONE 11, 1–17 (2016).
26. Davis, D. A. & Taylor-Vaisey, A. Translating guidelines into practice: a systematic review of theoretic concepts, practical experience and research evidence in the adoption of clinical practice guidelines. Can. Med. Assoc. J. 157, 408–416 (1997).
27. Salem, H. et al. A multicentre integration of a computer led follow up in surgical oncology is valid and safe. BJU Int. https://doi.org/10.1111/bju.14157 (2018).
28. McMullin, S. T. et al. Impact of an evidence-based computerized decision support system on primary care prescription costs. Ann. Fam. Med. 2, 494–498 (2004).
29. Bell, C. M., Jalali, A. & Mensah, E. A decision support tool for using an ICD-10 anatomographer to address admission coding inaccuracies: a commentary. Online J. Public Health Inform. 5, 222 (2013).
30. Haberman, S. et al. Effect of clinical-decision support on documentation compliance in an electronic medical record. Obstet. Gynecol. 114, 311–317 (2009).
31. Berner, E. S. Diagnostic decision support systems: why aren't they used more and what can we do about it? AMIA Annu. Symp. Proc. 2006, 1167–1168 (2006).
32. Kunhimangalam, R., Ovallath, S. & Joseph, P. K. A clinical decision support system with an integrated EMR for diagnosis of peripheral neuropathy. J. Med. Syst. 38, 38 (2014).
33. Martinez-Franco, A. I. et al. Diagnostic accuracy in Family Medicine residents using a clinical decision support system (DXplain): a randomized-controlled trial. Diagn. Berl. Ger. 5, 71–76 (2018).
34. From Invisible to Visible: IBM Demos AI to Radiologists. https://www-03.ibm.com/press/us/en/pressrelease/51146.ws. Accessed Aug 2019 (2016).
35. Rosenbloom, S. T. et al. Triaging patients at risk of influenza using a patient portal. J. Am. Med. Inf. Assoc. 19, 549–554 (2012).
36. Dowding, D. et al. Nurses' use of computerised clinical decision support systems: A case site analysis. J. Clin. Nurs. 18, 1159–1167 (2009).
37. EHRIntelligence. 5 Ways States Mandate Health Information Exchange. https://ehrintelligence.com/news/5-ways-states-mandate-health-information-exchange. Accessed Aug 2019 (2015).
38. Ash, J. S., Sittig, D. F., Campbell, E. M., Guappone, K. P. & Dykstra, R. H. Some unintended consequences of clinical decision support systems. AMIA Annu Symp. Proc. AMIA Symp. AMIA Symp. 2007, 26–30 (2007).
39. Kilsdonk, E., Peute, L. W., Riezebos, R. J., Kremer, L. C. & Jaspers, M. W. M. Uncovering healthcare practitioners' information processing using the think-aloud method: From paper-based guideline to clinical decision support system. *Int. J. Med. Inf.* 86, 10–19 (2016).
40. Harrison, J.E., Weber, S., Jakob, R. *et al.* ICD-11: an international classification of diseases for the twenty-first century. *BMC Med Inform Decis Mak* **21,** 206 (2021). https://doi.org/10.1186/s12911-021-01534-6
41. Wood PH. Applications of the international classification of diseases. World Health Stat Q. 1990;43:263–8.
42. World Health Organization. World health statistics. 2020. http://www.who.int/gho/publications/world_health_statistics/en. Accessed 12 April 2022
43. World Health Organization. International Statistical Classification of Diseases and Related Health Problems—10th revision: Volume 2—instruction manual (2nd ed.). Geneva: World Health Organization; 2004.

44. World Health Organization. ICD-11 coding tool. https://icd.who.int/ct11/icd11_mms/en/release. Accessed 12 April 2022
45. Damen W, Kilsdonk A, Vander WA. Information Networks, Hospital Management, Sterling Publications Ltd., Netherlands, 1991; 568.

Chapter 8
An Intensive Care Unit Design of the Future

Anil Kumar Chillimuntha, Kashipa Harit, and Sushman Sharma

In the era of pandemics, ICU is the most critical department in a hospital. It is a specialized and self-contained place where critically ill patients, whose life hangs in the balance of life and death, are lodged and cared for. It is a highly specialized and sophisticated area furnished, equipped, and manned by unique skilled expert personnel who handle very complex machinery. Based on the capability of an ICU to handle the varied medical complexities and the level of clinical expertise, ICUs are segregated into different levels of care such as level 1, level 2, and level 3. Consideration of standards and specifications in each level varies, so while designing the ICU, care needs to be taken for accommodating future upgrade of lower levels.

An intensive care unit is a separate self-contained area within the hospital equipped with highly specialized facilities designed for bedside close monitoring and rapid intervention of staff. Intensive care unit represents the highest level of care, which is a multidisciplinary and inter-professional specialty, treating patients with potential recovery from life-threatening diseases. The patients in ICU either have developed an organ failure or are at a risk of developing one. The capacity to temporarily support or if need be replace the function of these organs such as lungs, kidneys, and cardiovascular system is the critical care medicine domain. Since these critical patients are housed in a designated unit, the planning and designing go a long way in facilitating their recovery.

The planning and development should be futuristic and applicable to the working needs and demands. Designing with requisite standards and specifications to create optimal size cubicles that house the patient bed which is surrounded 360° by complex equipment, personnel, and hand hygiene stations is to be planned appropriately. Providing the right electrical, civil, and engineering controls is of paramount

A. K. Chillimuntha · K. Harit
METAS Adventist Group of Hospitals, Surat, Gujarat, India

S. Sharma (✉)
Department of Hospital Management, H.N.G. University, Patan, Gujarat, India

D. Bhatia et al. (eds.), *A Guide to Hospital Administration and Planning*,
https://doi.org/10.1007/978-981-19-6692-7_8

importance. Integrating information technology into the planning of medical records will enable proper monitoring in ICU and at home. Designing a robust critical care system capable of interfacing, collating, and analyzing information and providing connectivity envelope with the patients, relatives, staff, and doctors is a real need.

A good ICU operates on standard operating procedures and policies having complex quality controls and infection control protocols and facilitates training and research. Therefore, planning and designing an ICU with optimal space design, environment-friendly patient flows, and easy staff maneuverability are very intricate and crucial for a futuristic ICU. Before designing an ICU, it is important to understand the departmental relationships for critical care units as shown in the figure below:

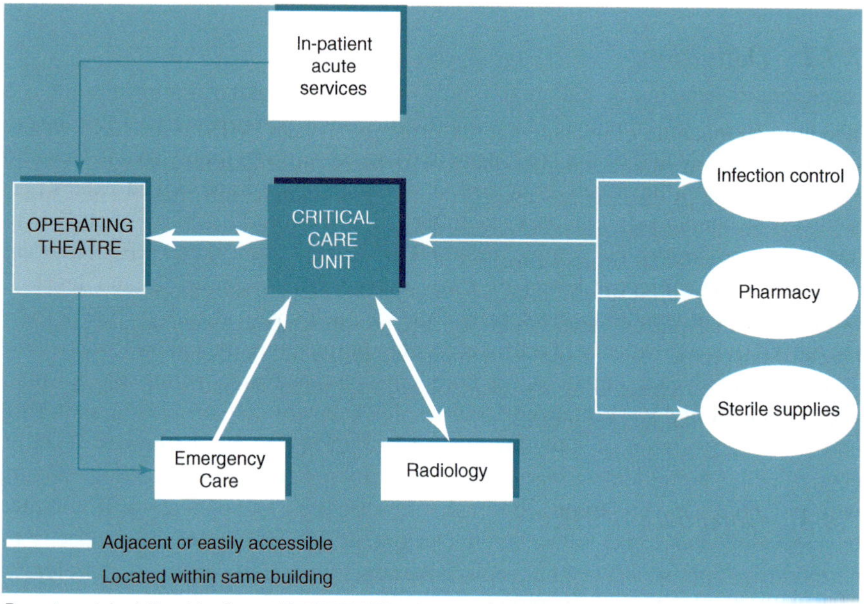

Departmental relationships for a critical care unit

The key result outcome of a well-designed ICU lowers morbidity and mortality; facilitates a lesser length of stay; minimizes the cost of care delivery; and results in higher revenue per bed and a high happy quotient for all stakeholders.

A well-designed ICU with structures and processes will provide a good work environment. It should support the care processes and relationships within the unit. This results in job satisfaction and motivation of staff, thereby providing high-quality care for patients. A conducive work environment is brought through appropriate ICU planning and design, which is directly proportional to the satisfaction and productivity levels of staff. Therefore, establishing a well-planned modern ICU is imperative in today's modern-day healthcare scenarios.

8.1 History of Critical Care

The concept of ICU has started with the Copenhagen polio epidemic in 1952. Many patients that time were experiencing respiratory paralysis and bulbar palsy. The mortality rate was historic 85–90%. More than 300 patients needed artificial support or ventilation for many weeks. To facilitate manual hand ventilation of lungs through tracheostomies, more than 1000 medical and dental students were used. In the year 1953, after a year into the polio epidemic, Bjørn Ibsen, an anesthetist from Copenhagen working in Blegdam Hospital, suggested that the treatment of choice is positive-pressure ventilation for the polio epidemic-struck patients. He devised the first ICU in Europe in December 1953 by gathering physicians and physiologists to manage these patients. Thus, the specialty of intensive care was born. After this intervention, the mortality dropped from 80 to 40%. Many today consider him to be the father of intensive care. Dr. Henning Sund Kristensen took over as the in-charge of this unit. Adjusting ventilation parameters as per blood gas analysis (pH, pCO_2, pO_2) electrodes which are invented by Astrup, Siggaard-Andersen, and Severinghaus. The pH monitoring technology was invented by the Danish Carlsberg brewing company, which greatly helped Dr. Henning and his team in the ICU. Max Harry Weil is widely known as the father of modern intensive care since he established in 1960 a four-bed "shock ward" in Los Angeles County, University of Southern California Medical Center, USA. The first microprocessor-controlled ventilator was invented in the year 1971. With the development of many new equipment and drugs, the rapid growth got stimulated for intensive care medicine. Intensive care units got a huge metamorphosis since its inception 68 years ago. Many emerging trends are bound to be seen in the coming years creating an ICU of the future.

8.2 Planning and Development Team

To develop an ICU, we need to meet the aspirations and demands of patients and staff using it. Therefore, a multidisciplinary approach in planning and developing an ICU is needed. A team should be formed to do this. Usually, an intensivist or an administrator heads the team. The team members are intensivist, administrator, senior experienced nurse, respiratory therapist, chief finance officer, and architects and engineers. The team coordination is vital. The team should determine the budget needed, location of ICU, level of care in ICU, number of ICU beds, engineering and safety, design for infection prevention, central nurse station and utilities, manpower needs, case mix of ICU, etc. If there is a renovation of the existing ICU, then temporary relocation should be planned.

8.2.1 Types of ICU

Intensive care units can be classified as per the pathologies or conditions treated. It can be medical intensive care unit, surgical intensive care unit, cardiac intensive care unit, neurological intensive care unit, transplant ICU, trauma care unit, burns intensive care unit, etc. It can also be grouped as per age criteria such as geriatric ICU, adult intensive care unit, pediatric ICU, and neonatal intensive care unit.

The department of health in the UK produced a document in 2001 called "Comprehensive Critical Care" in which the levels of care are summarized. Level one is ward-based care where the patient does not need organ support. For example, the patient might need IV and oxygen support through face mask or nasal prongs. In level two, there is a high dependency unit where single-organ support is required and ventilator not warranted, e.g., renal dialysis or invasive BP monitoring or inotropic support. Mostly, the nurse:patient ratio here is 1:2. In level three, care is intensive where a patient will need support for two or more organs and need mechanical ventilation. The nurse:patient ratio here is 1:1 with a duty doctor with RMO or intensivist or a registrar round the clock. The Indian Society of Critical Care Medicine (ISCCM) has used different levels such as Level I, Level II, Level IIIA, Level IIIB, and Level IIIC.

In India, there are usually four zones for an ICU such as patient care zone, observation area, support area, and lastly family support area. In patient care area, it includes all the area which is around the patient's bed. The observation area constitutes the central nursing station which is the nerve center of the ICU. Doctors' station and nursing stations are kept there. Usually, chairs with computers are placed here and quick investigations such as electrolytes with ABG and other investigations are performed. There are drug trolleys with crash carts too. Other support services are usually accommodated here. The support area usually includes doctor's duty room, counselling room, ICU office, discussion and teaching rooms, change rooms, stores, and toilets. The family support area constitutes the waiting area where they have access to relax and get water, food and beverages, and refreshments. Separate toilets with bath facility and sleepover couches with storage facility will make the life of family members comfortable. A prayer room is usually kept here. A social worker counselling room is good to have here.

8.2.2 Location of ICU

An ICU should be a safe place with easy accessibility and transport of patients. It should be well connected with spacious corridors, ramps, and large bed lifts. A critically ill patient should be wheeled in and out of ICU freely and safely. The ICU should be in close proximity to emergency, operation theatres, HDU, trauma wards, and diagnostic facility with pharmacy. First floor is the most ideal location, but if lifts are present, then any top floor will be ideal. There has to be a single entry and exit with provision made for emergency exit points too. The ICU should have access to pneumatic tube system used to transport the samples, medicines, laundry, etc.

One of the main aspects of planning an ICU is to make sure that there is a cohesive movement of staff, patients, and visitors. Ensure that there is adequate space for equipment and medicine storage cupboards with crash carts and double-lock narcotic cupboards. Location of nurse station with hand-wash facility and medicine preparation area with clean and dirty utility rooms requiring adequate space arrangements will go a long way in workflow management. One of the ICU designs is a dormitory like ICU where all patients are in one single area. The second type is a single accommodation cubicle or room where a patient is lodged alone. The third type is a partition between two rooms or beds. The final one is the isolation-type design with positive and negative pressure.

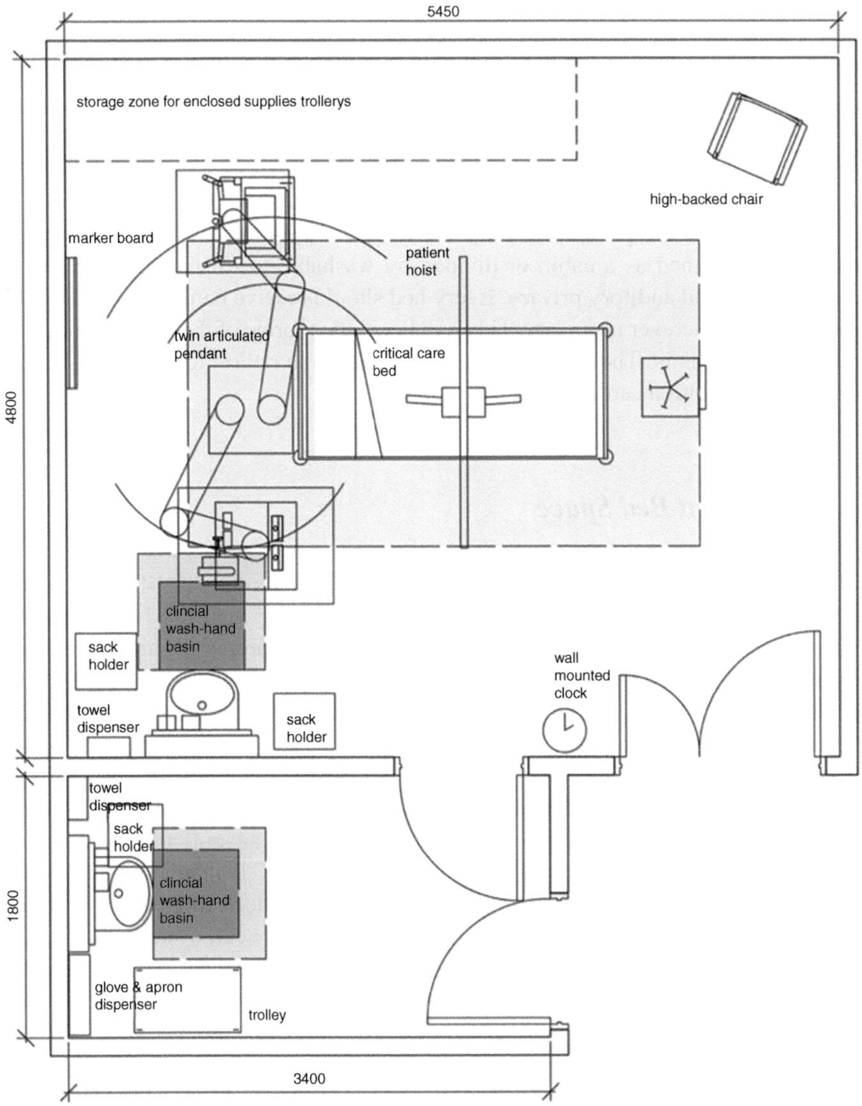

Critical care isolation room and lobby

While deciding the number of ICUs and number of ICU beds, a hospital should have it determined by a good brainstorming on space requirements and availability, trained manpower, budget, and need analysis. Usually, a tertiary hospital requirement of ICU beds is around 5–25% of total beds.

8.2.3 Bed Space

The bed space is a very critical parameter while designing an ICU. As per international standards, we need to have 25.5 m^2 for each bed to accommodate the patient bed and all accessories. The space per bed has been a contentious issue for planning an ICU. In the Indian context, it is recommended to have 150–200 sq. ft and even higher recommendation of 250–300 sq. ft per bed. The staff should be able to access the patient from all sides. The space should be such that the staff can handle all equipment and accessories safely. There has to be a space for minimum five persons around the patient, especially during an emergency code blue situation. Each bed should be designed as a cabin or divided by washable medical grade curtains to ensure visual and auditory privacy. Every bed should receive natural light and good outside view wherever necessary. This will boost the morale of the staff and positive outcome of patients. The ICU lighting should have the option to dim them so that surgical interventions are possible.

8.2.4 Patient Bed Space

The patient bed space should have an electric bed, which has chair and Trendelenburg positioning preferably with remote. A pressure-relieving mattress is essential. A UPS-powered ceiling-mounted pendant with two arms is preferable and can be easily used by staff of different stature. To accommodate the use of pendants and hoists, a minimum ceiling height of 3 m is mandated. The ceiling should have weight-bearing capacity. The pendants should be capable to accommodate medical gases, suction, data, and electrical wiring with UPS to house the equipment. The UPS and IPS points need to be color coded. The pendants need to have a minimum 3–4 oxygen outlets, 2 air outlets with 4 bar pressure, one 7 bar air outlet to use surgical instruments, and 2–4 medical vacuum for suction outlets. If inhalation antibiotics are administered, then anesthetic gas scavenging points need to be enabled in the pendants. There needs to be a patient and staff emergency call systems with crash call system. Telephone outlets and TV connection outlet need to be kept. Data points to house the IP camera need to be in place. The equipment placed on pendants are computer with flat screen, patient monitor, 3–6 infusion pumps, 4–10 syringe pumps, feeding pump, blood warmer, ventilation, and humidifier equipment. Positioning of the pendants is important to provide proper access to staff. To achieve infection control at each bedside, a washbasin to facilitate hand-washing is a must.

A ceiling-mounted hoist is needed to lift the patient. Patient bedside locker or storage cabinets are needed to store drugs and consumables. Some personal items such as family pictures or God's pictures are kept at patient bedside to provide emotional support.

An ICU should create and adopt a minimum sound environment to facilitate faster healing of the patient. When we have a normal conversation in an ICU, it produces 55 dB of sound, and while using a vacuum cleaner, it produces 70 dB. International sound council recommends sound levels during daytime and evening hours to be not more than 40–45 dB and in the night not more than 20 dB. This has proved to be a significant contributor towards the recovery of the patient.

8.2.5 *Heating, Ventilation, and Air-Conditioning (HVAC)*

There are different technologies used to control temperature, humidity, and purity of air in the ICU. Usually, if air changers are there, then we need to have six air changes per hour per room. If cubicles are there, 15 air changes per hour are advisable. Facilities for temperature and humidity regulation need to be facilitated. Neonate and pediatric patients need to be placed where higher temperature is facilitated. The high heat gains from medical equipment need to be factored to ensure that sufficient cooling is available and adjustable in patient areas. All the air is filtered 99% till the least size of 5 μm. The passages of ICU patient rooms and isolation rooms should also be adequately ventilated.

In negative-pressure isolation rooms, they have a higher level of exhaust than fresh air supply. A pressure difference of 2.5 pascals is advisable. A clean to dirty airflow is designed. The exhaust air is reused provided that there is a HEPA filter available.

8.2.6 *ICU Power Supply*

The ICU power supply should be planned very meticulously. In a well-designed ICU, the main electrical circuit breaker should branch out to all the individual ICU feeder lines in the hospital. There has to be a generator power backup with stabilizer and uninterrupted power supply (UPS) facility. The number and capacity plug points should be planned as per the number of envisaged equipment and their electrical rating. The light switches should be strategically located at appropriate places for staff comfort and convenience and patient control if needed. The lighting distribution board should be different from the power supply board.

An ICU should be designed to get more natural light through windows. This will elevate the staff morale, and patient recovery will be faster. Usually, while examining a patient, lighting should be a minimum 350 lux and during a procedure approx. 1000 lux. During night, while the patient is sleeping, just 5 lux is sufficient. Dull blue light in the night is known for contributing to good sleep and patient outcome. Maintaining the circadian rhythm will help in patient healing too. Providing blinds with blackout curtains will facilitate the patient to rest during daytime too. Emergency lights should be appropriately located with electrical connection for its battery recharge.

8.2.7 Bedside Equipment

The intensive care unit equipment are mostly aimed at life support and support of various organs in the body (e.g., lungs, heart, and kidneys). The equipment used in ICU vary from general simple instruments such as BP apparatus and glucometer to specialized equipment such as ventilators and bedside multiparameter monitors. These equipment are used to monitor and treat the illness of patients. Each patient has one or two nurses dedicated to him/her for constant monitoring and care.

There is a continuous or intermittent need for some of the bedside equipment which can be used on patients. Some of these equipment are defibrillators, invasive and noninvasive ventilators, ECMO machine, hemodialysis, peritoneal dialysis machine, hemofiltration machine, portable X-ray machine, electrocardiography (ECG) machine, echocardiography machine with sonography, electroencephalogram (EEG) machine, bronchoscopes and endoscopes, invasive cardiac output monitoring devices, and gamma cameras. Provision should be made for dialysis within the ICU. A wall-mounted renal dialysis unit needs to be kept with reverse osmosis (RO) water supply and drainage system. A digital clock is placed with elapsed time control visible at each bed.

8.2.8 ICU Beds

The ICU beds differ from the common ward beds in their design and functionality. As per the critical care unit planning and design notes of the Department of Health and Social Care Guidelines, U.K., an ICU bed should include "an electric bed capable of attaining chair and Trendelenburg positions, and fitted with a pressure-relieving mattress." Therefore, the bed preferably needs to be electric and connected with a UPS power supply. It can be operated with a handset or control panel that provides options to maneuver the bed positions. The cardiac chair and Trendelenburg positions facilitate for improving respiration and circulation of patient and help in the bodily functions. A pressure-relieving mattress with foam or air should have a pressure-redistributing ability, which enables to evenly disperse the weight of the patient on bed surface. It prevents bed sores on a chronic long-standing patient in the ICU.

8.2.9 Emerging Trends

Significant changes are happening in ICU design due to changes in medical informatics, equipment, and technology. Despite a need for patient-centered approach, technology still rules the decisions taken for the ICU design. That is the single most consideration brought about while considering and developing an ICU design model. Technology progress and greater versatility are possible. This accommodates the most important concerns of patients and designers of modern ICU. Merging all ICUs into one single area will be the trend of the future to save costs and give quality care through incorporation of proper planning and design of ICU. Same ICU bed is adjusted to the level of care needed. For example, Bellevue Hospital in New York City boasts of 55 ICU beds capable of flexing into any acuity levels of care. This helps the staff to be cross-trained to handle different levels of care where the medical team can transform into lesser or greater levels of care. This helps the patient's relatives deal with single team all through different levels of care. The staff will get to know the family and their needs. This resolves the most important feedback of non-familiarity with a myriad of medical and nursing staff at different levels of care.

With a glimpse into the potential future, the intensive care is transforming into a digital ICU. Today, many research projects in the lab are showing promising results for the future. The emergence of bioartificial organ transplants and organ regeneration is going to transform the way critical care is given in the future, which warrants strict isolation and stringent design. Some other interventions at the immunological, cellular, and genetic levels will need the use of sophisticated technologies, and ICU design parameters will change.

8.2.10 Decentralized Charting

The emergence of paper charting to electronic medical records has made the architects and designers of ICU to provide individualized configurations of ICUs. The focus on patient and family care has emerged from centralized nursing station to individualized decentralized nurse station, which is in close proximity to the patient. Electronic surveillance is supplemental but is not a substitute to a critical care staff. The centralized monitoring system is moving towards a patient-centered decentralized monitoring system to provide more patient safety. The medications, supplies, equipment, and documentation should be close to bedside to enable less travel within the ICU. The ability of physicians, nurses, intensivists, and other healthcare workers to visualize patients is of high priority. Therefore, the new ICU designs lay emphasis on patients' high visibility and flexibility.

With the support of telemedicine technology, artificial intelligence algorithms, and machine learning ability, the critical care staff can know the trends analyzed and predict patient status by minutes and hours. The proximity of documentation and caregiving enables the capacity of staff to predict and anticipate interventions.

The technology of the future will enable ICU at home to be a commonality and will use virtual reality and artificial intelligence. The future ICU will have two design approaches where there will be a physical space divided with transparent LCD glass for visibility and monitoring. Another design is to have a virtual space where you have multiple patients in one place with virtual walls of privacy. The ICU environment will have a programmed room control where there is automatic temperature control, light, sound, and air controls too. Automated surveillance systems flag the airborne microbes present in the devices, equipment, skin, and furniture, which activates targeted decontamination, sterilization, and purification systems. Large visual displays with diurnal and seasonal graphics and sounds with family or home pictures will be displayed all around the patient to make him/her feel homely. Holographic interactive displays of family can also be incorporated to make the patient believe that he/she is interacting and communicating to family members.

The bed will be like an environmentally controlled ICU biosphere capsule with biometric display using noninvasive sensing technology. Diagnostic, imaging, and therapeutic management will be done through mini robots, holographic nurse, and doctor all directed and instructed by an advanced informatics system. Patient communication and interaction will be through virtual reality visor display. The mattress and the exoskeletons will be reprinted with 3D computing and printing. There will be automated biomedical waste management where the waste is put into closed evacuation system and elimination chambers. Advanced cameras and holographic systems with a human touch capacity will be introduced to enable virtual visitation by relatives resulting in adherence to infection control protocols. The visor will bring pictures and sounds of home to make the patient oriented and not get into delirium. The patient beds will be linked to artificial intelligence (AI). Many critical care datasets, current research and experiences, and algorithms of care will be used. This provides deep learning and data analytics.

The patient needs to wear a customized suit, which has embedded sensors that will provide noninvasive monitoring for the external and the deep internal organs. Physiological imaging devices monitor the blood and organs at cellular, genetic, and plasma levels. 3D printers will provide individualized implants, devices, and stents. Manpower with highly trained nurses with complete knowledge of computers and informatics is needed for a hospital. Most of the doctors and specialists will do remote consultation, and they rely heavily on bedside techs, virtual reality, and mini robots. The biosphere capsule looks like the early 1950s' ventilator capsule called "iron lung" box. The irony is a return to the past to achieve the future.

8.3 Conclusion

As the debate over critical care unfolds, while designing a new ICU, we need to recognize the need for patient-centered, family-conscious approach that will care for the physiological, psychological, and spiritual needs. The future ICU promises to be a true place of healing and rejuvenation where all 360° dimensions are met and advanced technology will accommodate the subtle needs of patients, family, and staff.

Chapter 9
Transportation in Hospitals

Divya Rao, Averil Rebello, H. K. Mamatha, N. Shalini, and Arehally M. Mahalakshmi

Objectives

This unit on transportation fulfills the following objectives:
1. Need and development of patient transportation system
2. Enumerate the types of ambulances and their role in the care of patients
3. Ambulance design, staffing pattern, and essential equipment of an ambulance
4. Enumerate the types of intramural transport system for patients and materials within the hospital

9.1 Introduction

The process of transportation explains the ways and means by which men or material is transported from one place to another. Transportation is essential to access goods, services, and activities such as emergency services and healthcare. Patient transportation is the service of transporting patients to and from medical facilities in emergency and nonemergency situations. Hence, patient transportation not only encompasses ambulance but also a wide range of mechanical systems and transports in and outside the hospital used to lift and carry the patients. Ambulance, lift, escalator, trolley, stretcher, train, ambulance train, car, truck, rickshaw, bicycle, bullock

D. Rao (✉) · H. K. Mamatha · N. Shalini · A. M. Mahalakshmi
Department of Health System Management Studies, JSS Academy of Higher Education and Research, Mysuru, India
e-mail: divyaraobj.dhsms@jssuni.edu.in

A. Rebello
Department of Hospital Administration, Yenapoya Deemed to be University, Mangalore, India

D. Bhatia et al. (eds.), *A Guide to Hospital Administration and Planning*,
https://doi.org/10.1007/978-981-19-6692-7_9

cart, helicopter, aircraft, and animals like horses and mules are used for transportation of patients depending upon the location, type of patient, economic status, social strata, terrain, physical facilities, and degree of illness [1].

Hospitals have to pay attention to the planning and organization of the transportation service to and from the hospital as caring for the sick is the primary concern of a hospital.

In the current era, trauma is one of the main causes of emergency. In the event of an emergency, the patient is transported by emergency medical services to a facility that can provide a higher level of care or is more specialized. It can also be used to transfer patients from a specialty facility to a local hospital or nursing home when they no longer need this specialty care.

Medical transportation services allow patients to reach their destination rapidly and conveniently as all along the way, highly trained drivers, emergency medical technicians (EMTs), and paramedics provide reliable healthcare needed to ensure a safe arrival to the hospital and also ensure stress-free modern hospital logistics system.

Patient transport is the process of moving a patient to the medical facility which forms the extra mural form of transport, with ambulance playing a very vital role. In addition to this, the patient also moves from one area to another within the healthcare facility which forms the intramural form of transportation.

9.1.1 Types of Medical Transportation

- Nonemergency medical transportation
- Emergency medical transportation

The transportation system in the hospital can be divided basically into two types.

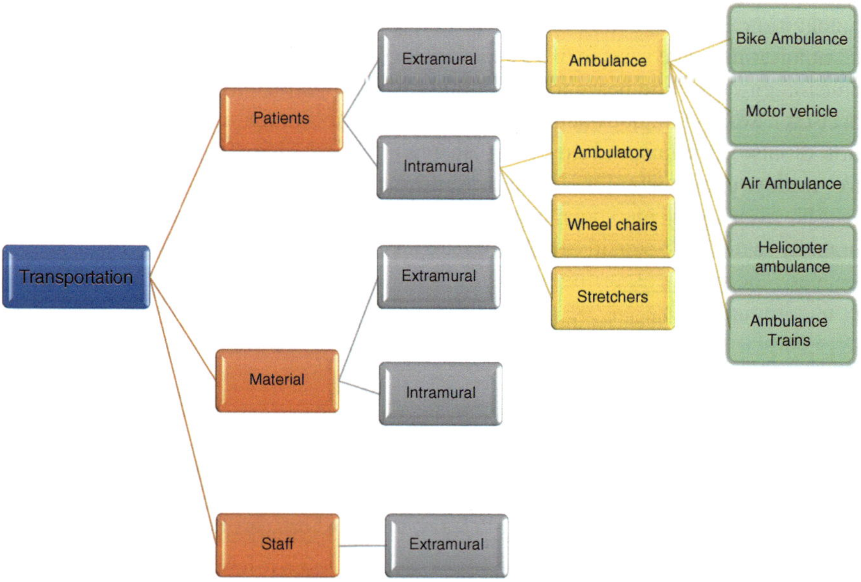

9.1.2 *Extramural Transport System*

The main form of extramural transport is the ambulance.

An ambulance is a medically equipped vehicle that transports patients to treatment facilities, such as a hospital [2]; usually, out-of-hospital medical care is provided to the patient.

"Ambulance is a specially equipped and ergonomically designed vehicle for transportation/emergency treatment of sick or injured people and capable of providing out of hospital medical care during transit/when stationary" (IGNOU Manual).

9.1.3 *Development of Ambulance Service*

Historical record has sparse documentation about transportation of patients. Animals like horses and carts were used to transport the injured to places to receive care.

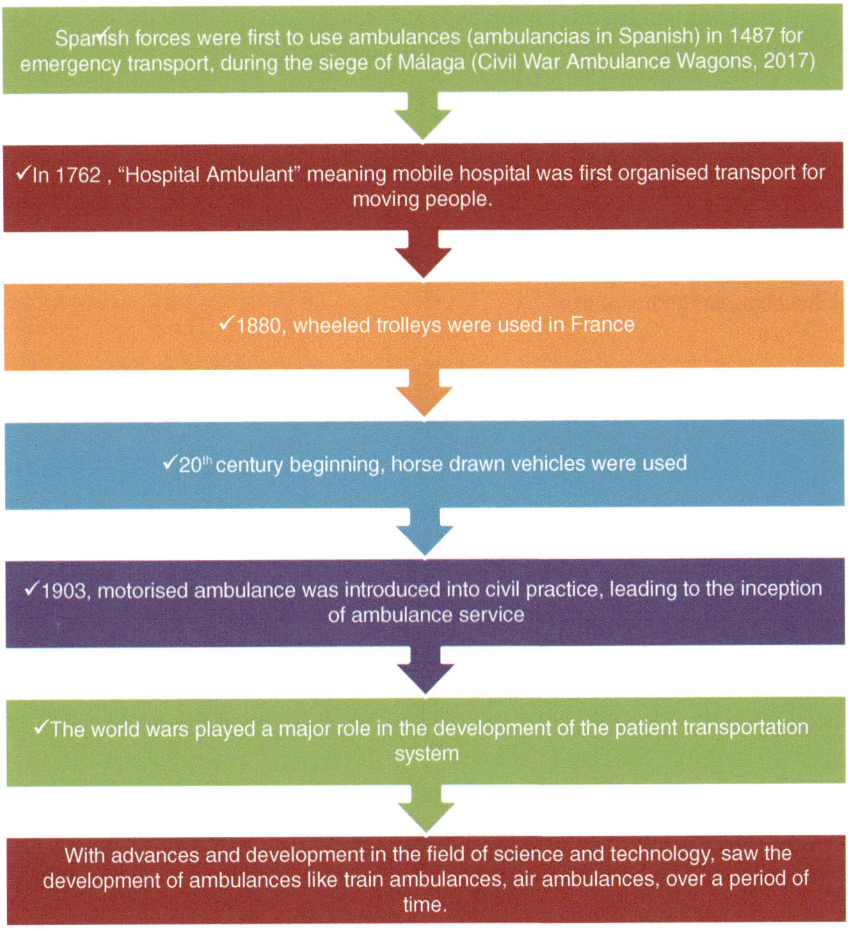

9.1.4 Definition of Ambulance

The term ambulance comes from the Latin word "ambulare," meaning "to walk or move about," which is a reference to early medical care where patients were moved by lifting or wheeling [3, 4]. The word originally meant a moving hospital, which follows an army in its movements [4] ["Essex Ambulance Response Cars," 2007].

Webster's dictionary defines ambulance as an "Organization for rendering first aid," leading to the use of it as a vehicle equipped for transporting those who are wounded, injured, or sick (Oxford dictionary).

Ambulance "is defined as a vehicle for emergency care, which provides a driver compartment and patient compartment, which can accommodate two emergency medical technicians and two lying patients, so positioned, that at least one patient call be given intensive life support during transit, which carries equipment and supplied for optimal emergency care at the scene as well as during transport, for two way radio communication, for safeguarding personnel and patients under hazardous conditions and for light rescue procedures and which is designed and constructed to afford maximum safety and comfort and to avoid aggravation of the patient's conditions, exposure to complication and threat to survival" [5].

9.1.5 Objective of Ambulance Services

The main objective of the ambulance service is to transport the sick and injured as quickly and comfortably as possible to the hospital so that they can receive prompt medical care at the hospital.

9.1.6 Types and Classification of Ambulances

Types of Ambulances

Ambulances were required for transporting not only accident and emergency trauma cases but also other emergencies like myocardial infarction, cerebral hemorrhage, foreign bodies, gunshot wounds, fractures, and associated injuries which require immediate treatment at the site by expert medical staff and a proper evacuation by trauma or critical care medicine trained staff of the ambulance, which forms a vital factor in saving the life of the patient [5] (IGNOU Manual).

Ambulances can be grouped into types depending on whether they transport patients and under what conditions [6].

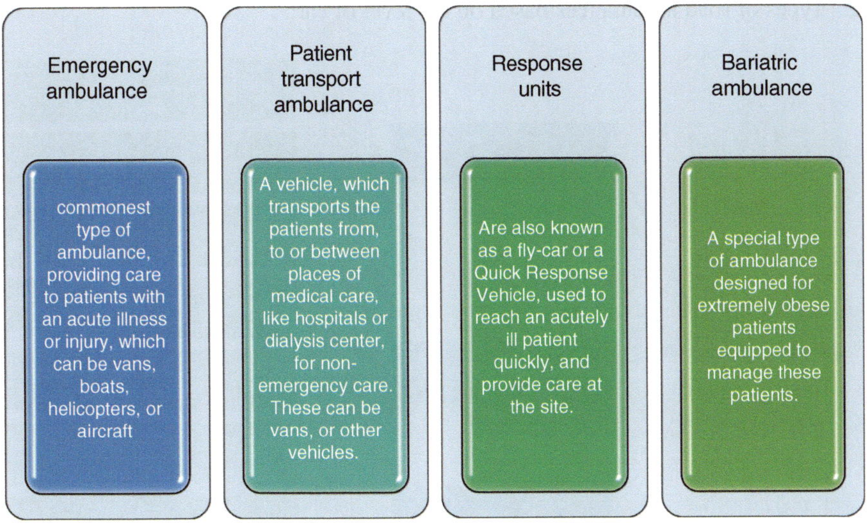

The classification of the ambulances is done on the basis of

1. Modes of ambulance
2. Level of care [7]
3. Structure [8]

1. Modes of ambulance

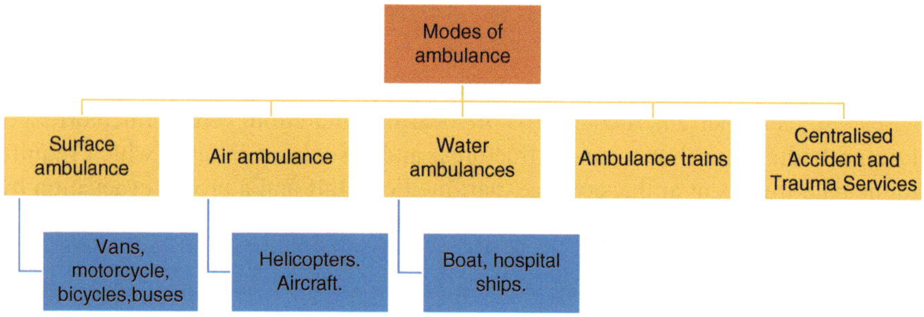

2. Types of road ambulances based on the level of care

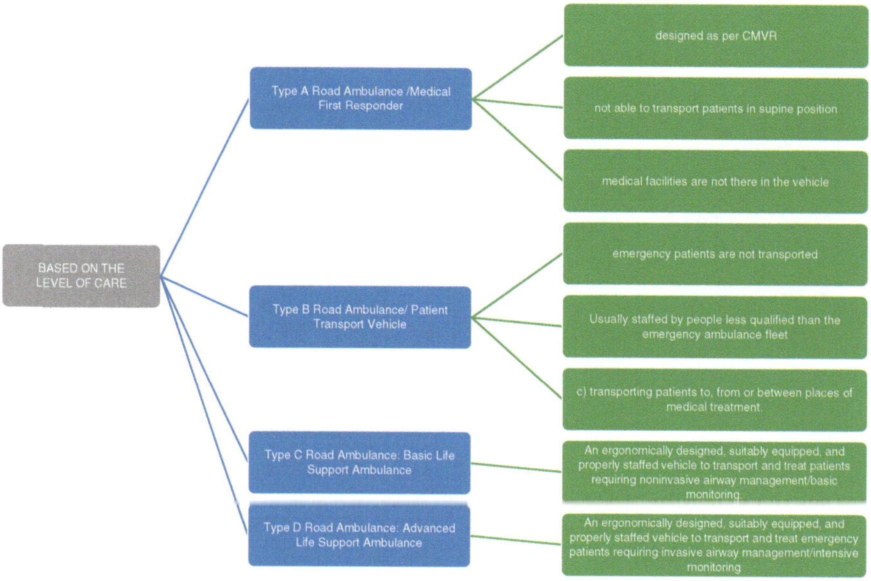

3. Based on structure

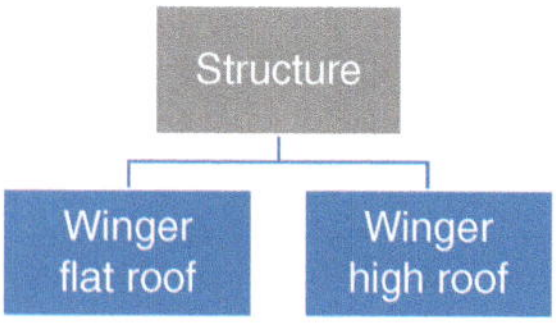

9.1.7 Role and Functions of Ambulance Service

The ambulance is part of the hospital's emergency medical service. Efficient, responsive, well-equipped ambulance service with a team of competent personnel is considered one of the essential elements of a well-organized emergency service. The survival of an injured patient after arrival at the hospital depends not only on the nature of the injuries, but also on the adequate first aid received and efficient transport from the scene of the accident.

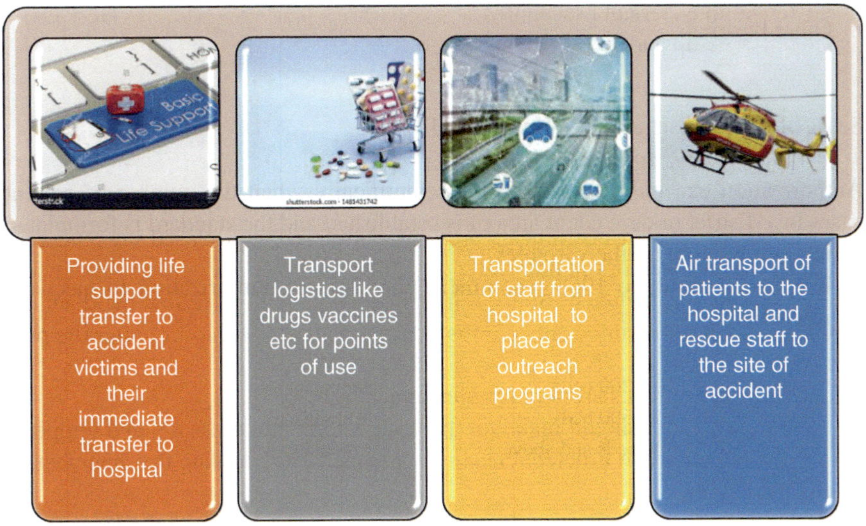

According to a World Bank report, India has only 1% of the world's vehicles, but 11% of the world's road traffic deaths occur in India. About 450,000 accidents happen in India every year, of which 150,000 people die [9] (World Bank Report).

"India has the highest number of casualties in road accidents," stated the report. "There are 53 road accidents in the country every hour and one death every 4 min." Indian roads generally witness 415 deaths/day due to accidents, the highest in the world, and 70% of these deaths are in the working age group of 18–45 years old [10] (Economic Times).

It was reported that in 2019, states and union territories (UTs) reported a total of 449,002 road accidents, killing 151,113 people and causing injury to 451,361 persons. 449,002 accidents and 151,113 deaths in 2019 translate into an average of 1230 accidents and 414 deaths every day and nearly 51 accidents and 17 deaths every hour [11] (Road Accidents in India 2019).

Mackay [10] emphasized in a research report that in 43.0% of motorcyclists and occupants who died, they could have a better chance of survival if they received immediate medical treatment at the accident scene within 10 min.

9.1.8 Utilization of Ambulances [12]

Ambulance service request can arise from different organizations, services, as well as individuals like:

- General practitioners
- Police control room
- In the hour of need by general public
- Nursing homes
- Polyclinics
- Other hospitals

Scale of Authorization of Ambulance [13]

Authorization can only be established scientifically when the number of patient cases in a district or dependent area of is established and the standard is formulated taking into account all the variables.

KN Rao Committee 1968 recommend the scale of authorization to meet the requirement at:

100–200 beds	3 Ambulances
200–300 beds	4 Ambulances
300 beds and above	6 Ambulances

Uses of Ambulance Services to Patients [14]

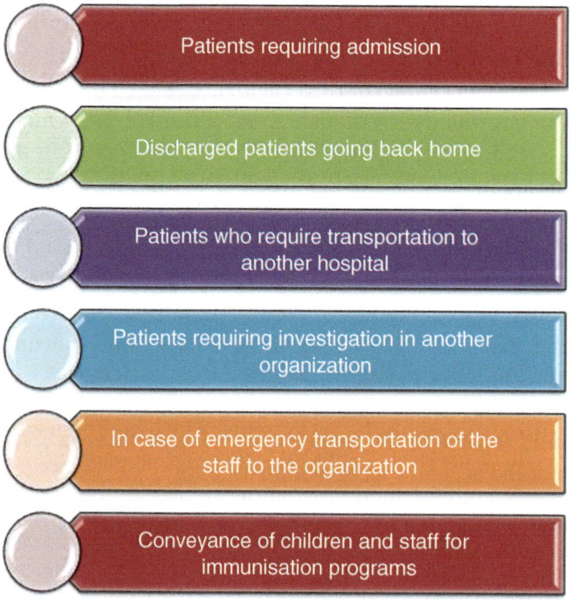

Priority for the Usage of Ambulance [1]

Ambulances, if used for other purposes than patient care and emergency, would lose patient time and lead to the wear and tear of the vehicle in the long run. Traditional priorities for the ambulance service in case insufficient transportation requests arise simultaneously are:

- Emergency call or accidents
- Patient conveyance to hospitals or clinics
- Transferring of patients between the hospitals
- Discharged patients returning home

9.2 Staffing Pattern, and Equipment of an Ambulance

As per the Committee on Ambulance Design Criteria (1973), an ambulance is a vehicle that has been designed, built, equipped, and staffed to cope with emergencies outside and en route to the hospital.

9.2.1 Ambulance Staffing Pattern [1, 5]

Ambulance	Drivers	Stretcher bearer/nursing orderlies at 4 per ambulance + leave reserve + staff for three-shift system
02	07	10
03	12	15
04	16	20
05	20	24

* requirements are for basic ambulances

Doctors: They may accompany the team in the ambulance depending on the type of emergency or accident or at times of disaster.

Critical care medicine (CCM) trained nurse: They can manage the emergency as well as supervision of the case.

Nursing orderly and stretcher bearer: They help in lifting the accident victims and seriously ill or comatose patients. They are trained in first aid, resuscitation procedures, as well as lifting of serious accident victims without causing further injury to the patients.

Call response time: The team with the ambulance should be in a position to move in less than 2–3 min once the call is received.

All the different categories of staff must be available in all the shifts around the clock. Periodic rehearsing must be carried out to keep the staff in readiness in times of need.

9.2.2 *Equipping of Ambulances* [15, 16] *(National Source: National Health Mission)*

The equipment in ambulance will depend upon the type of ambulance service.

Specifications of medical equipment for ERS ambulances under the National Health Mission and the type of ambulances:

S. no.	Medical equipment	Type of ambulance
1	Suction pump, portable electric	C and D
2	Suction pump, foot operated	A, B, C, and D
3	Suction pump, hand operated	A, B, C, and D
4	Laryngoscope	C and D
5	Flowmeter with humidifier bottle	A, B, C, and D
6	Oxygen cylinder "B" type	A and B
7	Oxygen cylinder "D" type	C and D
8	Bag and mask ventilation device (adult)	A, B, C, and D
9	Bag and mask ventilation device (child and neonatal)	A, B, C, and D
10	Trolley stretcher with back tilt facility and collapsible wheels	A, B, C, and D
11	Canvas stretcher folding	A and B
12	Stretcher scoop	A and B
13	BP instrument aneroid	A, B, C, and D
14	Stethoscope	A, B, C, and D
15	Pneumatic splints	A, B, C, and D
16	Cervical collar	A, B, C, and D

S. no.	Medical equipment	Type of ambulance
17	First-aid box	A, B, C, and D
18	Spinal board	A, B, C, and D
19	Double-head immobilizers	C and D
20	Fetal Doppler	D
21	Portable handheld glucometer	A, B, C, and D
22	Electric nebulizer	A, B, C, and D
23	Automated external defibrillator	A, B, C, and D
24	Monitors	C and D
25	Syringe pump	D
26	Transport ventilator, both adult and pediatric	D
27	Transport ventilator, neonatal and pediatrics	D
28	IV cutdown sets	C and D
29	Pulse oximeter	A, B, C, and D
30	Automatic noninvasive BP (NIBP)	A and B
31	Supraglottic device (LMA), all sizes	A, B, C, and D

9.2.3 Essential Accessories in the Ambulance [17]

According to NHRM the essentials accessories in the ambulance are:

(a) Head light, tail and rear light, reversing light, and turn signals
(b) Cabin lights
(c) Speedometer/odometer
(d) One spare wheel with tire and tube
(e) Suitable jack and handle
(f) Seat belt for driver and co-driver
(g) Front seat belt for driver and co-passenger
(h) Stretcher
(i) Siren
(j) Flashing light on top (as per standard)
(k) Oxygen cylinder holder
(l) Saline bottle holder
(m) Anti-skid floor

9.2.4 *Additional Equipment Required in the Ambulance Other Than for Patient Treatment (Emergency Ambulance)* [15, 18, 19, 20]

Two-way radio	•Forms one of the most important devices in modern emergency care, allowing communication with the hospital regarding the priority and arrival of a critical patient and the condition of his status
Mobile data terminal	•Mobile data terminals are connected to central computer at the hospital, are installed in some ambulances to pass on information
Tail lift or ramp	• The ambulance may be equipped with a tail lift or a ramp to facilitate the loading of the patient into the vehicle without the need for lifting. This is especially important a when the patient is obese or when intensive care vehicles require large and bulky equipment.
•Trauma lighting	□ In addition to normal working lighting, ambulances may be equipped with special lighting (usually blue or red) to be used if the patient becomes photosensitive.
•Air conditioning	□ Ambulances are often equipped with a separate air conditioning system in the work area, which helps to maintain an appropriate temperature for the patient being treated, but may also include additional features such as-filtration. against airborne pathogens.
•Data recorders	□ They are often placed in ambulances to record information such as speed, power and braking time, activate active emergency warnings such as lights and sirens, and use seat belts. They are often used in conjunction with GPS units

The report of the World Health Organization's National Committee on Macroeconomics and Health on India states that an average person in India, who does not own a motor vehicle, has to travel more than 2 km to get paracetamol tablet, more than 6 km for blood tests, and nearly 20 km for hospital care [17].

9.3 Intramural Transportation

Transporting patients, material, and staff within the healthcare facility is called intramural transportation.

9.3.1 Wheelchair Transportation

The World Health Organization defines a wheelchair as "a device providing wheeled mobility and seating support for a person with difficulty in walking or moving about." Wheelchair transportation is necessary for patients who are confined to a wheelchair or who are unable to walk independently [21].

Wheelchair Designed for Temporary Use

These are the most commonly used wheelchairs in hospitals and clinics called as the orthopedic or "hospital" wheelchairs (Fig. 9.1). They have a basic design and function that is simple to maintain while still being durable enough to last for years. These wheelchairs are self-propelled, making them ideal for short-term uses like postoperative care, transfer of patients from wards, or occasional use by people with minor mobility limitations. They are not designed to give a close fit, postural support, or pressure relief to the user [22]. A wheelchair requires a space of 1.0 m sq. ft [23].

Wheelchair Designed for Long-Term Use

A wheelchair must fit well and provide appropriate postural support and pressure relief for long-term users (Fig. 9.2). A variety of seat widths and depths, as well as the ability to alter at least the footrest and backrest height, are essential for proper wheelchair fitting. Cushion kinds, postural supports, and a changeable wheel position are all standard adjustments and possibilities [21].

Wheelchair Designed for User with Postural Support Needs

Long-term users with particular postural needs require wheelchairs that are highly adaptable or specially adjusted (Fig. 9.3). Additional components are frequently added to such wheelchairs to aid in the user's support [22] (Fig. 9.4).

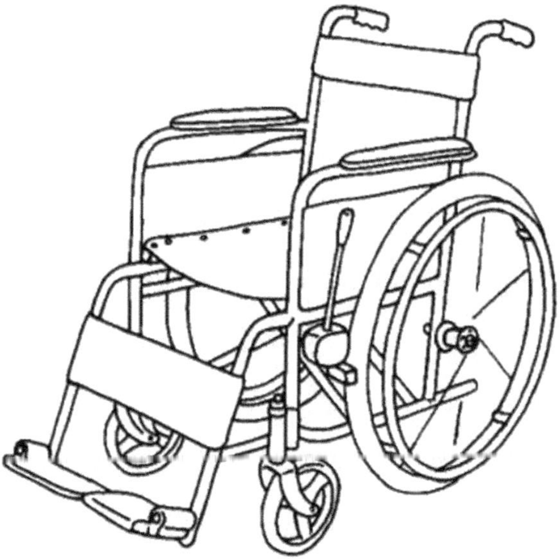

Fig. 9.1 Wheelchair designed for temporary use (Source: adapted from Who.int. [22])

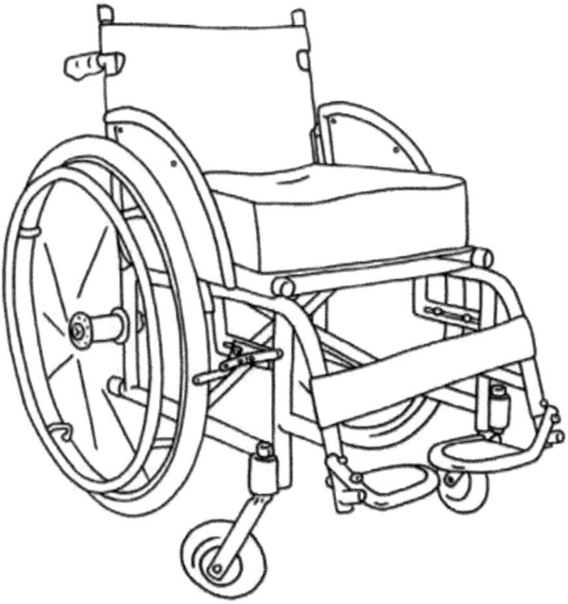

Fig. 9.2 Wheelchair designed for long term use (Source: adapted from Who.int. [22])

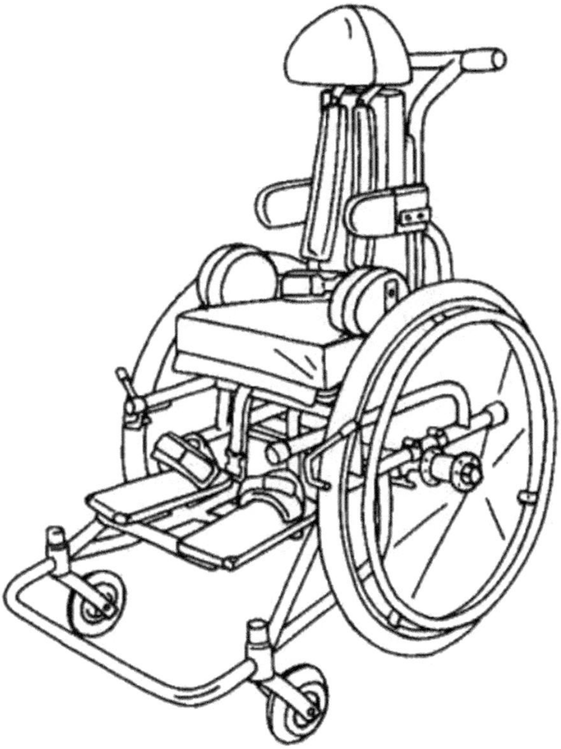

Fig. 9.3 Wheelchair designed for user with postural support (Source: adapted from Who.int. [22])

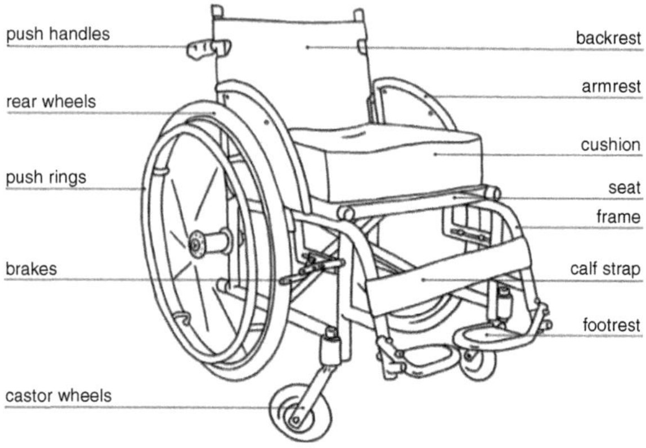

Fig. 9.4 Parts of a wheelchair (Source: adapted from Wheelchair Design) [24] Physiopedia

9.3.2 *Stretcher Medical Transportation*

Stretcher medical transportation is designed for patients who are unable to rise up or move into a sitting posture because they are bedridden.

Hydraulic Stretchers

Within a healthcare facility, mobile stretchers are utilized to carry a patient safely and quickly. A mobile stretcher is often constructed out of steel, aluminum, or plastic patient platform installed on a wheeled frame with mechanical, electrical, or hydraulic mechanisms for regulating the platform's height. Adjustable-height stretchers are often lighter and less complicated than fixed-height ones, but the latter can match the elevation of other surface levels, making patient transfers easier and safer. Intravenous poles, patient monitors, oxygen tanks, articulating headpieces, and other equipment can all be added to most stretchers. They can also be used as beds. Mattresses, adjustable side rails, and straps are included in most stretchers (Fig. 9.5).

The height of the stretcher platform can be changed in a variety of ways: some utilize a hydraulic pump or an electronic control, while others use a mechanical hand crank or support bars that fit into grooves to raise or lower the platform [22].

Scoop Stretcher

The scoop stretcher is an adjustable device with two hinged interlocking components that separate along its longitudinal axis. Each half is wedge shaped; they can theoretically be inserted beneath the patient without requiring the body to be rolled or lifted [25] (Fig. 9.6).

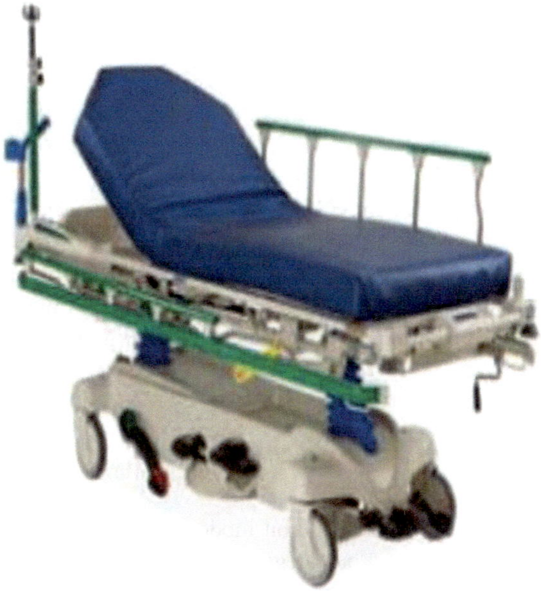

Fig. 9.5 Hydraulic stretcher (Source: adapted from Who.int. [22])

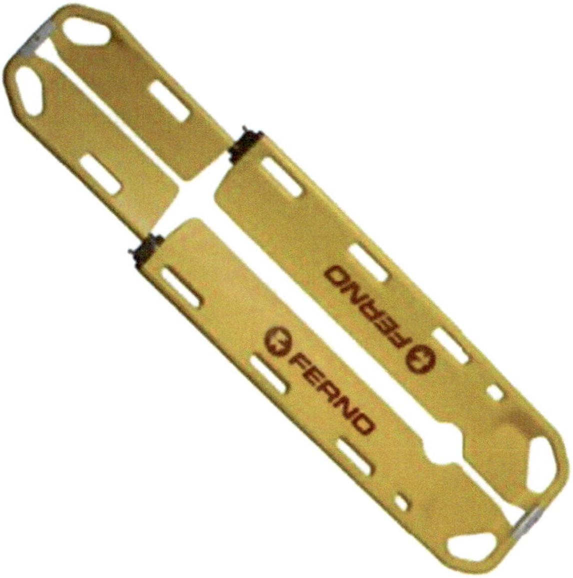

Fig. 9.6 Scoop stretcher (Source: adapted from Del Rossi [25])

Stretcher Trolley

In a hospital, a stretcher trolley is used to transport patients who are unable to move from a lying posture. The stretcher trolley requires two people to operate. Patient trolleys are designed to make it as easy as possible to move patients (Fig. 9.7).

Folding Emergency Stretcher

It is used by the rescue crew to rescue patients in the event of a fire, flood, or other disasters. One of the foldable support rails on the stretcher bed is included in the collapsible storage of the stretcher bed (Fig. 9.8).

9.3.3 *Lifts and Elevators*

Lifts are the most common mode of transport in high-rise building structures. In hospitals, lifts can be categorized and provisioned based on the function as below:

General Passenger Lifts

These lifts cater to all types of passengers, including wheelchair users. A general passenger lift serving clinical areas shall have a clear internal dimension of at least 2000 mm wide by 1700 mm deep, a minimum loading capacity of 1250 kg, and a

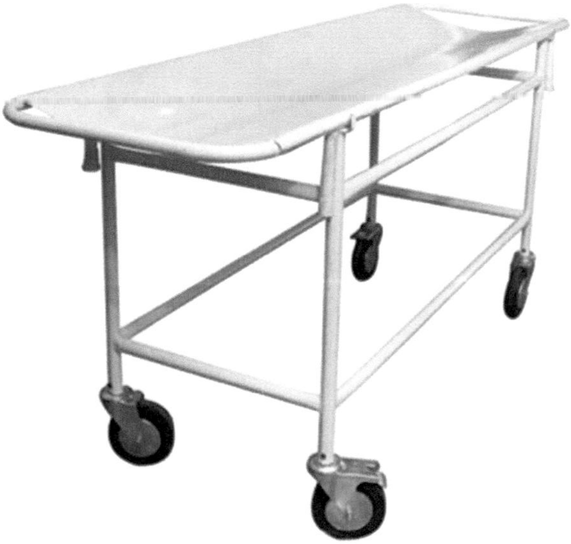

Fig. 9.7 Stretcher trolley (Source: adapted from Stretcher Trolley [26])

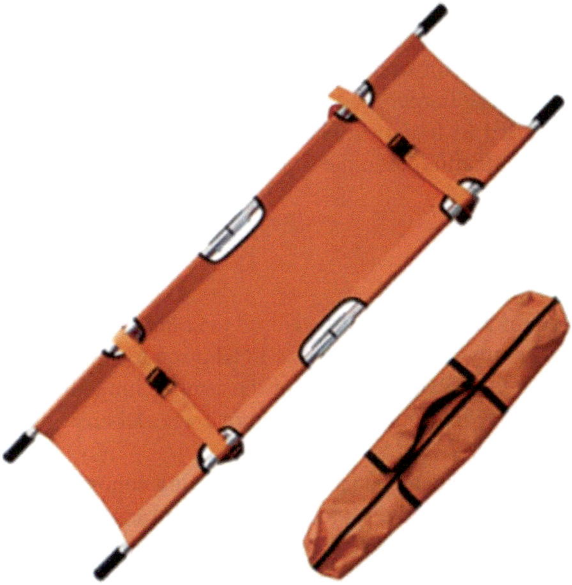

Fig. 9.8 Folding emergency stretcher (Source: adapted from Medical Emergency Folding Stretcher [27])

minimum clear door opening width of 1100 mm and clear height of 2100 mm. This is to provide adequate circulation room for wheelchair users and their companions. The lifts for cleaning services could be part of a larger group of passenger lifts. Housekeeping activities, on the other hand, should not be planned to coincide with general peak passenger demand. As much as is practical, public passenger lifts should be isolated from bed, service, and goods lifts, with distinct lift lobbies [28] (Healthfacilityguidelines.com).

Bed Lifts

These lifts are designed to transport patients on beds or stretchers, as well as the essential staff and support equipment. The bed lifts should have a rated load capacity of 2500 kg and a clear internal dimension of 1800 mm width by 2700 mm depth at a minimum. The width of the clear door opening must be at least 1400 mm and the height must be at least 2200 mm. The internal height of a lift car shall not be less than 2500 mm [28] (Healthfacilityguidelines.com).

Service/Goods Lifts

These lifts are designed to transport furniture, equipment, building materials, equipment maintenance supplies, and waste, among other things. The service/goods lifts should have a rated load capacity of 2500 kg and a clear car dimension of 1600 mm width by 2200 mm depth at a minimum. The width of the clear door opening must not be less than 1200 mm and the height must not be less than 2200 mm. The internal height of a lift car shall not be less than 2500 mm. Smaller goods lifts may be considered for smaller healthcare institutions (less than 50 beds) with adequate due diligence. Larger goods/service lifts with wider door opening sizes should be installed in facilities where heavier equipment is expected to be transported [28] (Healthfacilityguidelines.com).

Ramps

Ramps are a sloped surface used to connect two places of varying heights. They are frequently used instead of or in addition to stairs/steps to make spaces more accessible. Ideally, the entrance of the ramp is immediately next to the stairs. Ramps are primarily used in hospitals to move wheelchairs or stretchers in and out of the hospital [29].

Ramps can have one of the following configurations (Fig. 9.9):

1800 mm is the preferred width of a ramp. 1500 mm is the minimum to be provided with an unobstructed path of minimum 900 mm. Ramps shall have a maximum slope of 1:20. Ramps should be provided with landings for resting, maneuvering, and avoiding excessive speed. Landings should be provided every 10.00 m at every change of direction and at the top and bottom of every ramp. The landing should have a minimum length of 1.20 m and a minimum width equal to that of the ramp. A protective handrail at least 0.40 m high must be placed along the full length of ramps [29].

9.3.4 Material Transport

Material transport is one of the most challenging areas in the intramural transport services.

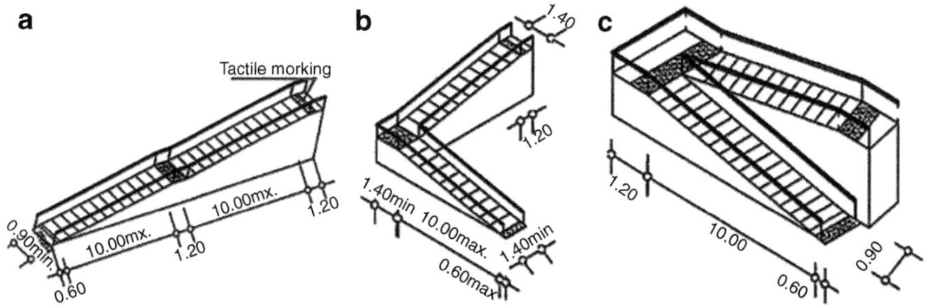

Fig. 9.9 (**a**) Straight run. (**b**) 90 turn. (**c**) Switch back or 180 turn. (Source: adapted from 9 Accessibility Design Manual: 2-Architechture [29])

It includes transport of

- Store equipment
- Medicines and other pharmacy goods
- Medical equipment
- Linen and laundry
- Biomedical waste
- Sterile instruments
- Medical records
- Laboratory samples
- Food and beverages

The most popular way of transporting materials from the source to the target department is the trolley system. A variety of trolleys are used in hospitals for this purpose.

Trolleys are goods vehicle with a platform body with four small wheels of equal size, mounted underneath it.

To transfer sterile items for CSSD or fresh linen from the laundry to the user departments, a closed shelved trolley is used (Fig. 9.10). Transfer of dirty linen to the laundry is done with a laundry hamper with a lid (Fig. 9.11).

Dressing trolley is used in a hospital to carry out dressing or cleaning of patients after a procedure (Fig. 9.12).

A food trolley is a cart that is used to provide hot and fresh meals. It features heating elements that keep the food hot and fresh for a certain amount of time. The trolley is propelled by its wheels. Food carts are used by hospitals to improve their food service and food quality. In hospitals, the trolleys are preheated. The food is separated by ward and transferred to large containers (Fig. 9.13) or packed in trays from the kitchen (Fig. 9.14).

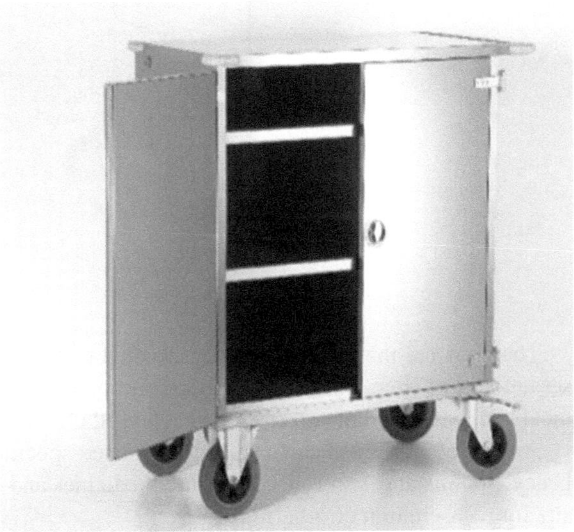

Fig. 9.10 Trolley for transport of clean supplies (Source: adapted from Trolley for clean supplies [30])

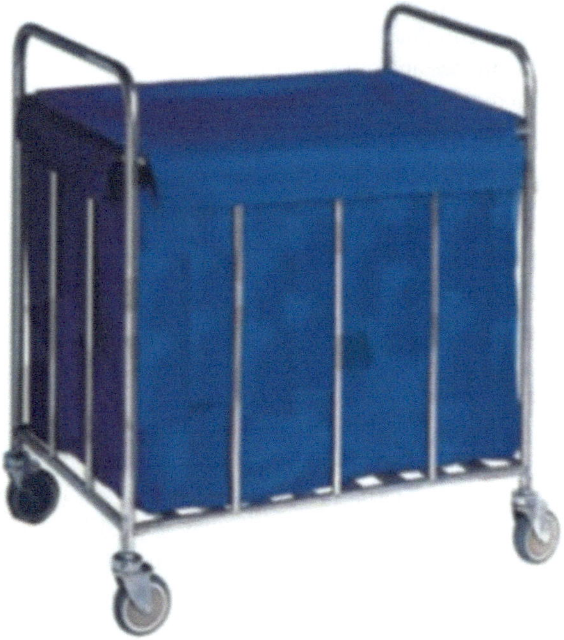

Fig. 9.11 Dirty laundry hamper (Source: adapted from Dirty laundry hamper [31])

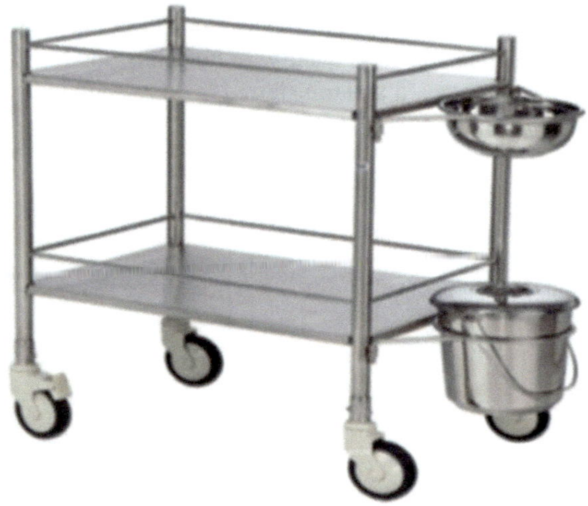

Fig. 9.12 Dressing trolley (Source: adapted from Dressing trolley [32])

The trays are then placed in the preheated trolley. The trolley is preheated for a set amount of time and then transported to each and every room. As a result, the meal is maintained hot and fresh throughout the process [33].

An emergency crash cart is a trolley created specifically for dealing with emergency circumstances. It is used to bring medicines and equipment to the emergency site for resuscitation efforts (Fig. 9.15).

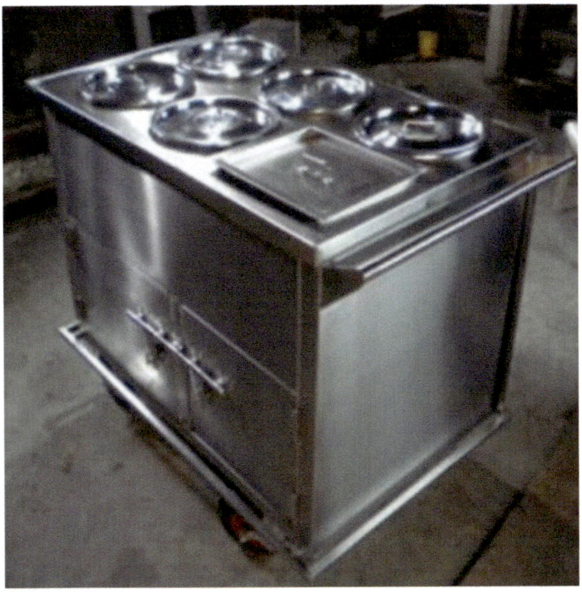

Fig. 9.13 Trolley for supply of food 34 (Source: adapted from Dressing trolley [Internet] [32])

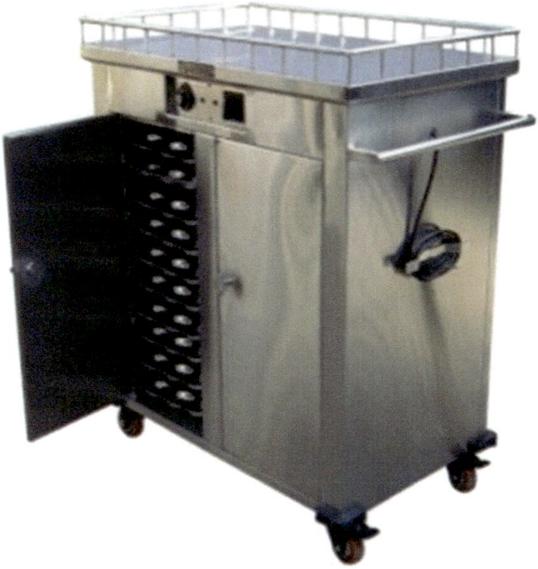

Fig. 9.14 Trolley for transport of packed food trays. (Source: adapted from food trolley for food tray [Internet] [35])

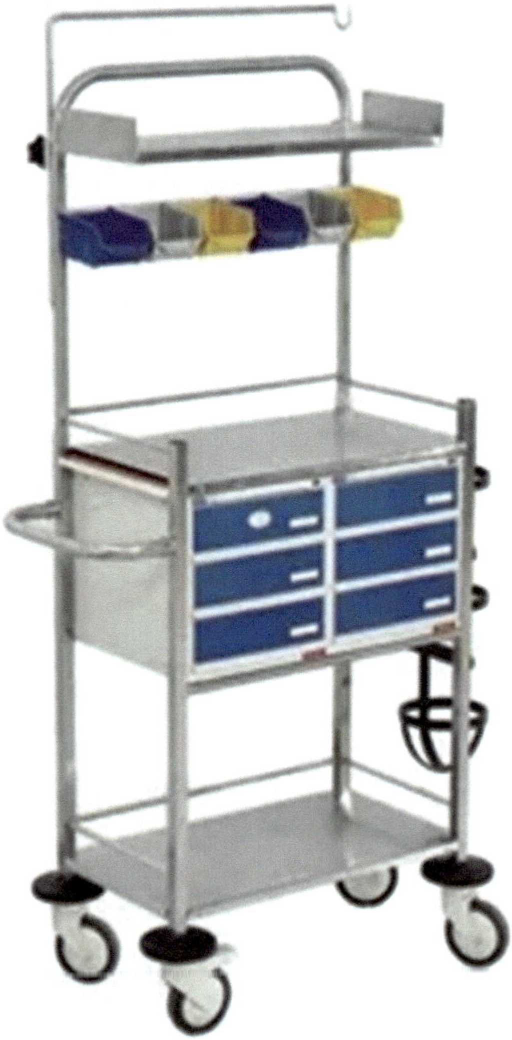

Fig. 9.15 Emergency crash cart (Source: adapted from Emergency crash cart [Internet] [36])

9.3.5 Pneumatic Transport System

Pneumatic tubes (or capsule pipelines, also known as pneumatic tube transport) are systems that propel cylindrical containers through networks of tubes by compressed air or by partial vacuum. Pneumatic transportation system is a network consisting of pipes and receiving-sending stations that is used for mechanized movement of samples or documents using compressed air force [37].

Components of the PTS:

- Blowers
- Three-way diverter
- Carriers

- PVC tubes
- Delivery stations
- Computer control center (Fig. 9.16)

9.3.6 *Dumbwaiters*

Dumbwaiters are small freight elevators designed to transport goods rather than people. Dumbwaiters are used to transport people between floors.

Dumbwaiter lift delivers quick, cost-effective, and comfortable vertical transportation for small freight elevators in a variety of buildings. It saves a lot of time and labor resources [38] (Fig. 9.17).

They are generally installed in the CSSD to transport sterile instruments to the OT, and in the laundry to carry clean linen to the wards and OT.

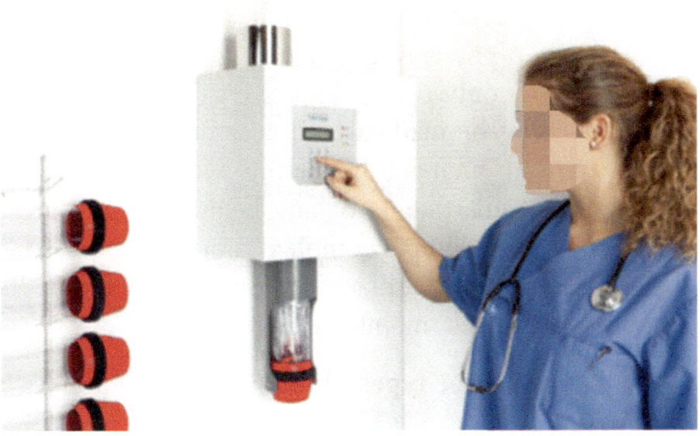

Fig. 9.16 PTS carrier and delivery station [Source: adapted from 18 (Pneumatic transport tube [Internet] [37])

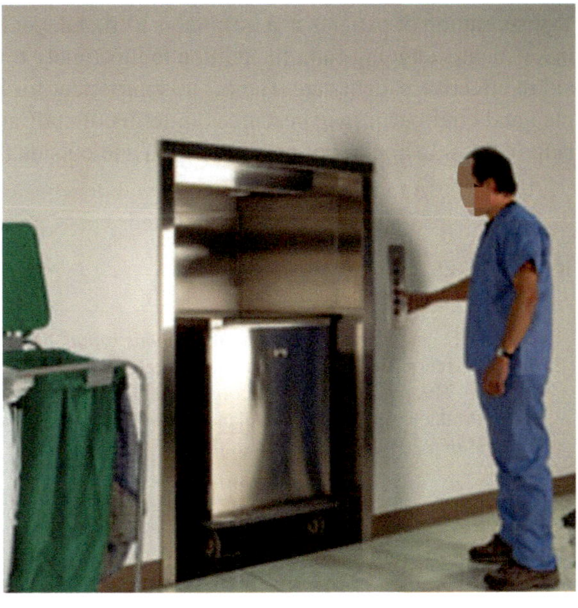

Fig. 9.17 Electronic dumbwaiter [Source: adapted from 19 (Electronic dumbwaiter [Internet] [39])]

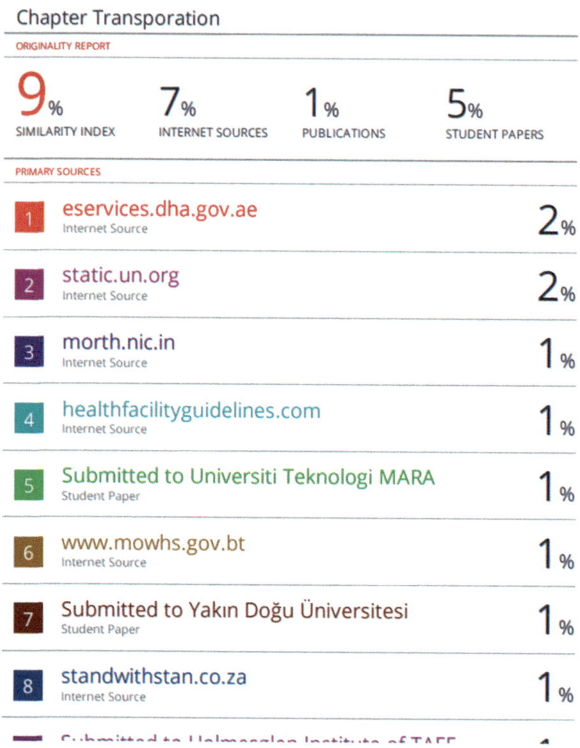

9.4 Conclusion

Transportation of patients in a hospital is a crucial, yet frequently overlooked, stage in a patient's ongoing care. In addition to this timely transportation of materials too aid in effective patient care. Hence, it is important for hospitals to ensure that they plan and equipment their resources in terms of staff and infrastructure that would help in the safe transfer of patients within and outside the hospital premises.

References

1. Joshi, D. C., and Mamta Joshi. *Hospital Administration*. Jaypee Bros. Medical Publishers, 2009.
2. Skinner, Henry Alan. "The Origin of Medical Terms:" Southern Medical Journal, vol. 42, no. 12, Dec 1949, p. 1110. https://doi.org/10.1097/00007611-194912000-00026.
3. "How Products Are Made: Ambulance". *How products are made*. *Archived from* the original *on 25 March* 2007. Retrieved 23rd March 2022.

4. Barkley, Katherine Traver. The Ambulance: The Story of Emergency Transportation of Sick and Wounded through the Centuries. 1st ed, Exposition Press, 1978.
5. IGNOU, Block-2 Support and Utility Services-II, Unit-2 Transportation System - Ambulance Services, 2017, http://hdl.handle.net/123456789/33710
6. Following the Rear: Travails of the Union Army's Ambulance corps: https://circulatingnow.nlm.nih.gov/2019/08/02/following-the-rear-travails-of-the-union-armys-ambulance-corps/
7. Pollock, A. Corbett Bell, The Ambulance: A History (Switzerland: Springer International Publishing, 2015), 17-26
8. "How Products Are Made: Ambulance". How products are made. Archived from the original on 25 March 2007. https://web.archive.org/web/20070325025913/http://science.enotes.com/how-products-encyclopedia/ambulance
9. https://en.wikipedia.org/wiki/Ambulance
10. Mackay, G. M. "Some Features of Traffic Accidents." BMJ, vol. 4, no. 5686, Dec. 1969, pp. 799–801. DOI.org (Crossref), https://doi.org/10.1136/bmj.4.5686.799.
11. Report of Hospital Review Committee (Delhi Hospitals), 1968, https://indianculture.gov.in/report-hospital-review-committee-delhi-hospitals-1968
12. https://nhm.gov.in/images/pdf/programmes/ERS/Specification_of_Equipments_for_ERS_Ambulance.pdf
13. (http://joshipurmun.gov.np/sites/joshipurmun.gov.np/files/Ambulance%20Technical%20Specification.pdf)
14. "Handheld radios for Emergency Ambulance Service". Emergency Ambulance.com. 16 January 2003.
15. "CCTV to protect ambulance staff". *BBC News*. 26 July 2004.
16. "Ambulance Lifts". Ross and Bonnyman. Archived from the original on 1 July 2007.
17. Report of the National Commission on Macroeconomics and Health MINISTRY OF HEALTH AND FAMILY WELFARE GOVERNMENT OF INDIA, 2005 https://ruralindiaonline.org/en/library/resource/report-of-the-national-commission-on-macroeconomics-and-health/
18. "New technology closes gap between accident victims and ER". CNN News. 7 April 1999.
19. "Motorola and Tetra Ireland Consortium Deliver National Public Safety Network" (PDF). Motorola. Archived from the original (PDF) on 16 September 2012.
20. "MDT Market Sectors". Microbus. Archived from the original on 27 March 2010.
21. [Internet]. Who.int. 2022 [cited 15 March 2022]. Available from: https://www.who.int/disabilities/publications/technology/English%20Wheelchair% 0Guidelines%20(EN%20for%20the%20web).pdf
22. [Internet]. Who.int. 2022 [cited 9 March 2022]. Available from: https://www.who.int/medical_devices/innovation/hospt_equip_34.pdf
23. Putsep E. Modern Hospital. [Place of publication not identified]: Lloyd Duke; 1979.
24. Wheelchair Design [Internet]. Physiopedia. 2022 [cited 15 March 2022]. Available from: https://www.physio-pedia.com/Wheelchair_Design
25. Del Rossi G, Rechtine GR, Conrad BP, Horodyski M. Are scoop stretchers suitable for use on spine-injured patients? The American journal of emergency medicine. 2010 Sep 1;28(7):751-6.
26. Stretcher trolley [Internet]. Amazon.in. 2022 [cited 19 March 2022]. Available from: https://www.amazon.in/SMARTCARE-HF10-Stretcher-Trolley/dp/B07FSP6YM4
27. Medical Emergency Folding Stretcher [Internet]. 2022 [cited 19 March 2022]. Available from: https://www.amazon.in/Medical-Emergency-Stretcher-Aluminum-Portable/dp/B081MYQL76
28. [Internet]. Healthfacilityguidelines.com. 2022 [cited 18 March 2022]. Available from: https://www.healthfacilityguidelines.com/ViewPDF/ViewIndexPDF/Vertical_Transportation_System
29. Accessibility Design Manual: 2 Architecture: 1-Ramps [Internet]. Un.org. [cited 14 March 2022]. Available from: https://www.un.org/esa/socdev/enable/designm/AD2-01.htm
30. Trolley for clean supplies [Internet]. 2022 [cited 19 March 2022]. Available from: https://www.indiamart.com/proddetail/cssd-trolley-21937520188.html

31. Dirty laundry hamper [Internet]. 2022 [cited 19 March 2022]. Available from: https://www.hospitalsstore.com/asco-linen-laundry-trolley/
32. Dressing trolley [Internet]. 2022 [cited 19 March 2022]. Available from: https://www.medicalservicesystem.co.in/product/dressing-trolley/
33. Anuraj NP, Ravichandran V. Design of a food trolley for hospitals in India. SASTech-Technical Journal of RUAS. 2013;12(2):90-8.
34. Food trolley [Internet]. 2022 [cited 19 March 2022]. Available from: https://www.exportersindia.com/product-detail/hospital-trolley-india-1560159.htm
35. Food trolley for food tray [Internet]. 2022 [cited 19 March 2022]. Available from: https://www.singhrefrigeration.co.in/hospital-trolley.html
36. Emergency crash cart [Internet]. 2022 [cited 20 March 2022]. https://www.indiamart.com/proddetail/hospital-crash-cart-14645255791.html
37. Pneumatic tube - Wikipedia [Internet]. En.wikipedia.org. [cited 20 March 2022]. Available from: https://en.wikipedia.org/wiki/Pneumatic_tube
38. Pneumatic transport tube [Internet]. 2022 [cited 20 March 2022]. Available from: https://www.air-log.com/en/hospital.html
39. Electronic dumbwaiter [Internet]. 2022 [cited 20 March 2022]. Available from: https://www.indiamart.com/proddetail/hospital-dumbwaiter-lift-9180722433.html

Further Reading

Oxford English Dictionary ambulance definition 1
https://economictimes.indiatimes.com/news/politics-and-nation/road-accident-scenario-more-serious-in-india-than-covid-19-with-415-deaths-daily-nitin-gadkari/articleshow/80771875.cms?utm_source=contentofinterest&utm_medium=text&utm_campaign=cppst
"Press Releases". Archived from the original on 13 July 2011.

Chapter 10
Central Service Sterile Department

N. Shalini, R. Sathish, M. V. Anitha, H. K. Mamatha, B. J. Divya Rao, and Arehally M. Mahalakshmi

10.1 Introduction

Central sterile supply department (CSSD) is a service unit in a hospital that processes, issues, and controls the sterile store supply to all departments of the hospital.

> Bhattacharjee defined CSSD as that service, within the hospital, catering for the sterile supplies to all departments, both to specialized units as well as general wards and OPDs [1].

CSSD is an independent department in the hospital with facilities to receive, clean, pack, disinfect, sterilize, store, and distribute instruments as per well-delineated protocols.

The essentials of CSSD are:

- Correct design
- Appropriate equipment
- Skillful operators
- Workflow

N. Shalini (✉) · M. V. Anitha · H. K. Mamatha · B. J. D. Rao
Department of Health System Management Studies, JSS Academy of Higher Education and Research, Mysore, India
e-mail: shalini.dhsms@jssuni.edu.in

R. Sathish
Department of Health System Management Studies, JSS Academy of Higher Education and Research, Mysore, India

Department of Oral Maxillo Facial Surgery, JSS Dental College and Hospital, Mysuru, India

A. M. Mahalakshmi
Department of Health System Management Studies, JSS Academy of Higher Education and Research, Mysore, India

Department of Pharmacology, JSS College of Pharmacy, Mysuru, India

D. Bhatia et al. (eds.), *A Guide to Hospital Administration and Planning*,
https://doi.org/10.1007/978-981-19-6692-7_10

10.2 History of CSSD [2]

- The Second World War led to the modern concept of practicing CSSD.
- The history of CSSD starts in 1928. The American College of Surgeons introduced the word CSSD.
- Regular CSSD was established in the United Kingdom in 1955 at the Cambridge Military Hospital.
- In 1965, the first CSSD was established in India at Safdarjung Hospital, New Delhi.
- Now every hospital has CSSD unit.

10.3 Objectives of CSSD

- To supply the sterile instruments, linen pack basins, and other sterile items.
- To record and maintain an accurate effectiveness of the cleaning, disinfecting, and sterilizing process.
- To enforce necessary controls to prevent cross infection according to infection control policies.
- To constantly update the practices to improve the quality or service provided.
- To provide services to all departments requiring sterilization process.
- In hospitals, CSSD plays a vital role in infection control.

10.4 Functions of CSSD

See Fig. 10.1.

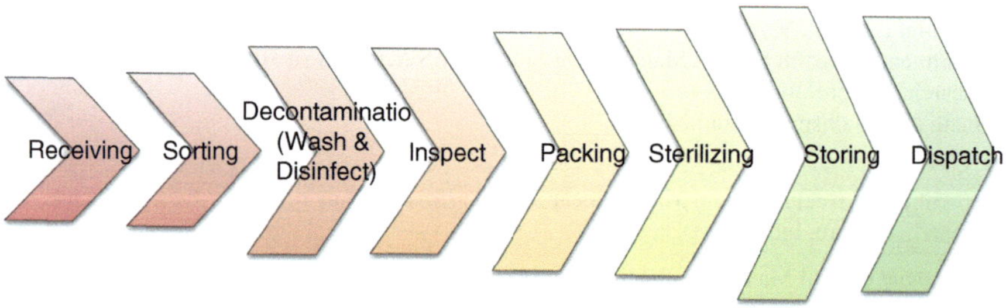

Fig. 10.1 Functions of CSSD

10.5 Planning of CSSD

The CSSD is broadly classified into two. See Fig. 10.2.

10.5.1 Central Unit

The following activities take place here:

- Receives dirty utilities
- Cleansing of dirty utilities
- Processing them
- Sterilization
- Storage
- Supply

10.5.2 Peripheral Unit

Sterile instruments are supplied to the different areas of the hospital (Theater Sterile Supply Unit).

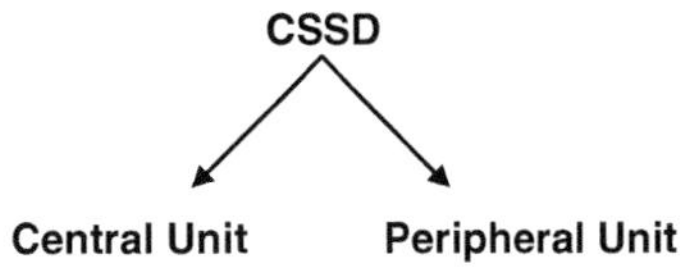

Fig. 10.2 Classification of CSSD

10.6 Division in CSSD

See Fig. 10.3.

CSSD is divided into

Functional areas:

- Receiving area
- Decontamination area
- Packing area
- Sterilization area
- Storage area
- Distribution area

Administrative area:

Space for routine clerical procedures
Space for write-up and storage of stationeries

10.6.1 Receiving Area (Red Zone Area)

- Contaminated/soiled instruments are sent to the CSSD in closed bins wherein they are prewashed in running water.
- Prewashed instruments are soaked in disinfectant solution (follow the disinfectant protocol for disinfectant solution and protocol for procedure) after the procedure is completed.
- Later, the instruments are sent for ultrasonic cleaning.
- Ultrasonic cleaner should maintain the designated time, pressure, and temperature for effective and efficient cleaning to happen by following the manufacturer's guidelines.
- Validation of the ultrasonic cleaners is checked by using aluminum foil test based on the outcome of the result.

Fig. 10.3 Basic division in CSSD

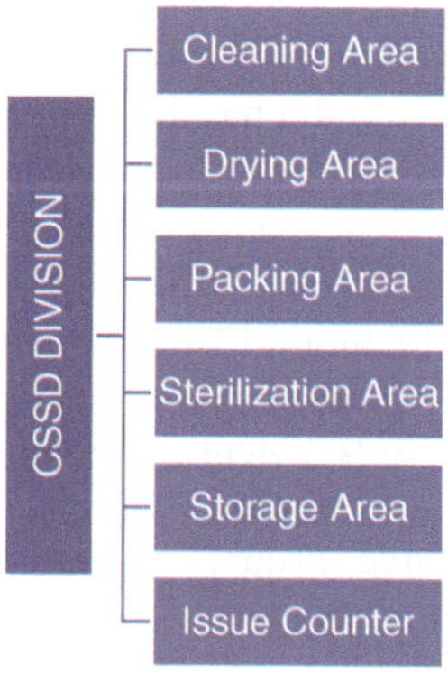

- **Good result**—(The ultrasonic bath is working effectively.) The pinprick holes, uniform in size, are seen evenly distributed throughout the foil.
- **Bad result**—(The ultrasonic bath is not functioning effectively.) There may be little or no holes on the aluminum foil.
- **"Hotspots"**—Missing/ineffective sweeping frequency.
- **Patchy holes**—Combination of large holes in some parts and minimal or no holes in the rest of the aluminum foil.

- Register is maintained at the department so that all the instruments along with their respected department names are noted.

  Requirements:

- Two sinks (washing and rinsing)
- Ultrasonic cleaner
- Tank/tub for chemical disinfection
- Solution for chemical disinfection of instruments
- Enzymatic solution for ultrasonic cleaner
- Scrub brush for removing the visible contamination of instruments
- Silicone gloves for the personnel working in this area, for washing and instrument handling in ultrasonic cleaner

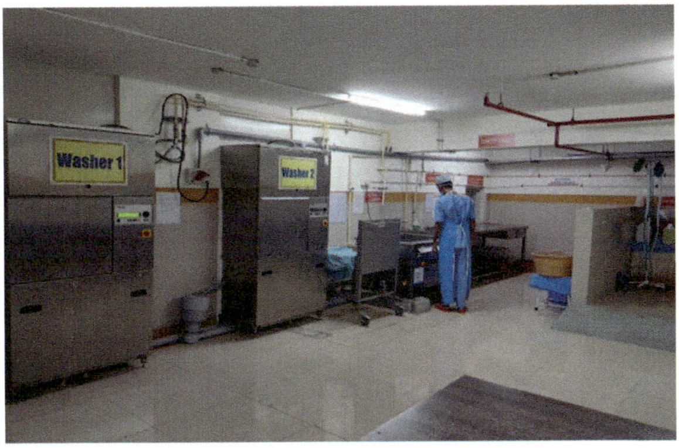

10.6.2 Packaging Area (Blue Zone Area)

Blue zone area is the area where there is restricted entry of work personnel; they need to follow a protocol while entering here like a dress code or wearing of PPE.

Care is taken to see that all the instruments are free of any air molecules and they are completely air-dried.

Instruments received in sets from their respected departments are put back in the same order and covered by use of linen/plastic pouch and paper (medical grade paper).

Three-line label (stickers) are placed on pouches; following are the details mentioned on the sticker:

- Batch number
- Machine number
- Date of sterilization
- Date of expiry
- Which department the instrument belongs to
- Person in charge for sterilizing that batch of instruments

Instrument wrapping/packaging should provide resistance to punctures and tears and should act as a barrier to microorganisms and moisture.

Requirements:

- Air dryer for drying washed instruments
- Material for wrapping of instrument (paper wrap, linen wrap)
- Sealing pouches with color indicators
- Sealing machines
- Three-line label with gun
- Ink to check the seal quality

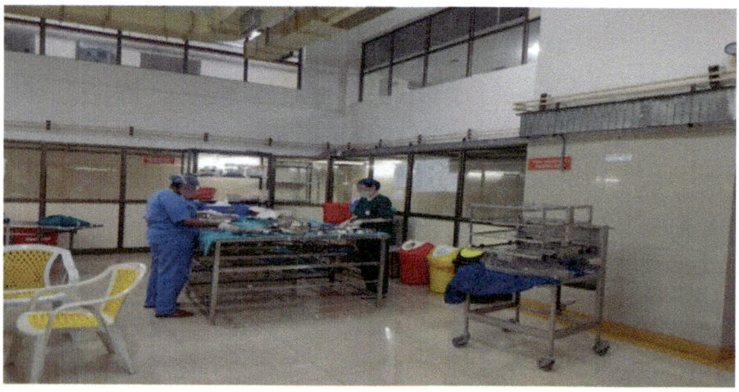

10.6.3 Sterilization Area (Green Zone Area)

This is a completely restricted area wherein only the people working at that department have access to remove the packed and sterilized (autoclaved) instruments from their respective sterilizers and stored before they are distributed to their respective departments.

Sterilizers which are present in their respective organization use their manufacturer's guidelines on temperature, pressure, and time duration of each cycle along with their maintenance guidelines for effective and efficient working process and procedures.

Sterilization is a process wherein an article is free from all living organisms including bacteria, fungal spores, and viruses.

Heat Sterilization

Various methods of sterilization are as follows:

1. **Dry heat sterilization**—Here, sterilization is carried out at about 160 °C for 1 h, e.g., glass syringes and cutting-edge instruments.
2. **Sterilization by steam**—Steam destroys microorganisms by irreversible denaturation or heat coagulation of cellular proteins.

Types of steam sterilizers:

(a) **Gravity displacement or downward displacement sterilizer**—The air from the chamber and load is displaced by gravity.
(b) **Pre-vacuum sterilizer**—The air from the chamber and load is removed by vacuum pump (IGNOU study material).

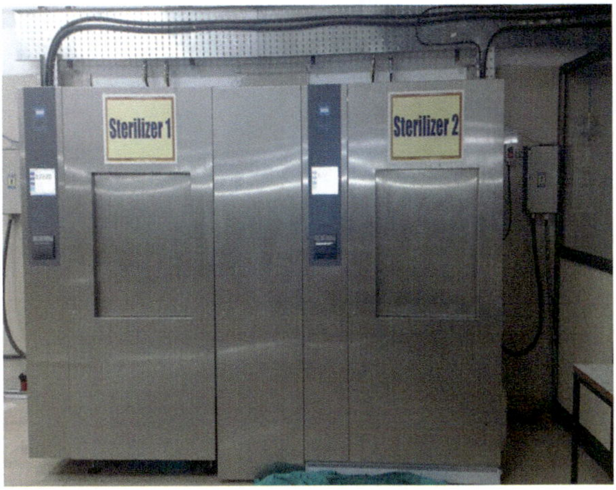

Ethylene Oxide Sterilization [2]

Ethylene oxide kills microorganism by altering the DNA by alkylation process:

- Gas is used here for sterilization.
- Very time consuming, usually lasting until 12 h.
- If the instructions are not followed properly, it can lead to toxicity from the gas used.

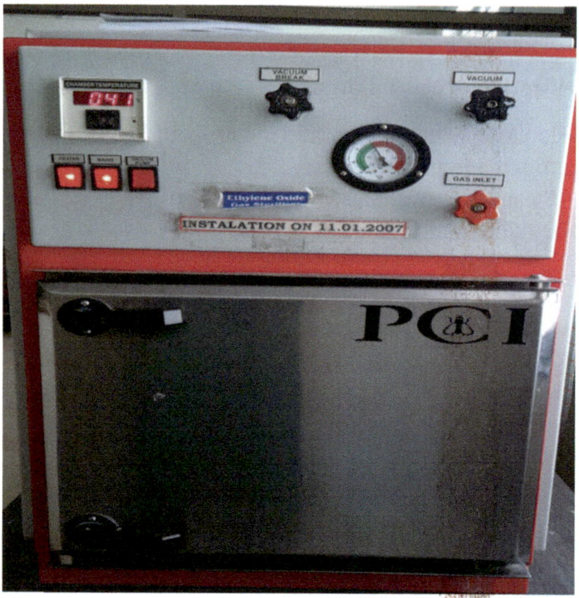

Flash Sterilization

Underwood Perkins defined **flash sterilization** as sterilization of an unwrapped object at 132 °C for 3 min at 27–28 lbs. of pressure in a gravity displacement sterilizer.

Time and temperature of sterilization depend upon the manufacturer guidelines along with the items that need to be processed [3] (Table 10.1).

Table 10.1 Type of flash sterilizers

Type of sterilizer	Features
Gravity displacement	• Nonporous instrument (metal instruments without lumen) • 132 °C (270 °F) • 3 min
	• Nonporous, porous instruments (instruments with lumen, rubber, plastic all is sterilized together) • 132 °C (270 °F) • 10 min
Dynamic air removal (e.g., pre-vacuum)	• Nonporous instrument (metal instruments without lumen) • 132 °C (270 °F) • 3 min
	• Nonporous, porous instruments (instruments with lumen, rubber, plastic all is sterilized together) • 132 °C (270 °F) • 4 min
Steam flush pressure pulse	• Nonporous and porous items V • 132 °C (270 °F) • 4 min

Chemical Sterilization [2]

Chemicals are used here as a means of sterilization; this is an absolute process, wherein spores are also destroyed along with the vegetative form.

Chemical agents used here are:
Cidex
Hydrogen peroxide
Formic acid
Chloramines (combination of chlorine and ammonia)

Radiation Sterilization

The gamma ray's sterilization is used for sterilization of articles and is one of the most effective methods of sterilization. This method is not used much in hospitals because of high cost of equipment and safety standard requirements.

Requirements
- Front-loading autoclave (preferably double door)
- Trolley for carrying and loading of instruments into the autoclave
- Chemical indicators with devices for ensuring the working condition of the autoclave (e.g., process challenge device)
- Biological indicator
- Silicone gloves for the operator's safety

10.6.4 Storage Area (Green Area)

Once the instruments are out of the sterilization machine, they need to be stored in a place where they have maintained a relatively adequate temperature, pressure, and proper air exchange:

- Maintain proper ventilation; it should be dust free and pest free.
- Clean and dry closed cabinets can be used.
- Stainless steel perforated racks can also be used.
- Instruments should be stored in such a way that instruments which are near expiring should be used well before the ones that are going to be expired later.
- If there is any tear in the packaging, the whole set must be sent again for re-sterilization following the entire steps again.
- Register is maintained regarding the issue of instruments to their respective departments.

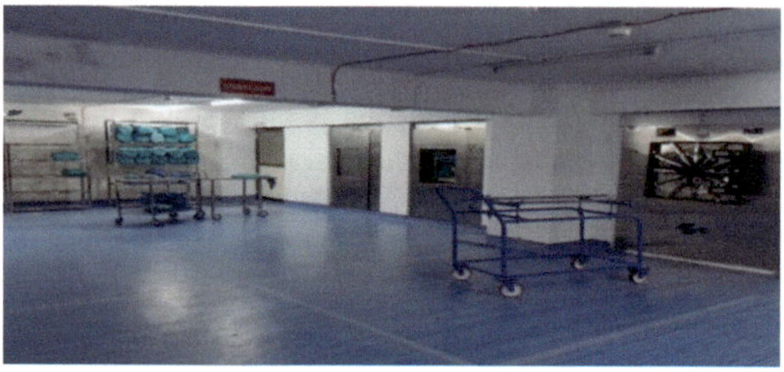

10.7 CSSD Design/Layout [4]

Layout of the department should have a linear workflow pattern, wherein all the contaminated/soiled instruments are brought into the CSSD in a separate entry point and the exit point in which the packed and sterilized instruments leave the department in a different exit point to their respective departments.

10.7.1 Linear Flow Instrument Processing Layout

See Fig. 10.4.

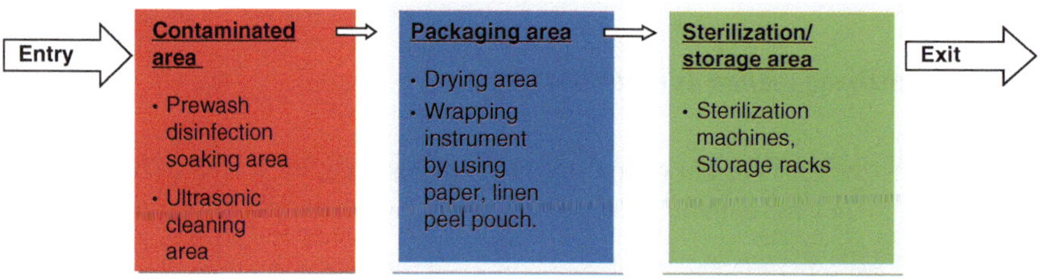

Fig. 10.4 Linear flow instrument processing layout

10.7.2 U-Shaped Instrument Processing Layout

See Fig. 10.5.

10.7.3 Designing of the CSSD

- CSSD is constructed in such a way that they follow a unidirectional flow, wherein contaminated instruments enter the department in one direction and exit in another direction to prevent any cross contamination.
- It serves the purpose of cleaning and disinfection.
- Flooring in the department should be nonskid, smooth, and robust.
- Ceiling should be of flush type and sealed to the walls.
- Air filtration—proper air pressure should be adapted in CSSD so that there is no room for any cross infection, HEPA filters along with air conditioners are maintained in the department, and air changes are usually done in relation to the size of the hospital along with how many cycles of sterilization are carried out.
- Fixtures should be easy to clean.
- Relative humidity should be maintained.
- Maintain the proper air pressure within the department such that there is less chances of infection/contamination. Clean zone maintains a positive air pressure.
- Regular cleaning of the department is preferred along with deep cleaning, which is done at a regular interval which enhances better working of the department.

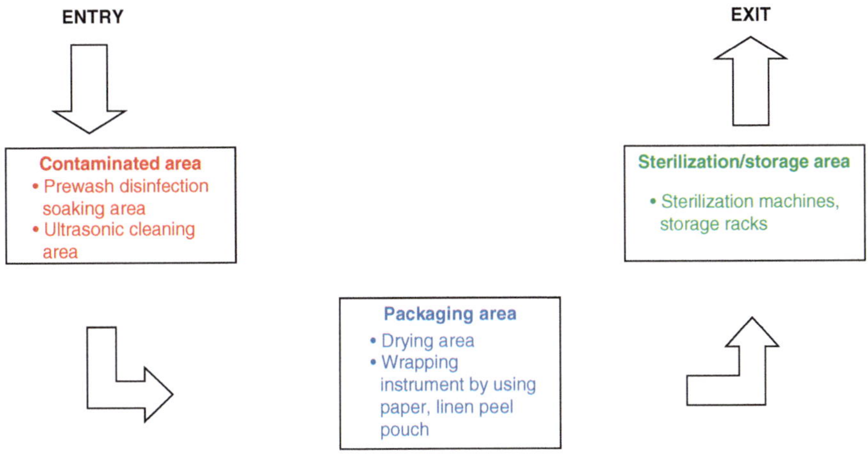

Fig. 10.5 U-shaped instrument processing layout

Lighting

Lighting fixtures should be such that they are closed so that they prevent insects and dust accumulation; light level should be at least 400 lux.

Signage/Displays in Functional Areas

The functional areas of the department should have the following displays:
- Manufacturer's manual of the equipment used.
- Standard operating procedure.
- Material safety data sheet should be displayed near to their respective instruments so that the working staff will be benefited in case of need.
- Signage regarding postexposure management.
- Proper signage along with directions should be made available at the department for easy access and to prevent any misdirection, and a restricted entry board should also be displayed.
- Physical separation/barrier should be present between soiled zone, clean zone, and sterile zones.
- The risk of cross infection spread by staff working in CSSD should be minimized.

10.8 Sterilization Monitoring

10.8.1 Physical Monitoring

Latest sterilizers are equipped with a digital printout at the start of each cycle wherein the parameters such as

- Temperature
- Air pressure
- Time

are noted down in a printed format/cycle and done on a daily basis.

10.8.2 Biological Indicators/Spore Testing

They are inexpensive and easy to use and provide a positive result; it is one of the most accurate means as it measures sterilization process directly by using the most resistant microorganism.

Table 10.2 Biological indicators

Spores	*Geobacillus stearothermophilus*
Monitors	• Steam • Hydrogen peroxide gas plasma • Liquid peracetic acid
Number of spores	10^5 spores
Method of use	• Ampoule is placed at the center over one or more packs within the chamber • Ampoules are later sent to laboratory for culture to obtain results
Incubation	• Done at a temperature of 55–56 °C for 14 days • Check for turbidity • Along with that incubate an unexposed spore ampoule simultaneously

Ideal properties of a biological indicator:

- Nonpathogenic
- Well characterized
- Easily procurable
- Cost effective
- Easy to handle
- Sterilization resistant compared to human pathogens
- Should give rapid results
- Should provide positive results when the sterilization parameters are inadequate to kill microbial contaminants
- Should be standardized (Table 10.2)

10.8.3 Chemical Indicators

These are the indicators which are placed on the packed units before they are subjected to sterilization.

Change in temperature and pressure confirms that the sterilization process has taken place or not; they are visible on the packed unit as they change their color once they are out of the chamber.

For example:

Autoclave tapes
Bowie–Dick test
Temperature tube
Ink seal test

10.9 Factors Affecting Efficacy of Sterilization [3]

See Table 10.3.

Table 10.3 Factors affecting the efficacy of sterilization

Factors	Effect
Cleaning	• Ensure that there is thorough cleaning happening which will reduce salt concentration, protein load, and bioburden, which increases the sterilization efficacy
Bioburden	• Around 100–103 organisms (primarily vegetative spores) are considered as natural bioburden for surgical devices, which is below 105–106 spores used with biological indicators
Type of the pathogen	• Sterilization-resistant spore-forming organisms are used as test organisms required for FDA clearance • Vegetative bacteria are the common contaminating microflora on surgical instruments
Protein	• The reason for decrease in the efficacy of sterilization is residual protein • Protein load can be removed rapidly by appropriate cleaning
Salt	• Other than protein load, residual salt also decreases the efficacy of sterilization • Salt load can be reduced by cleaning process
Accumulation of biofilm	• Sterilant exposure to microbial cell is impaired by biofilm accumulation, hence reducing sterilization efficacy
Length of lumen	• Sterilization penetration is directly affected by increase in length of lumen • More force flow is required through the lumen to achieve satisfactory sterilization
Diameter of lumen	• If lumen diameter is decreased also, there will be reduced sterilization efficacy • In that case, forced flow through lumen achieves satisfactory sterilization
Flow restriction	• Satisfactory sterilization is achieved when microorganism comes in contact with the sterilant used • Devices with sharp bends and blind lumen will prevent the contact of sterilant with microorganism, thus affecting sterilization efficacy
Design and construction of device	• Sterilization efficacy also depends on the compatibility of materials used in the construction of devices with various sterilization processes • Design issues (e.g., screws, hinges) will also affect sterilization efficacy

10.10 Special Consideration [3]

Processing patient care equipment contaminated with blood-borne pathogens (HBV, hepatitis C virus, HIV), antibiotic-resistant bacteria (e.g., vancomycin-resistant enterococci, methicillin-resistant *Staphylococcus aureus*, multidrug-resistant tuberculosis), or emerging pathogens (e.g., Cryptosporidium, *Helicobacter pylori*, *Escherichia coli* O157:H7, *Clostridium difficile*, *Mycobacterium tuberculosis*, severe acute respiratory syndrome coronavirus), or bioterrorist agents: Additional care needs to be followed while treating the instruments/equipment used for these patients, and they must be in harmony with the standard guidelines; follow the designated guidelines which are set in treating these instruments. Prion-related contamination must be handled cautiously as it can cause transmission of disease if not sterilized appropriately. Prion-contaminated instruments/equipment should be subjected for protein denaturation/sustained heat at high temperature for several hours along with standard sterilization protocol.

10.11 Quality Control [3]

- Conducting periodic training programs on the safety measures and procedures of doing things will help the staff enhance their knowledge about the department and improvise their skills on the effective methods of sterilization.
- Infection control should be conducted periodically.
- Maintenance of records.
- Periodic review of policies and procedures.
- Maintenance of incident reporting.
- Recall policy.

10.12 Documentation

Maintaining documents at CSSD is of prime consideration as it is a key factor of patient safety as well as infection control purposes (Fig. 10.6).

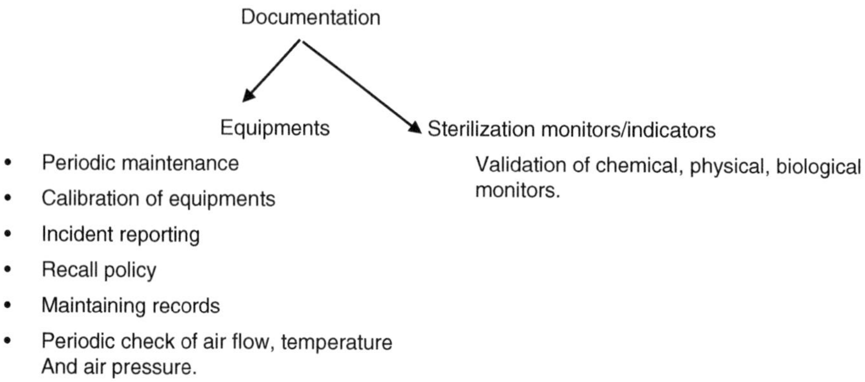

Fig. 10.6 Documentation

10.13 Incident Reporting

Incident reporting is usually observed at a workplace, wherein the process of recording worksite events, including near misses, injuries, and accidents, takes place.

A complete reporting along with documentation of all facts of incidents happened has to be done.

Usually, any accidents occurring at a workplace, leading to injury to any workers or any damage to equipment or property, are considered here.

10.14 Recall Policy

Registers are maintained at the department, which helps in easing the job of segregating the instruments as received from their respective departments; in case of any unacceptable situation, wherein there is a fault in the sterilization process or any of that sort, then by having a look at the register which mentions the date and batch number, the instruments are tracked and recalled back to the CSSD from their respective departments. After the problem is fixed, negative biological spore test is obtained, and the CSSD in charge after consultation with infection control can allow sterilization to be returned to operation.

10.15 Condemnation Policy

An expert in IT and biomedicine engineering must provide a report on the item after inspection of the following:

- Is the item reparable or does it need to be replaced?
- If it is reparable, can it be done in-house or does it need to be sent to the vendor?
- If the item is to be repaired by the vendor, is the cost below or above the cost of replacement?
- If it needs to be replaced, can the item be salvaged and used somewhere else or does it need to be discarded?

One member from the store and one resident medical officer/medical superintendent review the expert report, inspect items, provide approval sequence number (manual), and determine how to physically discard the items, and the details will be documented in the meeting minutes. Entry must be done in the inventory book regarding the condemned items, mentioning the number of items condemned and the total presently available items in stock.

10.16 Breakdown Policy

Breakdown of any equipment in hospitals will result in a lag in workflow; how we manage the situation without a lag in the workflow is of utmost importance for a CSSD personnel. Depending on the size of the organization, equipment are purchased. In case there are two steam sterilizers, if one breaks down also work can be managed by the other one left or if the organization is provided with only one equipment, then the organization can have a MOA with its sister concern till it is repaired.

Once the repaired equipment is ready and back to work, biological indicators are used on them to check the efficacy of the equipment.

10.17 Classification of Patient Care Items (CDC Classification)

A rational approach to disinfection and sterilization of patient care items and equipment was first introduced by Earle H. Spaulding almost 30 years ago.

Spaulding believed if instruments used for patient care are categorized as critical, semicritical, and noncritical based on the degree of risk for infection, then the type of disinfection procedures to be followed could be understood readily.

According to that, instruments are classified into

- Critical instruments
- Semicritical instruments
- Noncritical instruments

10.17.1 CDC Guidelines for Sterilization and Disinfection of Patient Care Items [3, 4] (Table 10.4)

Table 10.4 CDC guidelines for sterilization and disinfection of patient care items

S. no.	Category	Description	Instruments
1	Critical instruments	• High risk of infection is confirmed once they come in contact with microorganisms • Usually are the ones which penetrate soft-tissue bone • Have the greatest risk of transmitting infection • Heat sterilization is the method of choice used for such instruments	Instruments in this category are: • Surgical instruments • Cardiac and urinary catheters • Implants • Forceps • Scalpels • Bone chisels • Burs
2	Semicritical instruments	• Usually seen when there is contact with the mucous membrane or non-intact skin • Chances of spreading infection are comparatively low here	Instruments included in this category are: • Respiratory therapy, anesthesia equipment • Endoscopes • High-volume evacuator tips • Rubber dam forceps • Amalgam carriers • Cystoscopes
3	Noncritical equipment	• Here there is least risk of infection transmission as they contact only intact skin	List includes: • Bedpans • Blood pressure cuffs • Computers • Lead apron • X-ray unit tube head

10.18 Conclusion

Nosocomial infection is a big threat to humans; hence, CSSD plays a very vital role in reducing the chances of cross infection within the hospital and among individuals.

Department of CSSD ensures that a proper working process is followed so that effective and efficient results are obtained.

Staff employed in this department should have a thorough knowledge about the functioning of the department.

Regular training activities should be undertaken to improvise the knowledge and to upgrade their skills to overcome any difficulties in the future.

Periodic maintenance of all the equipment is to be done to enhance the working conditions so that there is no breakdown of them.

Maintenance of records should be followed on a regular basis.

Meticulous implementation of all types of sterilization indicators has to be carried out for the best outcome of sterilization process.

References

1. Banu A, Subhas GT. Central Sterile Supply Department-Need of the hour. J Pub Health Med Res. 2013;1(2):58-62
2. Text book on Hospital administration -Mamtha Joshi, D.C. Joshi
3. Guideline for Disinfection and Sterilization in Healthcare Facilities, 2008 Update: May 2019.
4. Textbook on modern dental assisting –Bird and Robinson.

Chapter 11
Engineering and Biomedical Engineering Department

Shubham Rathore, Dinesh Bhatia, and Sushman Sharma

11.1 Introduction

Any healthcare facility consists majorly two components: manpower and machine. To distinguish with other setups and to provide best of the medical treatment, state-of-the-art equipment are the foremost requirement for any hospital setup. There are two types of machines in any healthcare facility:

1. Nonmedical
2. Medical

Department which deals with nonmedical machines, for example civil assets, water, electricity, MGPS, and generator, comes under maintenance department, and all medical machines come under biomedical department. To maintain the proper working of all the nonmedical and medical equipment is the prime responsibility of engineering and biomedical department.

S. Rathore
Apollo Spectra Hospital, Jaipur, Rajasthan, India

D. Bhatia (✉)
Department of Biomedical Engineering, North Eastern Hill University, Shillong, Meghalaya, India

S. Sharma
Department of Hospital Management, H.N.G. University, Patan, Gujarat, India

D. Bhatia et al. (eds.), *A Guide to Hospital Administration and Planning*,
https://doi.org/10.1007/978-981-19-6692-7_11

11.2 Biomedical Engineering Department: Functions, Designs, Space Facilities, Utilities, Hospital Wiring System

The major aim of biomedical department is to maintain the proper working of all the medical equipment. If we broadly categorize the function of biomedical department, then we can divide it into four major categories:

1. Planning
2. Organizing
3. Directing
4. Controlling

Let us discuss these four major categories in detail:

11.2.1 Planning

This is the first and foremost important function of biomedical department. At the time of planning of any hospital setup, planning of medical equipment comes as an important step according to which only even the planning of room sizes, electricity points, backup power, etc. get finalized. The budgeting part also comes into this planning phase only.

The team of biomedical and user department decides the specification of any equipment with financial budgeting with the help of finance department. So basically, all the departments of any healthcare unit are closely interlinked and that makes healthcare setup a complex setup.

The second phase of planning comes when biomedical department needs to plan for all the machines' maintenance plan.

There are three types of maintenance plan:

(a) Preventive maintenance plan (PMC)
(b) Annual maintenance contract (AMC)
(c) Comprehensive maintenance contract (CMC)

(a) **Preventive maintenance plan (PMC)**: A periodical checking and calibration of the machine come into the preventive maintenance plan. It is normally decided according to the time or usage.
(b) **Annual maintenance contract (AMC)**: After the warranty period, the manufacturing company provides annual maintenance contract in which the service and maintenance charges are included, but if there would be any faulty part, then that would be chargeable extra.

(c) **Comprehensive maintenance contract (CMC)**: This kind of contract includes both service for repair and maintenance and change of any faulty part. CMC contract can be done for a year and can extend to 5 years if both the parties get consensus on this.

So, the major difference in AMC and CMC is that CMC includes the cost of change of faulty parts, whereas AMC includes only service charges.

The third phase for planning includes the upgrade of technology and condemnation of any equipment. For condemnation of any equipment, consensus of committee should be mandatory which will minimize the unethical activities.

11.2.2 Organizing

In day-to-day operations, biomedical department plays a vital role in organizing repair visits, spare parts, and coordination with the parent company and with the user department. The ultimate aim is to manage all the breakdown of machines, so that the patient will not get hampered.

11.2.3 Directing

All the instruction for any equipment handling comes under this. This is one of the major roles of biomedical department to teach handling of equipment to user department. All the handling instruction and manuals are the responsibility of biomedical department. For this, periodical training is one of the tools.

Other than the abovementioned categories, below are the simplified functions of biomedical department:

11.2.4 Functions

From the first day of hospital setup, the role of biomedical department comes into consideration. Whether it is about the selection of equipment or installation, biomedical plays a vital role in the coordination of other stakeholders. The major functions are listed as below:

- Planning and installation of medical equipment
- To suggest to go for more advanced technology or stay with the existing one
- Training of user department to handle the equipment
- Management of spare parts

- To manage the equipment with preventive maintenance plan
- Time-to-time calibration of the equipment
- To minimize the downtime for the equipment
- To maintain all the records related to a particular equipment
- To plan for (AMC) annual maintenance contract and preventive maintenance plan (PMC)
- To distinguish the machine which should undergo PMC and which should go to AMC
- Condemnation of any old equipment

11.2.5 Organogram

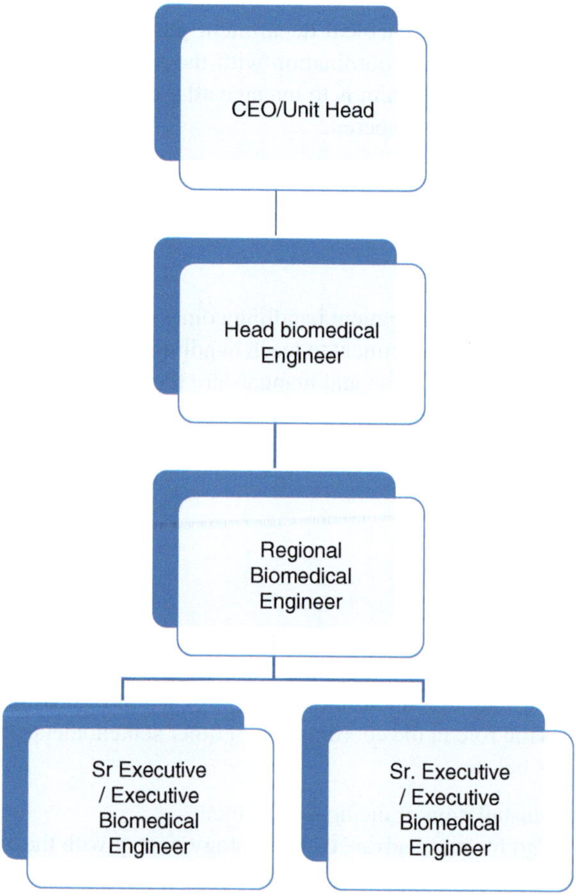

11.2.6 Location

This department does not come in contact with patients. The major coordination is with the user department and the external agencies. So, biomedical and engineering department comes under auxiliary services of a hospital. So normally, this department has been seen on the administrative floor or user-friendly floor. A spare store would be the requirement as per the bedded capacity to keep the new and essential parts and to keep used and faulty parts till the time of condemnation.

11.2.7 Hospital Wiring System

A hospital is a place which will be full of people always and that too including a variety of people like conscious and unconscious patients, visitors, doctors, nurses, and staff. There are so many machines and added oxygen and other medical gases with flammable material, which makes hospitals an extremely complex environment.

Because of these reasons, hospitals are difficult entities to be designed and planned as per the safety standards.

For doing hospital wiring system, one should use fire-resistant cables for the entire wiring system, which should be tested against the highest and lowest temperatures.

11.3 Engineering Department: Functions, Location, Design, Organization, Maintenance Management

Engineering department is one of the most vital utility departments in a hospital. Any civil tasks, electrical supply, water supply, medical gas supply, air-conditioning, lifts, TV, refrigeration, air compressor system, firefighting system, and communication units all come under the umbrella of engineering department. Any slightest malfunctioning of abovementioned areas can lead to serious and harmful events.

The major function of engineering department is to repair and maintain the existing facilities with alignment of a patient's safety and operationalization of the hospital.

Engineering department is directly and indirectly related to all other units of a hospital. The proper working of any other unit in the hospital depends largely on the smooth working of engineering department.

There are lot many expectations from engineering department than from other departments. At patient's level, at doctor's level, or at management level, maintenance department plays a vital role.

Patients expect uninterrupted power and water supply from Engineering Department and no failure of services which can hamper the line of treatment.

Medical team expect from engineering department that the services should be available in an absolute manner and that no interruption should happen and no discomfort is given to patients. There should be no compromise in the treatment of their patients. No delay in any treatment or investigation of patients should happen due to interruption in the work of engineering department.

Management has very high expectation from engineering department. For example, all the government compliances (lift license, etc.) should be in place, which are related to engineering department. There should be no complaints from internal and external customers regarding any of the tasks related to engineering department. Safety of patients and internal staffs should be maintained. Management would expect cost optimization.

11.3.1 Functions of Engineering Department

1. Providing a safe and hazard-free environment: This is one of the major tasks of engineering department to provide the safe environment to patients and staffs either by providing uninterrupted services or by managing the repair and maintenance.
2. Managing the preventive maintenance: All the machines and other resources demand regular servicing for which maintenance department has to maintain a calendar for all the preventive services.
3. To maintain legal compliances: Engineering department is responsible for maintaining all the legal compliances; for example, lift license and DG set license come under engineering department.
4. To maintain the inventory: Engineering department takes care of all the spare parts and other inventory related to any other machinery or of repair material.
5. Training of staff: It is one of the major responsibilities of engineering department to provide continuous training to user departments or the staffs who are handling those areas.
6. Managing the cost: The engineering department can reduce maintenance costs significantly by carrying out timely repairs and by strictly adhering to the maintenance schedules from time to time.
7. Helping hand to management: Engineering department can help authorities in new purchase or old condemnation and can save a lot of money with timely maintenance.
8. Prompt response to breakdown: In-house maintenance team can help to immediately rectify any sort of breakdown.
9. Maintaining records: Engineering department keeps record of all the daily data, history card of machines, etc.
10. To maintain safe and hazard-free environment by following proper processes and practices.
11. To provide documented manual and SOPs for maintaining quality program for engineering department.

11.3.2 Organogram

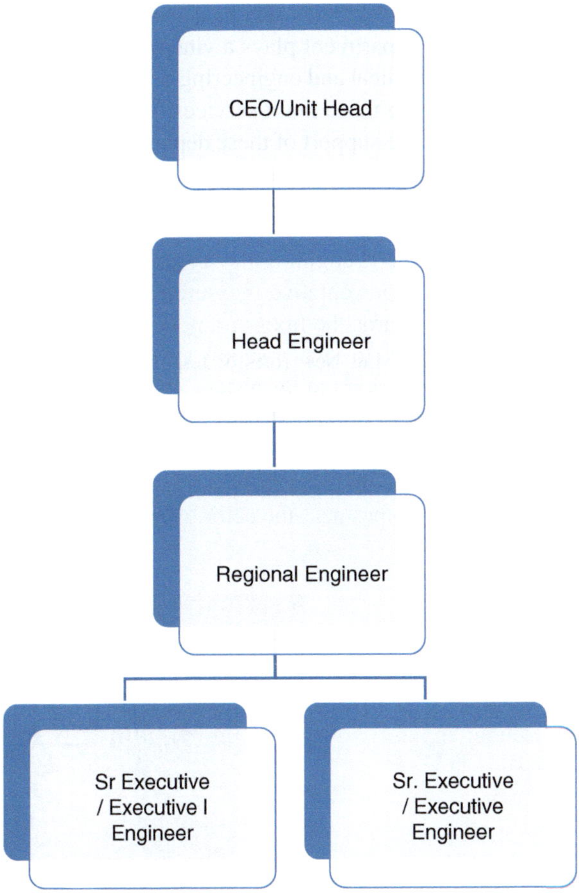

11.3.3 Location

The engineering department can be located in the admin block or may be in the basement or ground floor from where the user departments can access the department easily.

Department should have office area, store area for spare parts, and workshop area where minor repairs can happen.

11.4 Summary

Any hospital setup requires uninterrupted services, and for providing these services, biomedical and engineering department plays a vital role. Medical services are the pillars of a hospital, and biomedical and engineering departments are the supporting pillars for providing support to these main services, which may not connect with patients directly, but without the support of these departments, it is really difficult to maintain the smooth functioning of a hospital.

Further Reading

P H Frisch, B Stone, P Booth, W Lui New roles & responsibilities of hospital biomedical engineering

Biomedical Equipment Management and maintenance program https://nhm.gov.in/New_Updates_2018/NHM_Components/Health_System_Stregthening/Comprehensive_primary_health_care/letter/BMMP_Technical%20Manual.pdf

Chapter 12
Mitigation of Fire Hazards in Hospital

Sandip Bag and Karabi Ganguly

12.1 Introduction

Hospital or healthcare institution is the place where treatment is provided to the critically ill patient with the specialized healthcare staff and medical equipment using advanced health science. Therefore, safety is the utmost requirement for any hospitals [1]. But it is quite unfortunate that fire is the most common and devastating hazard in hospitals because complex hospital buildings are occupied by vulnerable people [2].

Problems in the electrical wiring as well as improper storage of hazardous and combustible materials can cause fire hazards, which intimidate the safety and security of patients and staff members alike and can transfer a hospital to a stalemate [3]. In comparison with the building used for office, school, and other general purposes, it is a tenacious responsibility to vacate the people from hospitals.

Fire safety norms for healthcare, one of the most crucial parameters, need to be followed strictly during planning and subsequently for the proper construction of a hospital. It is very regrettable that there are still some hospitals where fire management is still in written words fixed on the wall [4].

In most of the cases, the administration or management blames that a large number of hospital staffs do not know about or have awareness skills against the fire hazards as well as the steps essential to execute to combat the calamity. In addition, critically ill, bed-retained highly dependent and immovable patients make it a challenging task to clear the hospital building in a rush.

Therefore, mitigation of fire hazards in a hospital is a very serious and challenging task [5]. So, each and every healthcare facility needs more attention on the adherence of the safety rules and regulations. Furthermore, easy and safe move-out procedures in healthcare services are also essential for the life of the people inside the hospital.

S. Bag (✉) · K. Ganguly
JIS College of Engineering, Kalyani, India

D. Bhatia et al. (eds.), *A Guide to Hospital Administration and Planning*,
https://doi.org/10.1007/978-981-19-6692-7_12

12.2 Potential Fire Hazards in Hospitals

Prevention and management of fire are the most significant consideration in the premises of medical and healthcare facilities especially in hospital, care home, or medical practice of any kind because huge numbers of potentially vulnerable people are in the premises that may be at risk in the vicinity [6]. With the probability of numerous patients struggling with mobility and sickness, evacuation procedures become more complex and being ready to understand what the common hazards might be in these environments becomes all the more important [7].

There are several factors responsible for potential fire hazards in a hospital if we do not follow the safety norms properly within the healthcare premises such as the following [8]:

12.2.1 Medical and Surgical Equipment

Nowadays, some medical and surgical equipment utilize lasers and electrosurgical tools quite frequently, which causes an ignition hazard, especially near oxygen cylinders, surgical clothing, and flammable sterilizing liquids. Although fire safety norms are kept in mind during designing, many materials like gas cylinders and oxygen canisters used in hospitals are very combustible [9]. Therefore, such combustible materials should be reserved and managed properly and there should be strict adherence to protocols of electrical loading for energy-intensive equipment to minimize fire hazards [10].

12.2.2 Hospital Kitchens

Fire hazards in kitchen apparatus of hospitals are most common due to generation of flame from cooking fats, electrical ovens, toasters, open flames, etc. So, it is very vital to clean the frying pans, grills, utensils, and other equipment routinely, and cookhouse of the hospital building must be installed with the appropriate fire safety equipment.

12.2.3 Overused Sockets and Cables

In any hospital, there is a large number of electrical equipment which are repeatedly placed in overloaded sockets and cables. They sometimes use extension cords to make daisy chain together to plug more equipment at a time, which is a contravention and can cause serious problems after overheating, ultimately creating a sparking of fire. So, defective or overloaded electric appliances are one of the popular and leading logics behind fire in hospitals. In addition, due to tons of medical equipment required in each hospital, there are diverse risks involved such as circumvent, overloaded electricity points, and faulty or damaged wirings.

12.2.4 Smoking

Although most of the NHS hospitals have declared a complete prohibition on cigarette smoking, there is a significant fire risk as most of the people still evade them or, while smoking outside the building, do not dispose them properly. Unextinguished cigarette counterfoil can cause ashtray fires that can spread quickly if not addressed properly. Therefore, smoking zone in hospitals should be placed in a safe location away from the major buildings of the hospital.

12.2.5 Fire Door Compliance

As per the report and literature survey, it is clear that most of the fire violations in hospitals arise due to a number of fire doors not closing or latching properly. The presence of holes in fire doors would cause them to be no longer fireproof as earlier.

12.2.6 Gas Cylinders and Combustible Fluid

In any hospital, large number of gas cylinders and medical oxygen cylinders are available that need to be properly stored and secured. Hand rubs composed of alcohol that are highly flammable are used all over hospitals [11]. So, it is essential to have a minimum 6 ft breadth between the sanitation site and any flaming origin.

12.3 Fire-Prone Area of Any Hospital

Fire occurs in different sections of patient wards for various factors, and the most common sources are waste fires, combustible liquids and gases, cotton and curtains in wards and nurses' station, sparklers in central nurses' station, sparks from electric discharge lamps in warehouses, overuse of electrical sockets, defects in connection systems and heating gadgets, smoking in lavatory, kitchen fires, and intentional fires at the site of waste collection [12]. Some of the common fire-prone areas of a hospital are described below:

12.3.1 Central Sterile Supply Department (CSSD)

Central sterile supply department, commonly known as CSSD, plays a most vital role in patient safety and in reducing hospital surgical infection. This department of any hospital receives, stores, sterilizes, and provides sterile items in time to all sections including the wards, OPD, and other special units such as operation theatre. The primary attention of a CSSD unit is the castration of items like catheters, tubing, surgical appliances, treatment tray sets, and dressing materials. Although this unit aims to providing sterile items so as to prevent the spread of infection and in some ways to protect hospital staff and patients from biological hazards, it itself is prone to various hazards including electrical, mechanical, chemical, biological, environmental, fire, and physical. For sterilization, highly inflammable gas ethylene oxide (EtO) is used frequently as a gas-sterilizing agent. Improper air circulation system and fault in the gas line can cause accretion of EtO gas in CSSD, and the usage of smoking materials by staff in this unit may create a fire outbreak or even an explosion. Inappropriate stocking of flammable gases and liquids can lead to detrimental effects and may cause fire. Furthermore, erroneous maintenance of electrical machinery and aging electrical cables, in the presence of water, can be a origin of static electricity, sparks, or minor combustion, which can ultimately start the fire outbreak due to the presence of a large number of combustible materials such as gauze, linen cotton, boxes, and paper wrappers within this section.

12.3.2 Intensive Care Unit (ICU)

An intensive care unit, commonly known as ICU, is considered as either an intensive therapy unit (ITU) or a critical care unit (CCU). This unit is so special in any hospital or healthcare facility that dispenses intensive care medicine. So, ICU provides the demanding and life support care for acutely ill and injured patients.

An ICU setup in a hospital will have patient space, nurses' station, oxygen cylinder, and medication storage along with technologically advanced medical equipment such as physiological parameter monitoring device, IV stand, suction machine, alpha mattress, nebulizer, and DVT pump. Generally, 6–8 numbers of medical equipment are connected to ICU patient round the clock based on the current health condition. Therefore, in an oxygen-rich environment of positive-pressure ICU setup, there is a higher probability of fire mishaps to take place if fire safety norms are not followed properly [13]. The prospect of fire hazards is still high with extensive usage of alcohol-based hand sanitizer across ICU and considerable use of disinfectants like sodium hypochlorite solution for cleaning surfaces and equipment.

Though sodium hypochlorite is not combustible, it is a strong oxidizer that intensifies the combustion of other materials like paper and PPE kits. For example, a fire mishap would happen when ICU patient is resuscitated immediately from cardiac arrest using a DC defibrillator to deliver the desired electrical energy through paddle electrodes placed across the patient. The high-voltage electrical spark arises from paddles of defibrillator and will transmit to the patient if high-impedance gel is used mistakenly. These arcs from the electrodes can ignite body hair and spread to linens, i.e., patient gown and blanket, resulting as fire outbreak. The recently repeated hospital fire mishaps across the globe, especially in India, reported from hospital ICU, have raised the question mark regarding safe environment and safe work practice followed by hospital staff also [14].

12.3.3 Operation Room

Fire in operating rooms is a rare but disastrous incident that happens more than 500 times annually [15]. Three essential components of fire are always present in an operation theatre for all surgical purposes: an oxidizer such as oxygen or nitrous oxide, laser and electrosurgical equipment as an ignition source, and a fuel (alcohol, ether, etc.) [16]. The unwanted fire events inside the surgical room result in somewhat 2–3 patient deaths every year, and its impact not only alters the mental condition of a patient but also spreads to the whole team of the surgical section as well as the entire hospital arrangement. Therefore, safe utilization of surgical equipment, oxygen cylinders, and chemicals is required along with the functional firefighting system [17].

12.3.4 MRI Room

MRI machine is one of the most sophisticated and expensive equipment that are quite often used to provide critical diagnostic services to a hospital's mission. MRI machines enforce an exclusive fire protection challenge for a hospital because this machine requires tremendous energy, which is a potential source of fire, and also due to nonavailability of traditional firefighting techniques in the close vicinity of the machine's magnets. The protection of MRI machine from fire is very indispensable from a hospital point of view as its replacement cost is too high and it interrupts the hospital's productivity and profitability.

12.3.5 Kitchen

Hospital kitchen plays an important supportive role to provide good-quality food between mealtimes for patients, staffs, and visitors. The hospital cookery should be planned and equipped in the best possible fashion by which they can meet the special dietary demands with patient satisfaction and avoid contamination with common allergens. Blazes in kitchen facilities are quite familiar because of cooking fats, coiled heater, toasters, and open flames. So, there is a high chance of fire risks. Therefore, it is very vital to clean the frying pans, grills, and other utensils regularly, and canteen must be equipped with the appropriate fire safety like fire extinguishers and smoke detectors. Make sure that grease traps and fryers are cleaned regularly and cooks are well aware on fire safety.

12.3.6 Laundry Room

A reliable washing service is very crucial to any hospital as it provides acceptable, clean, and uninterrupted supply of linen to all sections. The primary functions of laundry system include sorting, cleaning, extricating, depleting, ironing, folding, mending, and supply in time. Ideally, hospital laundry room should be positioned away from the main service building but must be placed in a site having sufficient daylight and natural ventilation. Large hospitals with 500 beds and above should establish their own mechanism for laundry, and smaller hospitals should take the help of cooperative mechanized laundry.

This washing unit is another familiar part of a hospital complex that is highly vulnerable to fires due to generation of heat. All of us know that dryers get excessively hot when they are used for parched sheets and clothes. Mix that aggressive lint buildup in the lint trays and vents, and we have a potential fire waiting to happen. Make sure that laundry service room is kept away from the main building so that the chance of potential fire hazards is less. The NABH also endorsed a lint-cleaning chart that cleaners check and fill out to assure that dryers are always dredge and lint free.

12.3.7 Basement

Basement of any construction means one or more floors that are partly or completely below the ground floor, which is mostly used as a storage space for furnace, gas cylinder, water heater, air-conditioning system, car parking, etc. It is also utilized as a space for amenities such as the electrical system and cable television distribution point. Hospital basements are generally sluggish, dark areas where unused equipment, spare beds, oxygen cylinders, and inflammable liquids are stored. In addition, hospitals often utilize such basements as a shielding layer from the earth for their nuclear chemistry and radiation therapy and diagnostic resources. All the storage materials inside the basements are highly explosive, and the report on recent fire hazards in hospitals shows that basement is the most fire-prone zone of a hospital.

12.4 Basic Principles of Fire Safety in Hospital

Healthcare facilities like hospitals and nursing homes are normally operated on a 24 × 7 basis as there is a continuous flow of patients. Hospitals not only take care of patients but also ensure their safety on a priority basis [18]. Fire accidents at healthcare facilities are very common, but it is not desirable to force anyone to run for their life.

Attention on fire safety in hospitals becomes very crucial as hospitals provide a wide range of services including diagnostic and therapeutic functions, clinical testing, imaging, emergency rooms, and operation theatre for surgery. Beyond this, they have the role of hospitality such as food service and housekeeping. Its infrastructural houses consist of many heat-dissipating equipment, combustible gases and fuels, chemicals, electrical wiring, and so on, which facilitate fire mishaps in the hospital [19].

There are three fundamental principles that all hospitals could adopt to prevent fire accidents as well as recover the life of vulnerable people and also forbid the damage of the building property. The basic principles of fire safety are prevention, suppression, and evacuation.

12.4.1 Fire Prevention

The most suitable way to execute fire safety management in any hospital building is proper planning of fire prevention as prevention is better than protection. It is well established that a facility is neither 100% perfect nor hazard free and none of the plan can prevent every possible cause of a fire.

Primary focus on fire preventative strategy in a hospital includes (1) limiting the occurrence of fire, (2) reducing the magnitude of fires, and (3) delaying the spread of fires within the medical facilities [20].

Before consideration about fire prevention, first we have to grasp the three fundamental ingredients that establish fire, i.e., heat, fuel, and oxygen. These three components are attributed as "fire triangle" as they interact together and create a fire (Fig. 12.1).

Fuel: Any type of combustible material is known as fuel that can be used as the origin of ignited fire. The examples of flammable material include paper, oil, wood, ether, etc.

Oxygen: An oxidizing material that initiates the reaction with the fuel and extends the fire. The magnitude of fire depends on O_2 concentration. Therefore, lower concentrations of oxygen will turn down the fuel combustion.

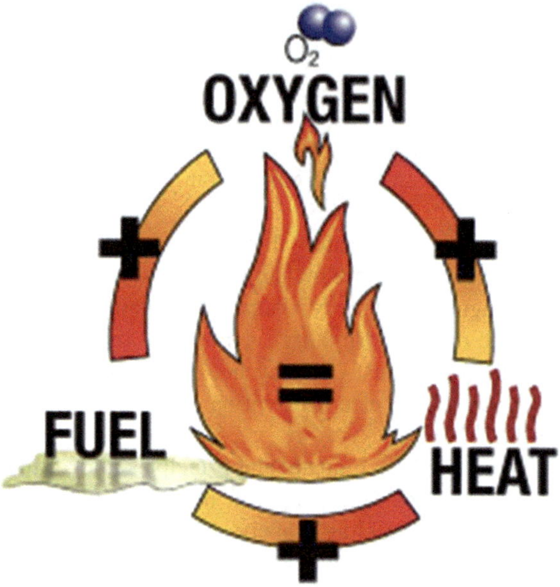

Fig. 12.1 The fire triangle (source: http://thesymbiont.blogspot.com/)

Heat: Heat allows fire to spread by drying nearby combustible materials and surrounding air near the flame. For fires, it is essential to interact with oxygen and they fuel each other at a temperature higher than the threshold value of ignition, which is known as the "flash point." Low flash point temperature means that flammable materials are easy to ignite.

Depending on the types of combustion materials, fires are categorized into **five classes**. These classes of fire include the following:

Class A: For such fire, ordinary combustible materials like wood, paper, plastics, textiles, and rubber are the main concern.

Class B: In this type, mainly flammable liquids such as petroleum, grease, ether, gasoline, oil based paints, tars, solvents like alcohols, and incendiary gases are involved that can be best extinguished by smothering.

Class C: This kind of fire involves electrical equipment like power tools, electrical wiring, circuit panel, electrical gadgets and motors, and computers that is caused by energized electrical elements like flawed power cords or overloaded electrical socket.

Class D: Combustible flammable metallic substances like sodium, potassium, magnesium, lithium, zirconium, and titanium are responsible for such fire, but this fire is not normally found in a medical center.

Class K: This is another category of fires mainly associated with vegetable and animal fat-based commercial cooking oils and greases that is unique to cooking. These types of fires are effectively contented with a Class K fire extinguisher.

(a) Planning Considerations for New and Existing Hospitals

One of the major attentions in an exorbitant hospital fire is to freeze the acceptance of incendiary architecture like carpet space, partitions, roofs, staircases, and fire escapes and some nonstructural components, mainly exits such as doors and windows, false ceilings, furniture, insulation, and mechanical and electrical pipeline, in a hospital structure [21].

For designing and developing new healthcare facilities, proper construction codes and guidelines for effective fire avoidance and suitable building goods having acceptable fire resistance category should be used. For both structural and nonstructural components of the facilities, the duration of fire resistance may range from ½ an hour to more than 4 h.

In case of renovation or refurbishment of a hospital structure, the drawing or plans of existing building are essential to resolve the fire-retardant backfit exigencies of the facility. This drawing or plan should be produced for modification of existing structure and/or creation of new furnishing for future correspondence and submitted to the fire service department for accident at the medical services; first responders will have prior familiarity of such a layout and part of emergency openings, fire compartments, etc. allowing for a more efficient response in saving lives.

(b) Construction and Design Considerations

(i) New Medical Facilities

In recent years, most of the hospitals' design and construction have been made of noncombustible materials that have satisfactory fire resistance ratings and do not release toxic smoke during a fire mishap. Firefighting ratings of the structural materials usually depend on layout process, occupancy technique, and utilization of the facility [22].

In case of newly constructed healthcare facilities, the architecture should consider the requisite fire rating of the structural elements of the building guided by building code standards. Construction codes may differ from country to country.

Considering a large number of fire accidents in hospitals, architects, designers, and engineers responsible for hospital building construction nowadays are paying more attention towards fire safety in healthcare building construction [23].

A fire-resistant building material means any material that withstands fire for a sufficient time without melt, and as a result, the residents of that complex can be safely removed from the campus. Therefore, attention towards fire safety is very vital especially in the construction of a healthcare building. To implement the much higher fire-resistant materials to a building construction, considerable screening should be paid on the properties of the materials used. The general data on the fire resistance ratings of some commonly used building materials for hospital building construction are illustrated in Table 12.1.

Table 12.1 Construction materials and their fire resistance properties

Materials	Fire Resistance
Timber 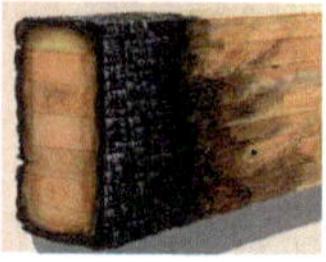	Timber has remained considered as major construction material since ancient civilization. It shows significant resistance to fire as it has low thermal conductivity and self-insulating nature. When timber snaps fire, first it is charred up to a certain depth and that outer charred layers behave like an active barrier and suppress the fire. This property of timber stops the fire by its own property similar to that of the self-insulating behavior of concrete. To make more fire resistant, sometimes such timber is impregnated with different fire-retarding chemicals known as ammonium phosphate, ammonium sulphate, borax & boric acid, zinc chloride etc. The amount of fire retarding chemical will vary depending on degree of protection. For example, in moderate preservation, 32-48 kg chemical is recommended while for higher stability as much as 80-96 kg chemical is mandatory. Currently, fire resistant dye is used on timber to make it more fire-resistant building material. Most common types of timber have charring rates of 20 mm in 30 minutes and 40 mm in 60 minutes. Some hardwoods such as oak, teak and green heart have slower char rates ranging from15mm in 30 minutes to 30 mm in 60 minutes.
Brick 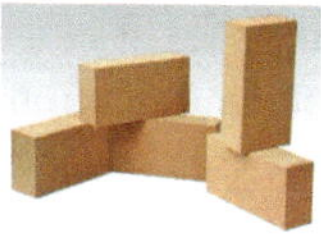	Bricks, one of the oldest and fundamental materials used as construction material since archaic civilizations, mainly used for the development of walls and pavement construction. Due to its poor heat conduction nature, bricks do not show serious damage till 1200-1300°C. The consideration of certain things makes the bricks as good fire resistance which includes Mortar type, Quality workmanship, Clay type and method of masonry construction. Fire resistant bricks are composed of fire kilns and have a high persistence value against much higher heat and temperature. Remember to know that a single brick offers extra fire-resistant property than a wall due to the incorporation of cement, sand and mortar. Walls constructed with bricks provide sufficient protection from fire based on the thickness of the wall during construction. A brick wall is considered as fire withstands material ranging from 60 minutes to 4 hours.
Concrete 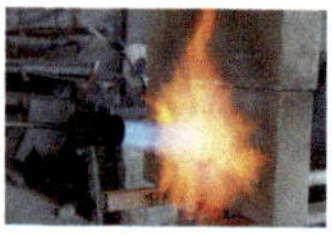	Concrete is the most extensively used fire resistant building element for industrial construction for quite a long time. Presently, its worldwide usage is more than double than that of combined usage of steel, wood, plastic, aluminium altogether because its fire resistance ability is quite outstanding. It offers greater resistance against fire to buildings as compared to steel due to its insulation nature in terms of transmission of heat. Poor thermal conductivity of such material makes the longer period of sustainability for structural, load-bearing capability. Concurrently, it also reduces the spread of fire further. Although, the concrete strength deteriorates noticeably at high temperatures but not much affected up to 250°C. Generally, reinforced concrete structures can repel fire for at least one hour at 1000°C. The fire resistance behaviour of reinforce concrete based on their marginal dimension and the concrete cover to reinforcement distance. For example, 25 mm cover to reinforcement can provide 60 to 90 minutes of stability and up to 45 mm reinforcement can contribute 2 hours of safeguard depending on the structural element.
Reinforcement Steel 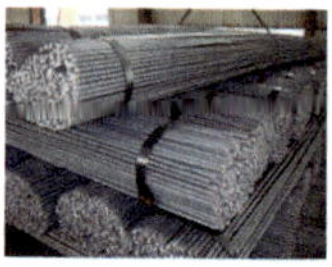	Now a day, reinforcement steel is a type of non-combustible fire-resistant material that is widely used in building structures as a beam, lintel, purlin, walls etc. Additionally, this steel is considered as suitable fixtures and fittings such as guard-rails, stairs, etc. However, this steel is non-combustible but softens as the temperature rises due to its low fire resistance value and this happens because of decreased capacity to resist tension and compression. If temperature rises to 600°C, its yield strength is reduced to 1/3 of its original value and starts melting above 1400°C or more. The molten steel tends to contract when it comes in contact with water spread through fire extinguisher. At that time twisting and distortion also begin because strength of steels already diminished due to melting. As a result, the stability of the structure is affected and prone to failure.
Glass 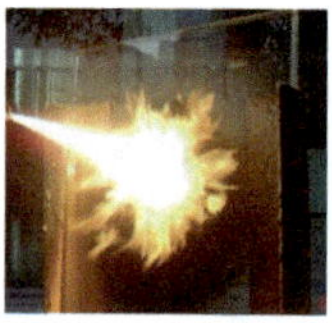	Due to poor conduction of heat and lower co-efficient of thermal expansion, glass become automatic choice as excellent fire resisting material but cracks may develop under soaring temperatures. Reinforced glass panes have been developed and used in glazed windows, doors to solve such problem. Wire interlayer glass, intumescent laminated glass, and pre-stressed borosilicate glasses are dual paneled fire-resistant glasses having high energy absorption rate that makes it four times as stronger than a normal glass window that can achieve a fire rating of up to 60 minutes. Nowadays, PVC or steel frames along with fire-resistant glasses are used instead of wooden frame will establish almost foolproof protection from fire.
Gypsum 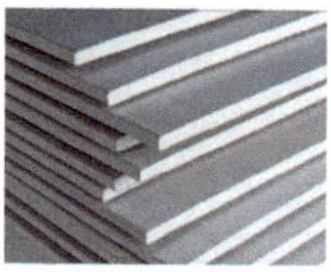	Gypsum, a wonder mineral, commonly used as fire-resistant material suitable for interior design of modern construction. Many structural constituents are put together to fabricate gypsum sheet to achieve good fire-resistant ratings for mitigate any type of fire hazards. The most useful gypsum derivative in the developmental stream is Gypsum Boards which is also known as "dry-walls". These boards comprise a gypsum sheet inserted between paper sheets which are processed through chemical modification to augment the fire-fighting capabilities of gypsum. Presently, architect utilized multiple coats of gypsum layer on dry wall boards to make sure their fire resistance properties of the underlying physical structure get enhanced.

(Source: https://civiconcepts.com/blog/fire-resistant-building-materials)

(ii) Existing Medical Facilities

Refurbishment of existing facilities may improve their fire resistance rating than earlier. For example, drywall gypsum board or reinforced concrete can be replaced with light-framed wooden walls and floors, which can have 60 min of fire rating depending on the board thickness [24].

Well-maintained fire compartment in a hospital building is very vital as it confines fire and smoke to a limited area in the building as well as prevents the spreading of fire vertically and laterally into the adjacent rooms. So, it is the primitive option of passive fire protection because in healthcare occupancies, the primary aim is to restrict the fire spread to the area of fire origin. Boards made of gypsum should be used to intersect the sturdy concrete floors, walls, and others to create uninterrupted fire-retardant barriers. Every fire compartment must have 2 h of fire resistance and also be detached by fire walls and doors. Hospitals are partitioned into several fire cells, and each compartment behaves as a self-sustaining entity through fire protection walls and flooring. In order to establish the integrity of individual compartment, no disparity between the doors, walls, and ceilings is allowed in the healthcare structure.

Fire doors and frames with fire resistance rating should be equipped between individual fireproof chamber and at every landing height of staircase and fire escapes because fire doors act as a passive fire prevention system for healthcare or hospital buildings (Fig. 12.2). During opening, this type of doors provide a passageway for occupants to evacuate to a safety place, and when closed it blocks the spread of fire, smoke, and toxic gases, which may consist of dangerous chemicals. So, a fire exit is

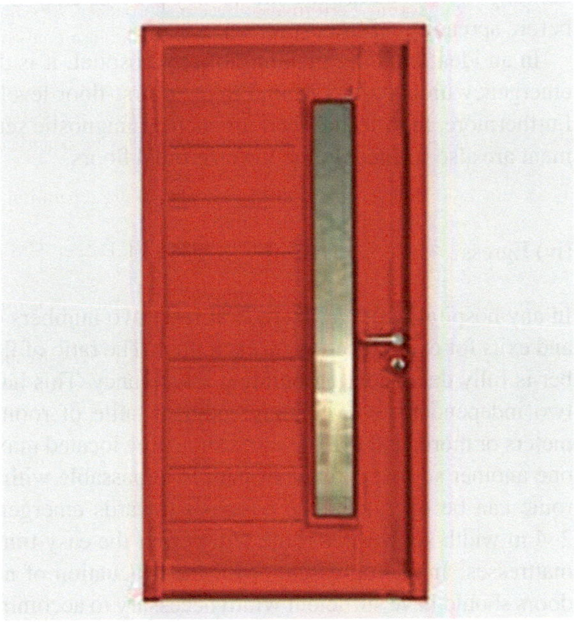

Fig. 12.2 Fireproof door used in hospital (source: http://ggfire-doorssolutions.com)

a key safety ingredient of any healthcare building providing an impediment to avoid or delay the escalation of fire and smoke while allowing a sufficient span to evacuate the incumbent to a safer zone. Since no one can predict when fire hazards will occur in hospitals, we must be prepared enough to respond against it. The presence or installation of fire-rated doors in hospitals and other healthcare facilities minimizes the fire outbreak and reduces the danger of a rapid fire spreading. It is desirable that most of the fire exits installed in each isolated area and section have a minimum 30–90 min of fire rating. Fire gates should have auto-closure.

Existing incendiary materials like wood, flammable liquids, electrical equipment and wiring, combustible metals, medical gases, and cooking appliances must be covered with fire-retardant varnish or other forms of fire-insulating, noncombustible materials; otherwise, discard altogether. Glass-based doors and windows should be fire resistant and durable. In addition, ceiling stoneware, wall, and carpet finishes should also be fire retardant.

(iii) Number of Floors

Number of floors is a major concern during emergency exit or evacuation as if the number of floors in hospital building is more; the evacuation (patients' evacuation in both horizontal and vertical movement) plan of such a building is more complicated.

If land space is not a constraint in healthcare premises, then design and construct a new medical facility by reducing perpendicular elevation and number of floors of the building. It is always preferable to build single-story or two-story, low-surge buildings spread across the site as they provide easy and quick access to evacuation before spreading of fire.

In an ideal building planning of any hospital, it is desirable to set up ICUs and emergency units on the ground floor or first-floor level with devoted ramp facility. Furthermore, high-traffic sections such as diagnostic services and outpatient department are also located on the lower/ground floors.

(iv) Egress

In any hospital building, there is at least two numbers of sovereign egress avenues and exits for every location on each floor. The ratio of floor space and opening number is fully dependent on building inhabitancy. This has endorsed to create at least two independent exits for any room or suite of rooms of minimum 230 square meters or more, and exit passages should be located maximum possible distant from one another so that if one exit path is impassable with smoke or fire, then another route can be operated. The passages towards emergency exits should be at least 2–4 m width so that this route will permit the easy transportation of hospital beds, mattresses, and so on essential for the evacuation of nonambulatory patients. Exit doors should have sufficient width necessary to accommodate a stretcher (minimum

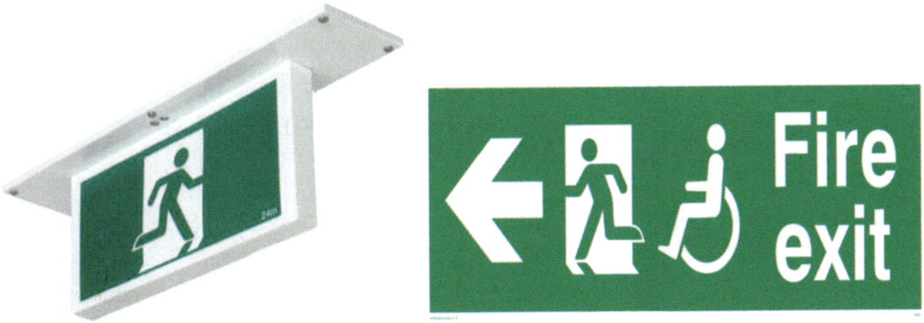

Fig. 12.3 Sign and direction to fire exit (source: https://www.protectorfiresafety.com/)

1.25 m width). Evacuation maps should be displayed at the hospital's main entry points and each floor to clearly describe the egress transmit and exits to all the occupants. Some of the internationally accepted identifying signs are shown below (Fig. 12.3):

The following approaches can also help to reduce the degree of fire hazards:

Prohibiting smoking within the facility—Nonchalance with cigarette flame and other dangerous smoking materials is a predominant cause of fire in healthcare facilities. Designated smoking area and incorporation of large metal ashtrays are the key design to prevent smoke fire. Furthermore, there should be strict prohibition of people from smoking near oxygen supplies and storage of gas cylinder. Proper care is also necessary for electrical cords and electricity-powered tools and equipment as they are one of the major causes for fire outbreak.

Periodical checking should be done to make sure that the electrical cables and sockets are in good, healthy condition with no catastrophe, nicks, or frayed areas. Do not utilize the electrical cables that are bent or carpets or overloaded electrical channels or extension cords. Additionally, reinstate any gadgets, devices, or parts of equipment that produce sparks, smoke, or unusual smells. Be cautious in the areas where fire occurs more frequently. Extra safeguard should be kept in kitchens, dining places, laundry rooms, and any other areas where fires are more likely to happen.

Proper cleaning of washer and drying of lint traps on a regular basis confirm that chances of accumulation of vegetable oil and other flammable materials on kitchen appliances are very little. Storage of flammable substances safely and securely in proper places ensures less possibility of fire hazards.

12.4.2 Fire Suppression

Fire suppression is very crucial to reduce the damage of the property or keep down the loss of human life. Fire response time in any hospital is challenged by limited resident mobility. In order to avoid the worst-case scenario, i.e., evacuation of the hospital, the prime consideration of fire safety system includes quick detection and extinguishing of fires in time. An active fire protection system is of utmost requirement to best protect the residents and other staff during fire in a hospital. The solution should cover several departments as a whole, and in some instances, it operates independently in fire-prone department from the property's electricity.

(a) Fire Alarm Systems

A hospital is a large, constructional complex which usually associates with multiple buildings spreading over a wide area and where various activities go on that cannot be disrupted, even by fire. If an evacuation process is still compulsory, then it is a very tedious and tough performance with many immovable patients.

Fire alarm systems are an utmost important part for hospital safety because they are usually used to notify staff and patients about a fire and also provide the instructions on what to do during this situation. Due to large and complex construction of hospital buildings, the installation of fire alarm systems for healthcare facilities may create a challenge. Fire alarm systems in any hospital typically include smoke detectors, heat detectors, and manual pull stations. The alarm system will activate while a fire is detected and makes a loud sound alarm to notify everyone in the hospital of the fire (Fig. 12.4).

Fires can be detected easily and conveniently by a number of ways. In such existing facilities, well-established and conventional modes of detection are present where when a person generally observes the fire and/or moldy smoke, a consternation system must be activated by him or her or a proclamation issued. In limited incidents, a designated "runner" relays the notification to others over voice messages. In few cases, manually activated alarming devices are used to create sound as fire alarm.

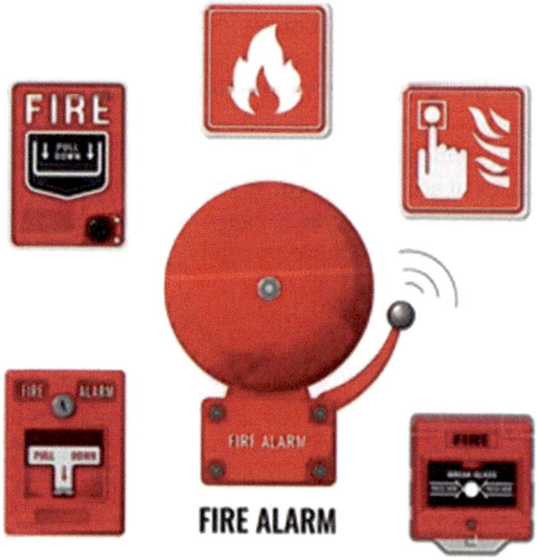

Fig. 12.4 Fire alarm system (source: https://www.istockphoto.com/)

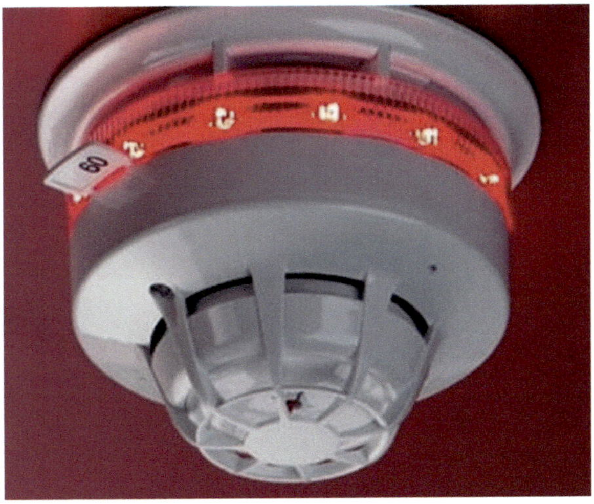

Fig. 12.5 Heat detector alarm (source: https://www.getkisi.com/guides/heat-alarm)

(b) Heat Detector

In any hospital, there are quite a large number of equipment starting from simple ECG machine to complex MRI scanners that engender a lot of heat when they are in operation. Sometimes, these instruments are extremely hot, so it is very crucial to make clear that they do not reach the precarious temperatures, which could make a short circuit. A heat detector will create an alarm sound when temperature goes beyond the threshold value set to indicate the dangerous situation (Fig. 12.5).

This system prevents the fire hazards initiating from overheating of equipment. Another substantive exposure is melting of electrical wire that occurs when the electrical wiring is in contact with heated devices, which make the environment precarious, and the wiring is liable for short-circuiting. A heat detector can fix such a problem by an alarming sound. As a result, mishaps and impairment of equipment are dissipated.

(c) Smoke and Heat Detectors

In a few places of hospital building, there is a lot of overlapping electrical wiring, which enhances the chances of short circuits and electrical fire risk. In those areas, it is very indispensable to have a detector that can easily pick up both, so a fire mishap is managed within a very short period of time (Fig. 12.6).

A range of smoke and heat sensors (ionized, photoelectric, and combined ionized/photoelectric) can be equipped with a fire alarm system to detect fires that begin in low-traffic areas away from personnel/staff. These sensors should activate the intelligent system with flashing visible light and ringing sound alert to signal all about the fire. Furthermore, these devices also identify the exact location where fire was exposed, through a remote-control panel that lights up to indicate the area where the fire detection device was triggered.

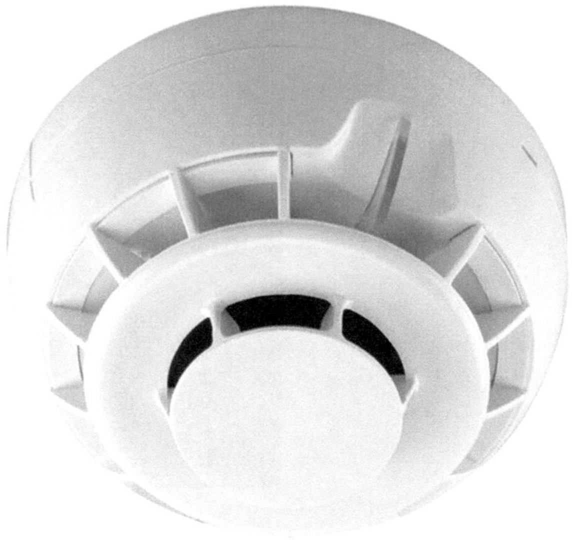

Fig. 12.6 Combined smoke and heat detector (source: https://www.indiamart.com/proddetail/combined-heat-smoke-detector-20529477112.html)

In general, smoke detectors will detect fire much quicker than the heat detectors. However, the designated personnel responsible for the explicit observation of smoke and heat detectors should consider the possibility of any erroneous or unwanted alarms. Otherwise, go for fixed-temperature heat detectors where a sudden rise in temperature is normal for fire. The position of such detectors depends on two factors, i.e., which kind of radar is being used and the geometry and control of the space. Customarily, the maximal covering ranges for smoke and heat detectors are 100 m^2 and 50 m^2, respectively.

(d) Fire Extinguishers

After detection of fire, a suitable elimination process to extinguish the fire is essential to diminish the accident and bypass expulsion. A number of firefighting equipment can be installed in different locations in any hospital to resist certain types of fires, with exceptional attention to the patients possessing various departments and the medical equipment residing within those areas. Six main types of fire extinguishers are available in the form of water, foam, CO_2, powder, water mist, and wet chemical. Each extinguisher is suitable for different classes of fire. Fire-extinguishing devices are labelled with accepted symbols and letters that indicate the classes of fires that they are equipped to fight. The brief description of each fire extinguisher with diagram is given below.

Water Extinguishers

Water extinguishers are called the most cost-effective extinguishers to fight type A fires involving paper, wood, and textiles. Some of these are very safe on electrical equipment although water is a good conductor. It has a red label and i considered as a Class A rating (Fig. 12.7). Four different types of water extinguishers are available in the market such as water spray, water jet, water with additives, and water mist or fog.

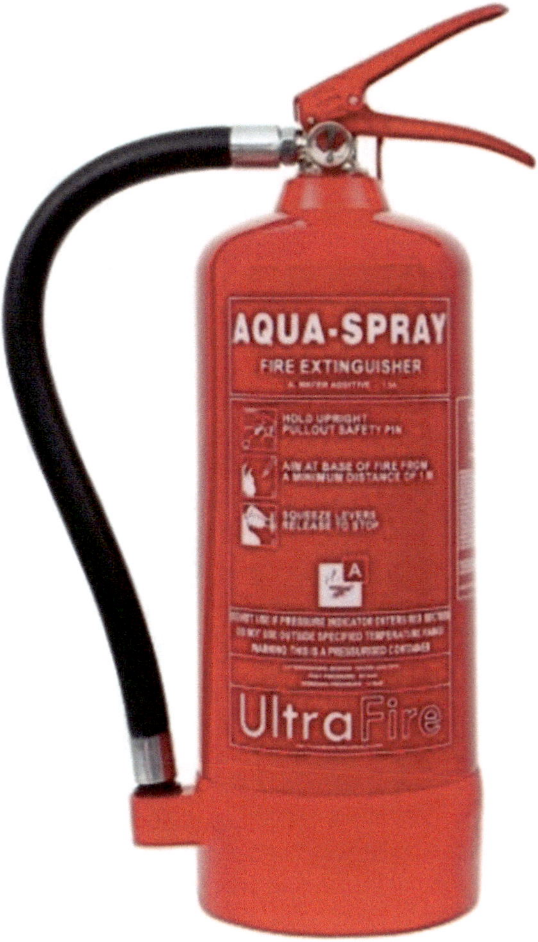

Fig. 12.7 Water extinguisher (source: https://www.safelincs.co.uk/ultrafire-6ltr-water-with-additive-fire-extinguisher/)

Foam Extinguishers

AFFF foam fire extinguishers having cream color label and that are highly impressive on type A and B fires as a foaming agent help to inhibit reignition (Fig. 12.8). They are highly competent in extinguishing fires involving combustible oil like petrol or diesel and more useful than water jet extinguishers as they are highly effective on solid materials like wood and paper. This device extinguishes liquid fires by enclosing the surface of the liquid, preventing flammable vapor from meeting the air, and starving the fire for fuel. They are not impressive against free-flowing liquid fires.

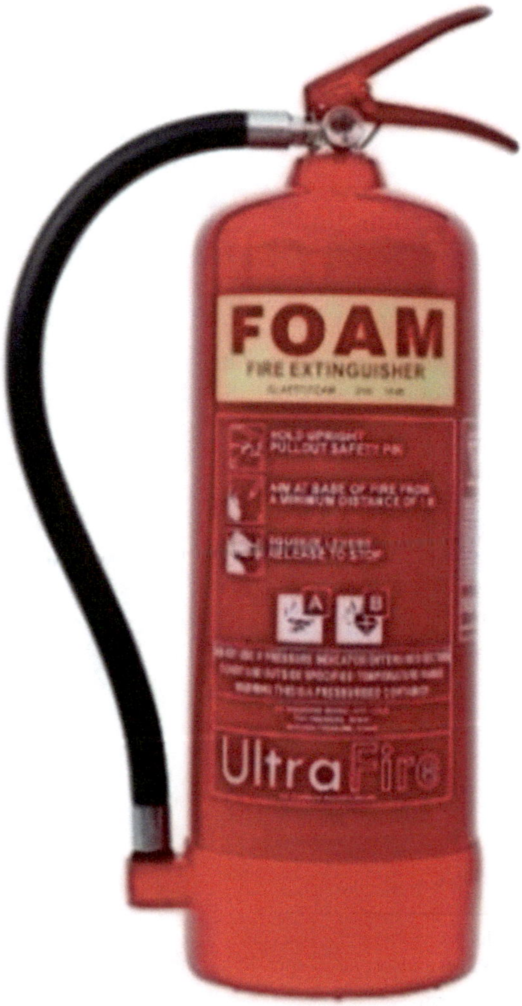

Fig. 12.8 Foam extinguisher (source: laoisfiresupplies.com)

Powder Extinguishers

Blue-labelled powder extinguishers are suitable for group A, B, and C fires and promised for Class D (metal) fires (Fig. 12.9). So, these extinguishers are known as multipurpose fire extinguishers. Although they are very effective on fires involving electrical equipment, they do not cool down the fire and that is why it can reignite. These extinguishers are either copper-based or sodium chloride-based powder that extinguishes fire by isolating and smothering it. These extinguishers are mounted on two-wheel carts and have an operating range of 3–6 ft.

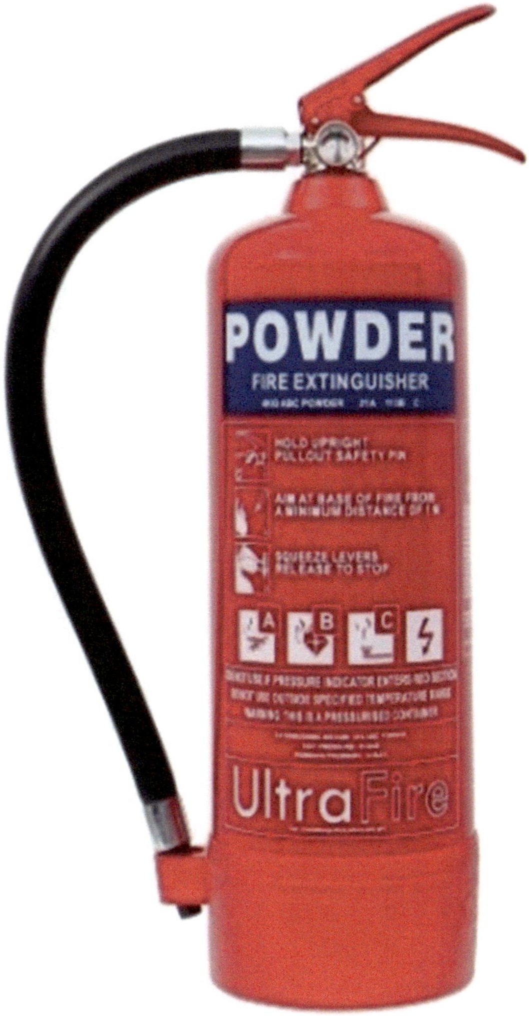

Fig. 12.9 Powder extinguisher (source: indiamart.com)

Carbon Dioxide Extinguishers (CO_2)

CO_2 extinguishers are ideal for places where lots of electrical equipment are there because they are safe to use on fires involving electrical apparatus and have a black label. Unlike foam extinguishers, these extinguishers do not leave any residue because it contains pure carbon dioxide which is a clean extinguishant. They can also be effective for Class B fires involving flammable liquids such as paraffin or petrol and therefore are considered to have Class B fire rating. CO_2 extinguishers work on the principle of smothering the fire and obstructing the supply of air to the fire (Fig. 12.10).

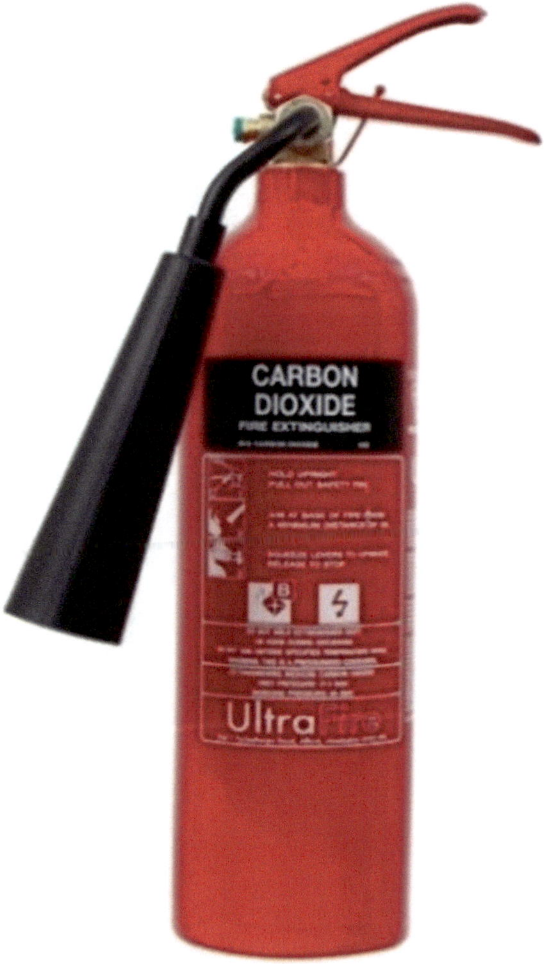

Fig. 12.10 CO_2 extinguisher (source: indiamart.com)

Wet Chemical Extinguishers

Wet chemical fire extinguishers have a yellow label and are designed specifically for use on Class F fires involving combustible cooking oil and deep fat fryers such as lard, olive oil, sunflower oil, maize oil, and butter. They can also be useful on Class A fires (wood, paper, and fabrics) and Class B fires (flammable liquids). If used properly, they are extremely effective. The wet chemical rapidly knocks the flames out, cools the burning oil, and chemically reacts to form a soap-like solution, which seals the surface to prevent reignition (Fig. 12.11).

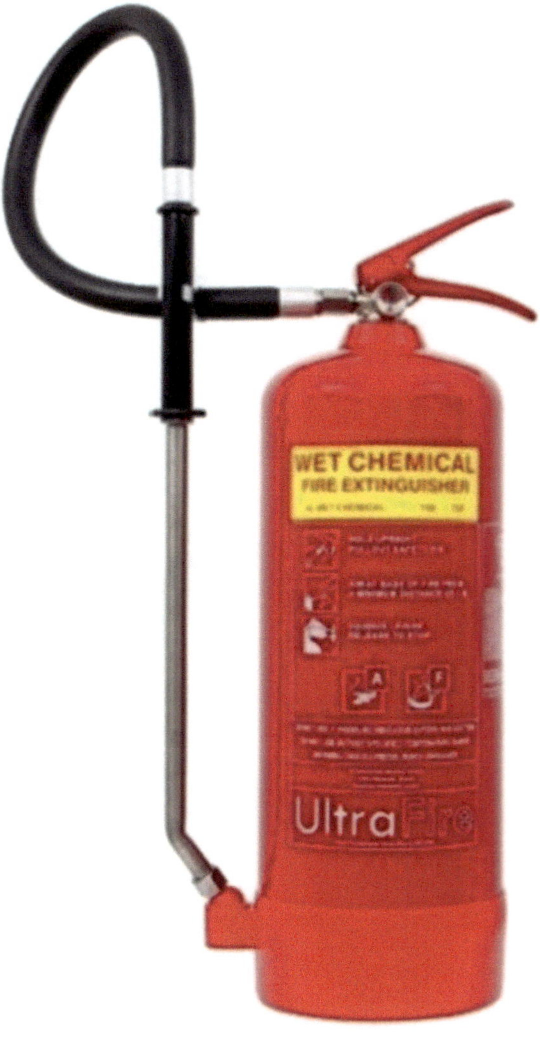

Fig. 12.11 Chemical extinguisher (source: safelincs.co.uk)

They are known to have Class F rating and have a special type of lance applicator nozzle. They usually have an additional Class A rating and are normally not designed for use on Class B fires (petrol, diesel, paint, paraffin, etc.), although the 3 L Gloria wet chemical fire extinguisher is an exception.

Water Mist Extinguisher

Deionized water mist fire extinguishers have a white label and are highly impressive on Class A, B, and C fires and burning electrical equipment (Fig. 12.12). The unique design of the water mist extinguishers having a supersonic patented nozzle creates

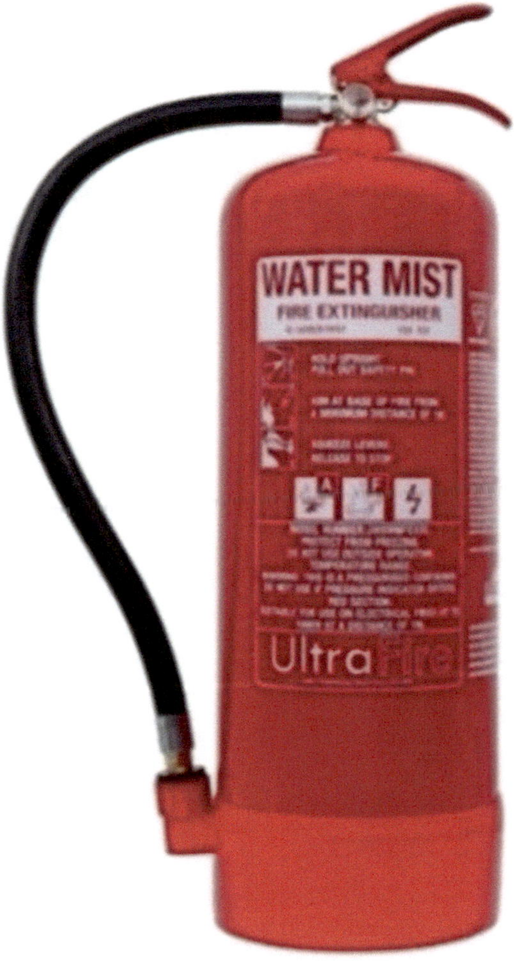

Fig. 12.12 Water mist extinguisher (source: https://www.justfiresafety.co.uk/shop/3-litre-water-mist-fire-extinguisher/)

a microscopic mist curtain by producing over 22 billion water droplets from only 1 L of water, reducing the oxygen content. The droplets are so fine at usually 25 μm in diameter and create an ultrafine mist which has superior firefighting capabilities. Water mist extinguishers are safe and well suited for use on burning electrical equipment as the deionized water mist does not conduct electricity and the water mist does not form puddles which could lead to electrocution. This leaves almost no trace and no collateral damage and leads to the extinguishers often being referred to as "dry" water mist.

Methods of Fire Extinguisher Use

Anyone from fire wardens and hospital staff who is likely to have to use firefighting equipment should be trained on how to use basic fire suppression devices. It is also imperative to select the right type of extinguisher to be used to suppress the fire. The four fundamental steps to be followed for using a fire extinguisher can be remembered through a simple acronym: **PASS** (Fig. 12.13):

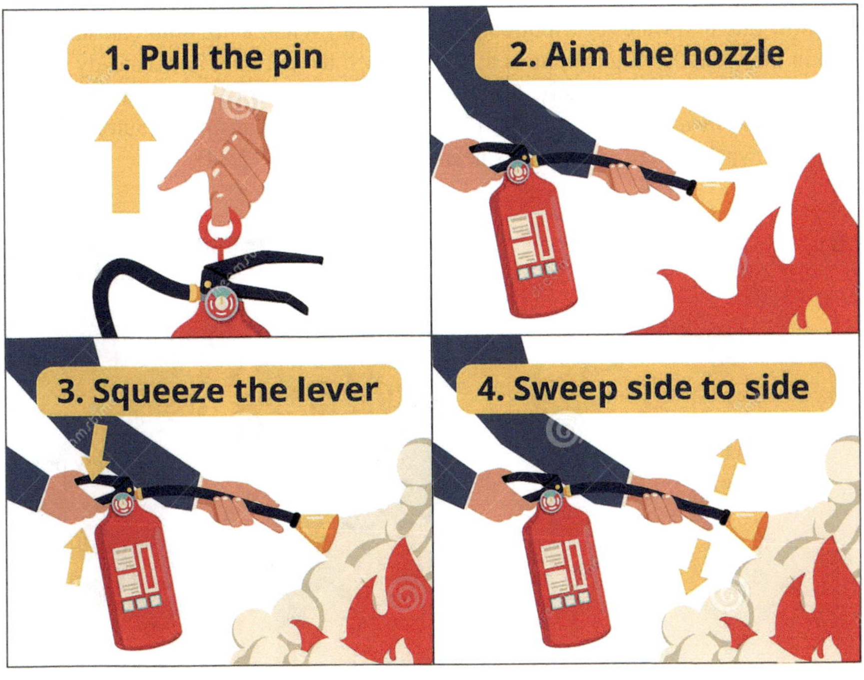

Fig. 12.13 Application techniques of fire extinguisher (source: https://www.dreamstime.com/how-to-use-fire-extinguisher-pass-labeled-instruction-vector-illustration-safety-manual-demonstration-visualization-all-image 204103504)

- **Pull:** Stretching the pin will break the tamper seal. Hold the extinguisher with the nozzle pointing away from the operator and release the locking mechanism.
- **Aim:** Aim low to point the nozzle or hose at the base of the fire. During operation, do not touch the horn on a CO_2 extinguisher as it gets very cold and can damage the skin.
- **Squeeze:** Compress the lever slowly and evenly to release the extinguishing agent.
- **Sweep:** Clear the nozzle from side to side at the base of the fire until the fire is stopped.

(e) Sprinkler System

Apart from fire alarm and fire extinguisher, there are other fire suppression devices that can be installed in a hospital to improve the facility's resilience to fire hazards. A sprinkler system is an active firefighting device that is installed in most of the buildings of any hospital as a preventative measure. The head of the sprinklers is fixed in the ceilings facing towards the floor or any fire hot spots. The other end of the sprinkler system is connected to a water supply system having adequate pressure and flow rate to a water distribution piping system. When a fire outbreak starts, the seal in the sprinkler head ruptures at a predefined temperature and a steady stream of water flows at high pressure. So, a sprinkler system implemented in fire control in a hospital means protecting a building against fire by causing an automatic discharge of water, usually from pipes near the ceiling (Fig. 12.14).

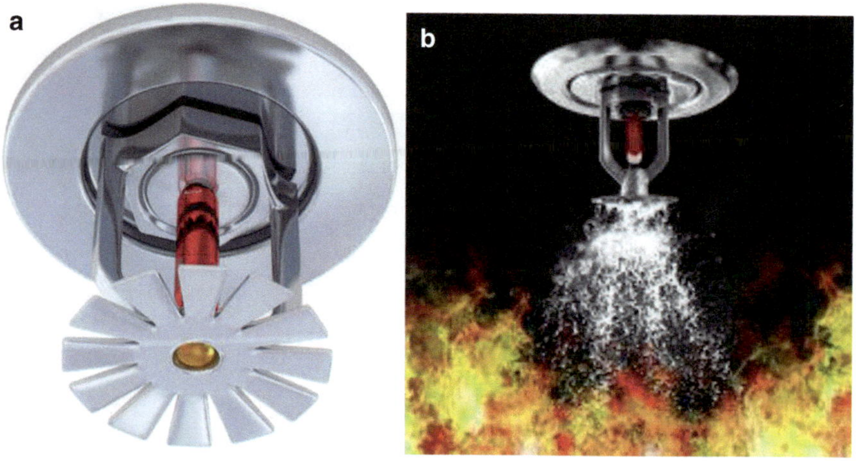

Fig. 12.14 Sprinkler system: (**a**) wall mounted and (**b**) operational procedure (source: https://www.123rf.com/photo_25658719_close-up-image-of-fire-sprinkler-on-white-fire-sprinklers-are-part-of-an-integrated-water-piping-sys.html)

Therefore, **sprinkler systems** are intended to either control the fire or suppress the fire in hospital buildings, and it is installed either by building codes or as per the recommendation of insurance companies to reduce potential property losses or business interruption. Automatic sprinklers are placed at specific locations after connected to the water pipeline system. A high-pressure water sprinkler system can turn down the effect of fire without requiring much water. In fact, they are reported to reduce injuries by up to 80% and reduce property damage by up to 90%.

Fire sprinkler systems (both water and mist sprinkler) are suitable for outdoor areas and spaces where electrical wiring is not too much. This system is also useful in the cafeteria, canteen, or terrace to save precious time and gain control over the fire.

The main drawback of sprinkler systems is its high cost; that is why they are quite expensive to incorporate into existing hospital facilities. A fire safety specialist should investigate the building's structural and architectural layouts to determine the feasibility of installing a sprinkler system.

(f) Fire Hose Reels

Fire hose reels are commonly installed in areas with a high fire risk to provide a reasonably accessible and controlled supply of water to enhance firefighting capacity compared to conventional fire extinguishers (Fig. 12.15). The length of a fully extended fire hose is typically 18–36 m with an internal diameter varying from 13 to 19 mm. These appliances are designed in such a way that it can deliver a minimum 330 mL of water per second. Depending on the size of the medical facility, the size of the hose reel is determined.

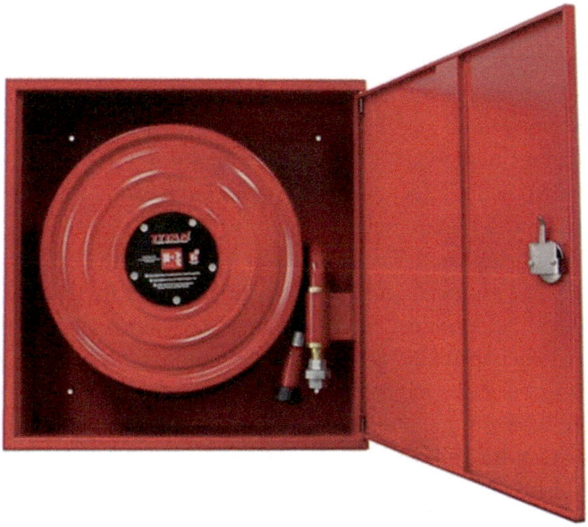

Fig. 12.15 Properly installed fire hose reel (source: https://www.indiamart.com/proddetail/fire-hose-reel-with-30-meters-hose-13724517973.html)

The direction and flow of water to the fire are controlled by attaching a nozzle to the end of the hose reels. All fire hose reels typically consist of a unique ball valve shutoff device, a plastic or solid brass hose reel nozzle, and mounting bracket. Fire hose reels are used to fight Class A fires only.

The operating procedure of fire hose reels is as follows:

- Make sure that the jet-type nozzle is in the closed position.
- Swivel the main valve.
- Turn the hose off the drum and direct towards the fire.
- Unlock the nozzle or valve and direct the flow of water to the fire.

(g) Smoke Extractors

In any event of fire, there are highest risks of human life due to the rapid spread and faster accumulation of smoke. One of the possible ways of minimizing this danger is by incorporating smoke extraction systems conventionally in the initial design of heat, ventilation, and air-conditioning (HVAC) systems.

Smoke extraction systems are basically mechanical systems, which can be manually or automatically activated after the triggering of the alarm.

These systems are specially designed to discard the hazardous smoke from the fire area and intercept the spread of smoke to other areas of the building through the vents and the high-pressure pumping of air to specified areas to arrest the ingress of smoke (Fig. 12.16). The incorporation cost of the smoke extraction system in the existing facility is quite high.

(h) Planned Preventative Maintenance

One of the most crucial features of an effective suppression system to mitigate fires is planned preventative maintenance. Inspection of fire suppression systems should be performed regularly and documented as a part of standard healthcare facility management system [25]. After checking, the equipment should be properly tagged and signed off for safe use with an indication of any action taken, and also mention the next scheduled check date.

The National Fire Protection Association (USA) endorses that smoke detectors must be replaced after 10 years. However, if they are battery operated, smoke detectors should be checked every month as part of standard hospital maintenance [26].

Water sprinkler systems should require both planned preventative maintenance and robust reactive maintenance procedures. Particularly, heads of the individual sprinkler are typically maintenance free. Therefore, costs are mainly related to maintaining the system through weekly tests and upkeep of water supplies and pump equipment.

Fire hose reels should be checked properly and signed off periodically.

The hospital administration should ensure that the ISO-certified hose reels are used to combat fire hazards by the fire service each year. Inspections of equipment should be carried out on an ad hoc basis after its use in a fire incident.

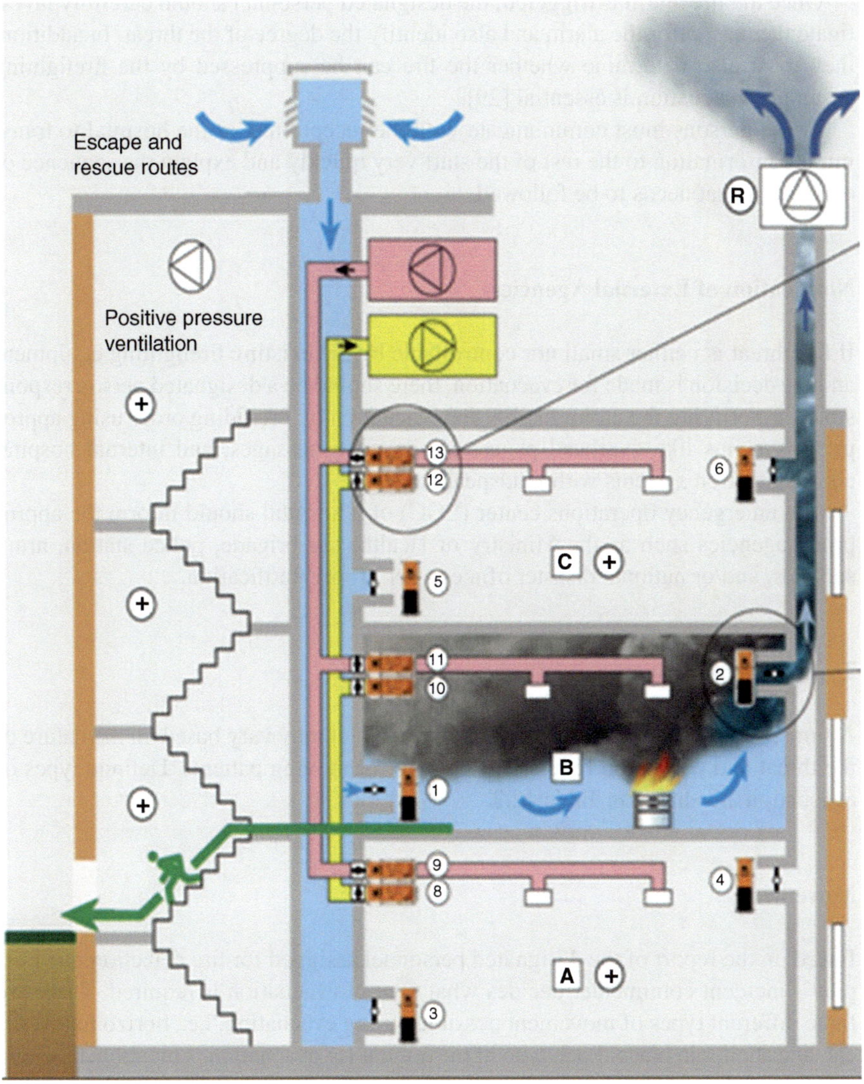

Fig. 12.16 Designing of smoke extractor (source: https://labmonline.co.uk/features/understanding-design-application-smoke-shafts/)

12.4.3 Evacuation

This is a crucial component that is aimed to save the life in extreme emergency situations like fire outbreaks in hospitals [27]. An exhaustive and clear evacuation plan needs to be placed in such a location where all staff members are aware of and are experienced in carrying out this procedure. The evacuation procedure will vary for every healthcare facility because there is no standard method of evacuation [28].

Once the fire alarm is triggered, the designated personnel should carefully investigate the reason for the alarm and also identify the degree of the threat. In addition, they must also determine whether the fire can be suppressed by the firefighting system or evacuation is essential [29].

Those persons must communicate with the receptionist of the hospital to transmit the information to the rest of the staff very quickly and explain the sequence of evacuation that needs to be followed.

Notification of External Agencies

If fire threat is neither small nor controllable by the existing firefighting equipment and the decision is made for evacuation, there should be a designated person responsible for notifying the entire facility for evacuation by providing order using appropriate systems like overhead pages, emails, text messages, and internal hospital communication systems with loudspeakers.

The emergency operations center (EOC) of a hospital should inform the appropriate agencies such as the Ministry of Health, fire brigade, police station, army services, and/or national disaster offices after proper notification.

Types of Evacuation

A time frame for evacuation is very decisive, and it may vary based on the nature of the threat and the period required to prepare for moving patients. Definite types of evacuation are shown in Table 12.2.

Movement

Based on the report of the designated personnel assigned for fire detection, the hospital's incident commander decides what type of evacuation is required. There are three different types of movement possible during evacuation, i.e., horizontal, vertical, and shelter in place. Each type of movement for evacuation is mentioned below:

Table 12.2 Types of evacuation vs. required steps

Types	Steps
Immediate	Emergency move means there is no time to prepare; evacuate the patients and staff immediately
Rapid	Evacuate the occupants as quickly as possible and safely from the area. There is very limited time to prepare, i.e., 1–2 hrs. Follow the evacuation procedure
Gradual	No immediate danger as there is sufficient time for evacuation process (many hours to several days)
Prepare only	Although patient movement is not required, begin to prepare for evacuation

Horizontal: The most fundamental way of evacuation is the horizontal type that involves eloquent patients in immediate vicinity of danger being taken away from the warning zone but kept on the same floor in a safe position.

Vertical: This movement usually concerns about the complete evacuation of a specific floor in the hospital. Patients and staff will be evacuated out of the hospital through such movement only if required.

Shelter in place: The staff may be instructed to "shelter in place," which means they remain in their units and wait for further instructions.

Evacuation Routes

Evacuation routes should be clearly established and displayed in each floor properly. All hospital staff should have a clear idea about evacuation routes and, based on the type of evacuation, take one route as instructed by the hospital's incident commander. After that, wardens or health and safety officer will direct patients and visitors to evacuate the area orderly and patiently. Proper evacuation planning must be considered for all the spaces surrounding the hospital premises, which will assist in the expansion of emergency transit routes, gathering areas, estate, and so on.

Level of Evacuation

The scale of evacuation during emergencies can be divided into two categories namely:

1. Full evacuation
2. Partial evacuation

In most emerging situations, a complete evacuation will not be essential. Due to the complex building setup and vulnerable condition of many hospital patients, evacuation is generally considered as the final step of rescue. Evacuation should be ordered only during extreme emergency and when there is a forthcoming or inherent unmitigated threat to patient/staff safety if there are serious hazards due to fire, smoke, and structural breakdown of the facility.

Evacuation Transport Equipment

For safe evacuation of patients having functional disability or mobility impairment from a hospital building during emergency, it is essential to have proper transportation equipment available for them. This evacuation transport equipment may include blankets, wheelchairs, beds, canvas stretchers, backboards, sked stretchers, etc. Some of the transportation equipment like backboards and sked stretchers are usually not kept in the hospital but provided by the national disaster office, the fire brigade service, or the defense force members.

There are some important practical points to be considered when using transportation equipment in a hospital for emergency evacuation such as the following:

(a) Adequate number of transportation aid should be available to evacuate each floor of the facility.
(b) Transit facility should be stored in areas that are easily accessible at all times; it should not be stored in locked closets.
(c) All the mobile carriers should be part of the regular facilities planned for preventative maintenance program.

12.4.4 The Important Safety Measures in Hospital to Mitigate Fire

Fire safety in a hospital is a prime benchmark that needs to be contemplated during the design and construction of a hospital building. In comparison with the normal buildings, it is a very tough exercise to expel people from the wards as most of the patients are in serious condition. It is so deplorable that there are some hospitals where fire safety norms and guidelines are not followed properly.

The hospital training and learning aim to criticize that most of the staff did not have any knowledge on fire safety and the steps that need to be applied to face the hardship. In addition, the highly reliant, immovable, and critically ill patients make it a harder and arduous task to vacate the hospital building in a scramble.

Hospitals and other medical premises need to concentrate more on the easy and safe evacuation methods as healthcare practices are responsible for the safety and security of the people inside the hospital wards and they are expected to adhere to the legally approved fire safety measures and codes.

Emergency management plan (EMP) against fire outbreak should be updated with national as well as international standard so that it can stand against the unexpected mishaps of a fire in a hospital. Some of the important fire safety measures of a hospital that are highly effective are shown below.

- **Detailed Action Plan**—During fire disasters in any places especially in hospital, there are no time and space for thinking. Comprehensive plan will save time for thinking and support us to react instantly in the right way. For a successful execution of the action plan, involvement and coordination between all the departments of the hospital are essential.
- **Establish the Incident Command Structure**—Proper transmission of command has an imperative influence in diminishing the catastrophe caused by a fire accident. Therefore, establishment of a functional incident command structure having groups and subgroups is a prerequisite to mitigate fire hazards. The people present in groups and subgroups will form an effective tree of communication and follow the instructions that are circulated from the group leader.

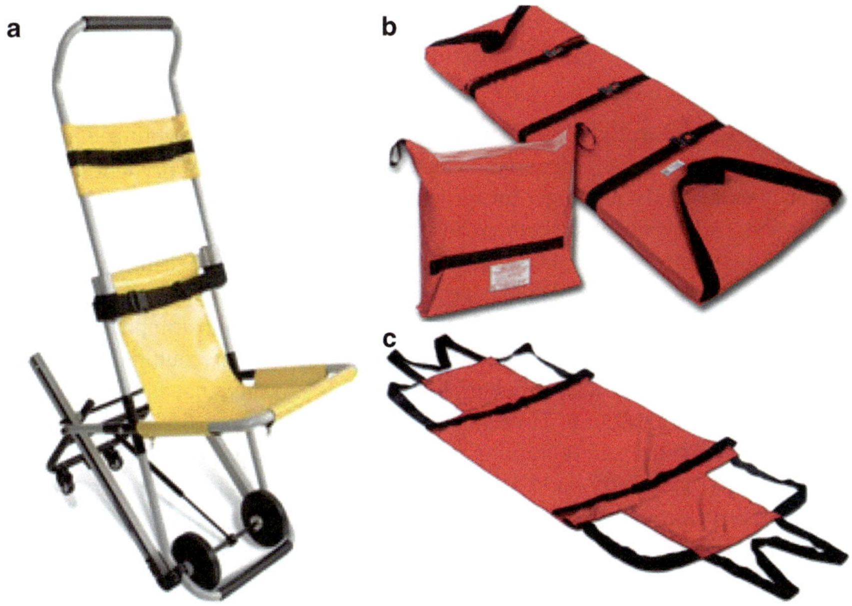

Fig. 12.17 Fire safety evacuation aids: (a) chair, (b) mattress, and (c) sheet (source: https://www.f1train.co.uk/Evacuation-Mattress/)

- **Instructions for a Fire Safety Management Team**—Fire safety management team should involve in the hospital planning from the very beginning, and opening the doors of conversation with this team well in advance will minimize the devastation caused by the fire mishap. Keeping the communication gates always open with the fire safety management team will keep the disaster to a minimum.
- **Fire Safety Evacuation Aids**—The fire safety evacuation aids will help us to evacuate the patient smoothly and safely as hospital evacuation procedure is a very challenging task due to immovable patients (Fig. 12.17). There are three variants of evacuation aids available in today's market such as the following:
  - ***Evacuation chairs***—This type of safety aid is ideal when electronic support is needed for the evacuation or rescue of people very fast on stairs, both up and down the stairs. They are convenient for all stairs except round stairs and stairs more than 40° steep. Evacuation is possible with one person, but there is no problem to evacuate two people at a time.
  - ***Evacuation mattresses***—It is a suitable alternative when evacuation chair is not available. With this, a patient is literally towed away from his or her immediate surroundings. Evacuation mattresses are suitable for all types of stairs for two people always.
  - ***Evacuation sheets***—This aid is ideal for evacuating bedridden patients. The evacuation process is successfully applied with the mattress of the hospital bed beneath which an evacuation sheet is attached. An evacuation sheet can be useful for vertical and horizontal evacuation, on all types of stairs.

So, the hospitals must be equipped with expulsion chairs, sheet, and mats that could grip the patient securely while sliding to a safer location within a short period of time.

- **Checking of Firefighting Equipment**—A number of firefighting equipment used in hospitals such as smoke detectors, fire extinguishers, fire alarms, emergency exit signals, and other fire-protecting devices should be checked regularly for satisfactory fire management to combat outbreak. Conduct a performance checking of all the firefighting apparatus while doing the fire drills to ensure the smooth function to combat the disaster.
- **Fire Safety Training**—Fire safety training is one of the most important considerations to reduce the damage and save lives during a fire outbreak mainly in healthcare premises. In any modern hospital, it is expected that all the staff members of this organization have sufficient knowledge about fire safety and also undergone the fire safety training programs and participate in mock drills. This program will not only build a responsive and reliable team against fire but also establish a safe and secured ambience that intercepts fire accidents.

  Prevention is always better than cure. So, prepare a list of hazards that can create fire accidents and make the system aware of those fire hazards and their preventive methods.

  A hospital should always carry a high-risk symbol of fire accidents for all its oxygen cylinders and medical equipment utilized for patient care. In the present situation, it should be ensured that the whole system of any hospital is intricate with fire prevention by taking proper safety measures, make sure that all the fire safety equipment are intact and operational, and all the staff members are reliable during emergency and have undergone the fire safety training.

12.5 Innovative Equipment for Firefighters

To mitigate fire hazards, some innovative equipment are evolving as new firefighting equipment that include firefighting robots, impulse firefighting gun, horn and strobe, etc. The details of some innovative equipment are explained here briefly.

12.5.1 Firefighting Robots

Firefighting robots can battle some utmost fires where people stay cautiously at a safe distance as they are unable to reach. A US-based company has designed such firefighting automatic devices that can be impressive against the fires which are too treacherous for human firefighters. Currently, two firefighting robots named **Thermite** and **FireRob** are fabricated using aluminum of aircraft-standard and high-quality steel, which is able to combat the exceptionally soaring fire

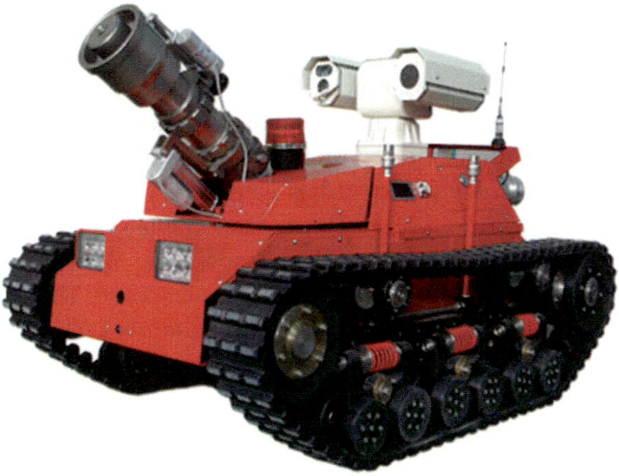

Fig. 12.18 Firefighting robot (source: https://www.indiamart.com/proddetail/fire-fighting-robot-22971638388.html)

temperatures. Both the robots can inject 2500 gallons and 1250 gallons of water per minute, respectively, which is a strength that is comparable with the aggregate force of as many as eight people to control.

Considering certain assignments in mind, robotic firefighting systems are designed, which include inspecting and finding fires, performing inquiry and relief, and investigating hazardous factors along with the most fundamental exercise of fire management and elimination (Fig. 12.18).

Firefighting robots are of two types: fixed robotic system and mobile robotic system. Fixed firefighting robotic systems are used in heavily populated and hazardous areas for rapidly extinguishing any threat which is just like a sprinkler and alarm. This type of robotic system is based on UV or IR sensors. On the other hand, mobile robotic firefighting systems are available in the form of remote-controlled vehicles affixed with fire suppression tools like water or foam hoses. They are competent to travel into those areas not safe for people through an array of sensors, visual camera, and more other technologies that transmit information for navigation to a remote operator. For example, Varun is an all-round compact unmanned ground vehicle specially designed to support the troops and firemen in the risk zone. This system is specially built for Indian condition that is able to move on all types of terrain. This robot will be actuated and monitored from a far distance from the fire zone and controlled by a remote control with multiple functions.

So, firefighting robot system is designed to supplement the function of fire workers by keeping them out of extremely dangerous situation but not to replace the human firefighters. This advanced technology can be operated from a quarter mile away and helps to reduce the people's exposure to extreme fires. Firefighting robots can run for about 20 h without refilling.

12.5.2 Impulse Firefighting Gun

As time is the most crucial factor during fighting against fire, the impulse firefighting gun can control the flames and smokes within a few minutes. The impulse firefighting gun fabricated by IFEX Technologies behaves more like a shotgun than a fire-eating device, but it has incredible power to control and diminish small and large fires (Fig. 12.19). Due to its portable shape, this system can be executed very fast to conceal the fires prior to spreading and it substantially lowers the reaction time between alarms and firefighting response. This instinct gun exploits a mixture of compressed air, water, and foam additives to smother the blazes from a secure length ranging between 20 and 52 ft, but it is most effective from a distance between 20 and 32 ft.

The impulse gun is featured with two cylinders, i.e., one cylinder is loaded with a fire-extinguishing material and the second cylinder is packed with compressed gas. Once firefighting gun releases the water valve, water is pushed into the pipeline for discharge. Pulling the trigger makes compressed air to expel the water or water-foam combination at a speed of about 400 km/h. Only water may be used to douse the fires caused by electrical machineries with high voltage, but foam additives can provide additional power to fight against liquid sparks.

Firemen operate this gun in consolidation with a backpack or trolley that enables an easy and faster attack on fires. This gun is different from traditional or typical firefighting arrangements due to higher pace of water. The tremendous kinetic energy of an instinct shot enables a firefighter to precisely invade into a large, cooling blast deep into the heart of a fire. The rapid variation in air pressure caused by the solidified air also refrains the fire of oxygen, annihilating it expeditiously.

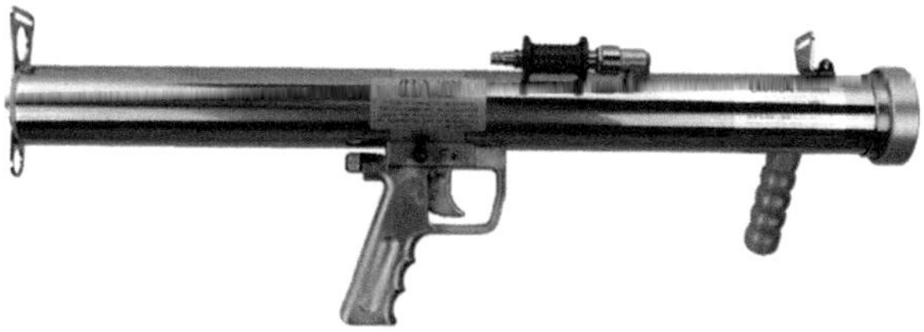

Fig. 12.19 The impulse firefighting gun (source: https://www.ifex3000.com/en/impulse-firefighting-gun/1-litre-impulse-firefighting-gun-3001/)

12.5.3 Horn and Strobe

The horn and strobe (sound and light) device is a fire alarm device that is a very crucial unit to any installed fire system. It is intended to notify the presence of fire to the occupants through high-pitched alarm along with a beaming light. This device is designed to be a part of reliable emergency evacuation and fire-alerting systems in high-rise buildings, hospitals, hotels, and public facilities (Fig. 12.20).

The horn produces a loud sound for a quick evacuation while the strobe flashes the light for people with hearing impairment. In addition, beaming lights can act as a guidance for the residents through the smoke during a safe evacuation. The strobe must be installed everywhere in the building like hallways, restrooms, and corridors to make sure that the alarming light is clearly visible. Horn and strobe fire alarms offer flexible application features that are installed with any desired system.

This modern fire alarm system can be set off either publicly or privately depending on the requirements. In a hospital, it should be set in public mode so that all the occupants of the target area are notified to self-evacuate. The visual intensity of the strobe is adjusted as per the need and situation. The strobe's light covers a wide area where the beaming light would be visible to the residents of that place. Horn-strobe alarm systems are ideal for people with hearing impairment during an emergency event because loud noise accompanied by beaming light will alert them about the fire. This alarm device is perfect for big buildings having many floors, units, sections, etc. Major advantages to this system include adjustable volume settings, low current requirement, and being economical to use.

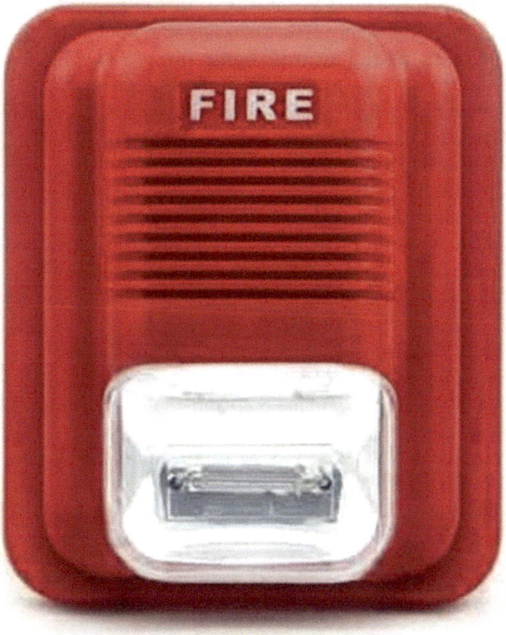

Fig. 12.20 Modern fire alarm system—horn and strobe (source: https://www.indiamart.com/proddetail/fire-alarm-hooter-21111761191.html)

12.6 Conclusion

In the present scenario, fire hazard is more common in hospitals because in the last 10 years there have been several large and medium fire mishaps in hospitals. So, prevention of fire hazards in hospital premises is one of the most challenging and tough jobs. To mitigate fire hazards, several steps are considered for existing facilities and new hospitals are planned by adhering to the NABH guidelines and maintaining rules and regulation with proper building codes and safety measures. Sufficient numbers of smart evacuation transport equipment should be kept in the hospital to save the life of endangered people. In addition, some innovative firefighting equipment such as firefighting robot, impulse firefighting gun, and horn and strobe are developed for rapid cushioning of fire that can be installed as a safeguard. Therefore, proper planning, suitable fire suppression equipment, and fire safety training to all the staff members will effectively mitigate the fire outbreak in a hospital.

References

1. Salamati Nia S P & U. Kulatunga U (2017): Safety and Security of Hospitals during Natural Disasters: Challenges of Disaster Managers. *Int. J. of Safety and Security Eng.,* 2017; 7(2): 234–246.
2. Francescutti LH, Sauve M & Prasad A S (2017): Natural disasters and healthcare: Lessons to be learned. *In Healthcare Management Forum 2017.* Sage Publications, Los Angeles, CA, 2017; 30(1): 53–55.
3. Sharma R, Bakshi H & Banerjee A (2020): Fire Safety Hazards: How Safe Are Our Hospitals? *Indian J Community Med.* 2020 Jan-Mar; 45(1): 104–105.
4. Nagral S (2012): Fire in a hospital. *Indian J Med Ethics.* 2012; 9: 76–77.
5. Quintiere J G (2016): Principles of fire behavior, *Chap. 10. CRC Press*, Boca Raton.
6. Moran FE (2017): Hospital Fires: *What are the Hazards*? 2017.
7. Danzi E, Fiorentini L & Marmo L (2021): FLAME: A Parametric Fire Risk Assessment Method Supporting Performance Based Approaches. *Fire Technology*, 2021; 57: 721–765.
8. Chowdhury K. Fires in Indian hospitals: Root cause analysis and recommendations for their prevention. *J Clin Anesth.* 2014; 26: 414–424.
9. Akhtar N, Ansar F, Baig MS & Abbas A (2016): Airway fires during surgery: Management and prevention. *J Anaesthesiol Clin Pharmacol.* 2016; 32(1): 109-11.
10. Cordero I (2015): Electrosurgical units - how they work and how to use them safely. *Community Eye Health.* 2015; 28(89): 15-6.
11. Rocos B & Donaldson LJ (2012): Alcohol skin preparation causes surgical fires. *Ann R Coll Surg Engl.* 2012; 94(2): 87-9.
12. Gavin Stormont G, Anand S & Christopher M. Deibert CM (2021): Surgical Fire Safety. *Stat Pearls*, 2021.
13. Muchatuta N A & Sale S M (2007): Fires and explosions. *Anaesthesia& Intensive Care Medicine,* 2007; 8(11): 457–460.
14. Dhaliwal N, Bhogal R S, Kumar A, Gupta A K (2018): Responding to fire in an intensive care unit: management and lessons learned. *World J. Emerg. Med.*, 2018; 9(2): 154-156,
15. Jones TS, Black IH, Robinson TN & Jones EL (2019): Operating Room Fires. *Anesthesiology.* 2019; 130(3): 492-501.

16. Choudhry AJ, Haddad NN, Khasawneh MA, Cullinane DC & Zielinski MD (2017): Surgical Fires and Operative Burns: Lessons Learned From a 33-Year Review of Medical Litigation. *Am J Surg*. 2017; 213(3): 558-564.
17. Hart SR, Yajnik A, Ashford J, Springer R & Harvey S (2011): Operating room fire safety. *Ochsner J.* 2011; 11(1): 37-42.
18. NPFA 550 (2007): Guide to the fire safety concepts. *National Fire Protection Association,* Quincy, MA.
19. Reiling J; Hughes R G & Murphy M R (2008): The Impact of Facility Design on Patient Safety. *Patient Safety and Quality: An Evidence-Based Handbook for Nurses*. 2008.
20. Mankar D (2019): Hospital Fire Safety Management: Review on Planning and Safety Measures. *Int. J. of Emerg. Science and Engg*., 2019; 6(2): 1-4.
21. Campbell R (2017): Structure Fires in Health Care Facilities, *National Fire Protection Association*, Quincy, MA, UAS, 2017.
22. Kobes M, Helsloot I, De Vries B & Post J G (2010): Building safety and human behaviour in fire: A literature review. *Fire Safety Journal*. 2010; 45(1):1-11.
23. Reinhardt T & Ottmar R (2004). Baseline Measurements of Smoke Exposure Among Wildland Firefighters. *J Occup Environ Hyg*. 2004, 1(9): 593-606.
24. ISO 16732-1 (2012): Fire safety engineering—fire risk assessment—part 1: general.
25. Banerjee N, Chatterjee S & Chatterjee S (2015): Fire Risk assessment in high rise hospital building in Kolkata: safety issues from ergonomics perspective, in *Proceedings of the 13th International Ergonomics Conference, Humanizing Work and Work Environment*, Mumbai India, 2015.
26. Sarsangi V, Saberi H, Malakutikhah M, Sadeghnia M, Rahimizadeh A & Aboee Mehrizi E (2014): Analyzing the risk of fire in a hospital complex by "fire risk assessment method for engineering (FRAME)," *International Archives of Health Sciences*, 2014;1: 9–13.
27. Boyd A, Chambers N, French S, Shaw D, King R & Whitehead A (2014): Emergency planning and management in health care: Priority research topics. *Health Systems*, 2014; 3(2): 83–92.
28. Wabo N C, Örtenwall P & Khorram-Manesh A (2012): Hospital evacuation; planning, assessment, performance and evaluation. *Journal of Acute Disease*, 2012; 1(1): 58–64.
29. Cagliuso, N V, Leahy N E & Sandoval M (2010): Developing the hospital emergency management plan. *Health Care Emergency Management: Principles and Practice'*, Jones and Bartlett, Sudbury, MA, 89–110

Chapter 13
Principles and Implementation of Quality Management and Patient Safety Systems in Hospital

Maheshkumar Patel and Kiran Harikumar

13.1 Healthcare Quality Management: Journey

Quality management in healthcare is a promise made to the public by various health sectors, working towards the goal of providing the best possible services for each patient. First, in 1914, Dr. Ernest Codman initiated a healthcare quality initiative and challenged physicians to take a responsibility for the patient [1]. He invited physicians for the compilation of information and data and analysis of surgical outcomes. Dr. Ernest recorded relevant patient information on a pocket-sized card, which he used to evaluate and study outcomes. After these next few decades, focus preliminarily remained on assessing the poor outcome and identifying deficiencies in healthcare practitioners and possible measures taken for improvement. During the 1960s, Avedis Donabedian created the Donabedian model framework for examining health services and evaluating the quality of healthcare. According to this model, the information about the quality of care can be drawn from three categories: structure, process, and outcomes [2].

This model influenced many practitioners to identify different ways to improve patient outcomes in the broad area of the structure, process, and outcome.

Quality management in healthcare has observed a paradigm shift from expecting errors and defects to considering that a perfect patient experience is achievable. Philip Crosby supports the same principle that the system for causing quality is prevention and not an appraisal. The literature suggests that the causes of death for many patients in hospitals are medical negligence and nosocomial infections. These deaths can be easily avoided by incorporating a quality management program.

M. Patel (✉)
Aster DM Healthcare, Dubai, United Arab Emirates

K. Harikumar
Primary Health Care Corporation Qatar, Doha, Qatar

D. Bhatia et al. (eds.), *A Guide to Hospital Administration and Planning*,
https://doi.org/10.1007/978-981-19-6692-7_13

Table 13.1 Deming's 14 points of quality management

1.	Create constancy of purpose towards improvement of product and service, with the aim to become competitive and to stay in business, and to provide jobs
2.	Adopt the new philosophy
3.	Cease dependence on inspection to achieve quality
4.	End the practice of awarding business on the basis of the price tag. Instead, minimize total cost. Move towards a single supplier for any one item, on a long-term relationship of loyalty and trust
5.	Improve constantly and forever the system of production and service, to improve quality and productivity, and thus constantly decrease costs
6.	Institute training on the job
7.	Adopt and institute leadership. The goal is to help people and equipment to do a better job
8.	Drive out fear, so that everyone may work effectively for the company
9.	Break down barriers between departments
10.	Eliminate slogans, exhortations, and targets for the workforce asking for zero defects and new levels of productivity to only create adversarial relationships, as the bulk of the causes of low quality and low productivity belong to the system and thus lie beyond the power of the workforce
11a.	Eliminate work standards (quotas) on the factory floor. Substitute leadership
11b.	Eliminate management by objective
11c.	Eliminate management by numbers and substitute leadership
12a.	Remove barriers that rob the hourly worker of his or her right from the pride of workmanship. The responsibility of supervisors must be changed from sheer numbers to quality
13.	Institute a vigorous program of education and self-improvement
14.	Put everybody in the company to work to accomplish the transformation. The transformation is everybody's job

Source: Deming, W. Edwards. Out of the crisis (MIT press) (1986:Pp. 23–24)

Shewhart highlighted that the aim of manufacturing companies shall move from inspection and specification to focus on reducing the variation in the production process and meeting customer product expectations [3]. Deming was influenced by Shewhart, recognized quality as a key driver of companies, and percolated these message methods to Japanese engineers and executives. His quality control methods helped post-World War II Japan rebuild its devastated economy and led to significant success during the 1950s and thenceforth. Deming's 14 Points [4] on Quality Management (Table 13.1), or the Deming Model of Quality Management, a core concept for implementing total quality management (TQM), is a set of management practices to help companies increase their quality and productivity. During the 1980s–1990s, contribution of Crosby [5], Deming [4], and Juran [6] was well known in manufacturing companies across the United States. Their effort took attention to overall system design, process management, and importance of the involvement of the entire team in improvement. Considering this hospital & healthcare governance team initiated using these concepts to drive organization leaders to look at quality from different lenses.

Concomitantly around 1985s, accreditation bodies and various organization forums got intensively involved in the collection and assessment of the quality of data. Chassin and Galvin highlighted the concerns of underuse, misuse, and overuse

Table 13.2 Clinical quality problems in health service provision

Overuse: The potential for harm from a health service exceeds the possible benefits
Underuse: A health service that would have produced a favorable outcome was not provided
Misuse: A preventable complication occurs with an appropriate service

Adapted from Chassin MR, Glavin RW. The urgent need to improve health care quality: Institute of Medicine National Roundtable on Health Care Quality. JAMA. 1998;280(11):1000–1005

in medication and called attention to practice variation in medicine and to the suboptimal patient outcomes associated with this variation (Table 13.2) [7].

To Err Is Human: Building a Safer Health System was a landmark report issued in November 1999 by the U.S. Institute of Medicine that estimated that thousands of people will die from medical errors every year. This report led to a significant increase in the awareness of US medical errors, and the push for patient safety that followed its release continues. The report was based upon an analysis of multiple studies by a variety of organizations and concluded that between 44,000 and 98,000 people die each year as a result of preventable medical errors [8].

The high-value clinical care results from the most efficient cost of achieving a high level of clinical quality. Successful implementation of Six Sigma results in virtually no defects. No model has proven to be the best in quality management. Healthcare providers want to continually improve the care they provide. However, different tools or models may work in different scenarios, and to succeed it is vital to have a commitment from the governance and leadership team. Healthcare systems need proper support and control methods. The quality of healthcare comes from its fundamental parameters. According to the Institute of Medicine, the services are of quality while they are safe, effective, patient centered, timely, efficient, and equitable.

13.1.1 Components and Elements of Quality Management Program in Hospital

The components of a quality management program are often grouped into three levels:

- The strategic or organizational level from governance and leadership team—dealing with the quality policy, objectives, and management and usually produced as the quality manual
- The tactical or functional level from the managerial level who are dealing with general practices such as training, facilities, and operation of quality management

- The operational level dealing with the standard operating procedure (SOP) worksheets and other aspects of day-to-day operations such as a nurse, paramedic, and support staff

The Quality Manual

The quality manual is composed of the management documents needed to implement the quality management program. Please refer to some common topics included in the quality manual:

- Quality policy statement
- Objectives and scope of quality management
- Organization and management structure and relationship between management, technical operations, support services, and quality system
- Job description for key staff members
- Reference to relevant organization policies, manual, and operating procedures
- Document control and maintenance procedures and processes to ensure tracking of all procedures, data, and reports

Departmental Policy and Manual

All concerned stakeholders such as physicians, nurses, paramedics, pharmacists, and support staff shall be appropriately involved in the development of the departmental policies and manuals, which are based on hospital quality policy and manual. The supervisory staff is responsible for the development and implementation, while the operational staff provides technical expertise and advice. All employees must be trained on organization quality management programs and departmental policies and manuals. Also, at all stages, service personnel must be consulted on the practical aspects of any proposed change. It is their responsibility to notify the management of any concerns, issues, or changes that may affect the organization's quality program. The management shall support the allocation of appropriate resources, approve projects, assign responsibilities, and maintain accountability.

Standard Operating Procedures

Standard operating procedures are an essential tool for gaining control over your daily operating system or processes. Standard operating procedures (SOPs) explain the subtle details in documents that describe all specific operations and methods, e.g., medication prescription, dispensing, and administration. They are an internal reference guide for a specific procedure, and each appropriate step should be described. Anyone with the appropriate skill level should be able to follow the SOP. They should cross-reference and refer to other SOPs as needed. The procedure should be written in short, clear sentences. Also, well-developed SOPs cater as an effective communication tool that contributes to employee understanding and job satisfaction. The most technically competent person should write an SOP to carry out the described procedure [9].

Training and Development

It is essential to train all staff on organization quality policies and its objectives and department policies, procedures, and SOPs. Each staff member shall receive ongoing training to maintain and advance his or her skills and knowledge. Training is crucial for any organizational growth and success, and it is essential for both employers and employees of an organization. There is much to be said for the role of practical education in a discipline dealing with the practical application of research; there is a great deal to be gained through providing those who will practice quality improvement with a sound knowledge of the theory behind it [10]. For developing a training plan, the hospital shall gather data from all relevant sources to understand its staff's ongoing education needs. Also, we need to consider the results of quality program activities as one source of information to identify staff education needs. Organization leadership supports the commitment to ongoing staff education, and adequate resource is deployed or arranged for facilities, educators, and time for ongoing in-service education.

Auditing and Maintaining Quality Assurance

When all quality assurance system documents are available, they should be tested. During this time, the quality assurance team should conduct a series of audits covering all aspects of the system. Quality consistency is achieved by defining the variables, including error definitions and their point values, and then applying the standard method for identifying errors. In order to maintain a quality management system, compliance in each area of the system should be checked periodically. This involves auditing the structure, process, or outcome to assess whether they continue to meet the defined standards or guidelines. The audit procedure should be documented formally. Data traceability is an important factor that can be verified by randomly sampling the data and tracking the data in all relevant documents before sampling. At the end of each audit, a system overview with clearly defined strengths and areas of improvement should be created. Reports of all audits should be made available to the leaders and concerned stakeholders who are responsible for the relevant work. A concerted plan should be developed to address observed deviations, and necessary corrective and preventive measures should be taken. The audit should be independent involving a multidisciplinary team where appropriate and should be comprehensive and preferably conducted at a regular workflow as an announced or unannounced audit. Feedback organizations must ensure consistency in the application of the program among all quality assurance staff. Collaboration and training of stakeholders are key to achieving and maintaining compliance.

13.1.2 Common Quality Improvement Methods and Tools

Process Mapping

Process mapping involves reviewing the entire process through a variety of techniques, including photography, video recording, field observations, interviewing and feedback from stakeholders, and role-playing as needed. Process mapping allows review and mapping of the entire patient journey or pathway with all stakeholders. It aids in identifying inefficiencies, non-value-added steps, duplication, variation, discrepancies, and opportunities for improvement.

Used for?

Map the process or pathway to identify process improvement opportunities.

When to Use It?

When the process or pathway is complex with associated inefficiencies.

How to Use Process Mapping Effectively?

Process mapping is key for any quality improvement project; hence, start with a high-level process map, outline the scope of the process and key issues step-by-step, and create a more comprehensive process map. This exercise provides all participants with broad insights into the process under consideration and, in contrast to the participants' ideas, shows exactly what is actually happening. Process mapping promotes ownership of employees in each phase of the process and allows all concerned stakeholders to share views to avoid the domino or adverse effect of changing one phase of a process to another phase. Mapping should be done between teams and departments, showing the entire process from start to finish, allowing quality improvements to flow between teams and departments. Below is the high-level map by a detailed process map, which looks at the MRI investigation process carried out in a major hospital (Fig. 13.1) [11].

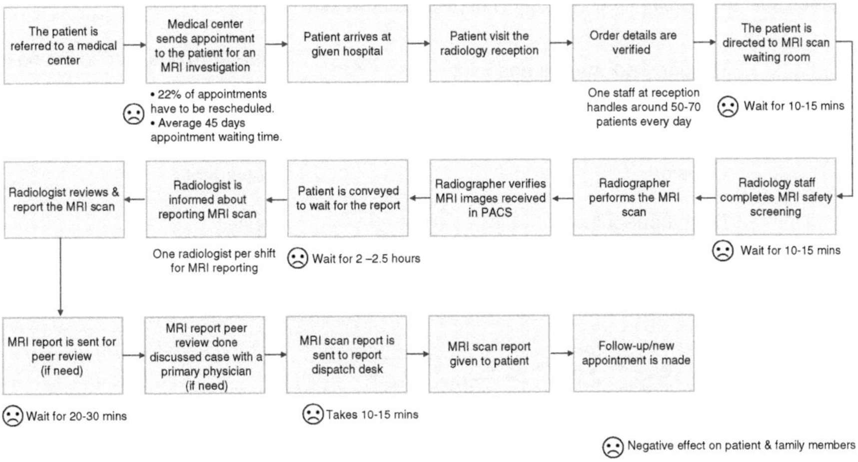

Fig. 13.1 Sample process mapping

Flowchart

The flowchart shows the individual steps of the process in sequence. A flowchart identifies the beginning, between, and end of the process and how one part of the process is dependent on another. It is a generic tool that can be used for different purposes and can be used to describe different processes, e.g., blood sample transportation process and admission process. It is one of the widely used analysis tools and also one of the seven basic quality tools. The elements that can be included in a flowchart are a series of actions, materials, or services that go in and out of the process, decisions made, stakeholders involved, time involved in each step, and/or process measurements.

Used for?

To identify or to know the actual flow of events in a process that follows.

When to Use It?

When any process needs improvement or to know the complexity and recognize the non-value-added loops and identify where simplification and standardization may be possible. It can also be used to weigh the actual flow of the process against the ideal flow to identify opportunities for improvement.

Table 13.3 Commonly used in symbols in detailed flowcharts

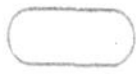	Use for mark start or endpoint	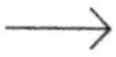	Flow from one step to the next one
	Process		Link to another
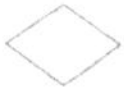	Decision	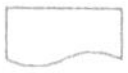	Document
	Data-Input-output		Delay

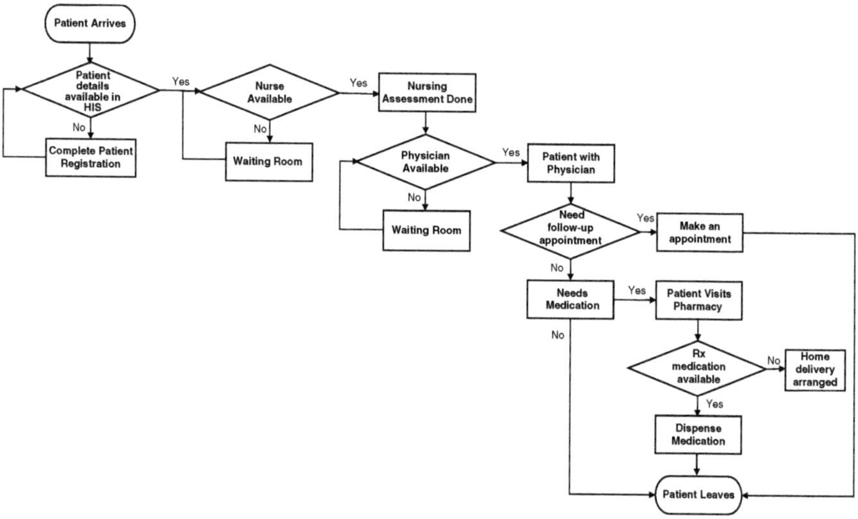

Fig. 13.2 Example of outpatient physician consultation visit flowchart

How to Use a Flowchart?

First, start with identifying the boundaries of the process, and clearly define where the process begins and ends. It is essential to identify and involve all concerned stakeholders in the charting process. This includes doctors, nurses, paramedics, managers, supervisors, biomedical engineers, pharmacists, housekeepers, etc. whoever are involved in the selected process. All stakeholders should decide on the level of detail to be included in the flowchart. To have a brainstorming session about the process and identify, then write each step of the flow and arrange the activities in proper sequence. Once all the activities are included, review the activities, have concurrence from all members that the sequence is correct, and draw arrows to show the flow of the selected process. Please refer to Table 13.3 to know what is commonly used in symbols in detailed flowcharts (Fig. 13.2).

Clinical Audit

A clinical audit is a quality improvement method that helps to measure the gap between ideal practices, which are determined from evidence and guidelines and actual practices. A clinical audit is not done to pinpoint the patient care team or individual practitioners but aims to improve the system in individual work. If it is applied correctly, the clinical audit can bring changes and improve practice and patient outcomes and enhance safety and clinical effectiveness.

Used for?

To check the delivered clinical care meets the defined clinical guidelines or protocol and monitor improvement to address identified noncompliances.

When to Conduct a Clinical Audit?

Clinical audit is often used on an ongoing basis to measure compliance against evidence-based clinical guidelines and standards or as a quality improvement initiative to assess the clinical outcome based on the care delivered.

How to Use It Effectively?

Clinical audit is a multidisciplinary team activity wherein aspects of structure, process, and outcome (Table 13.4) of care are selected and evaluated against the criteria derived from evidence-based clinical standards. The clinical audit process typically involves the following steps:

- Select the clinical audit topic based on the organization prioritization matrix.
- Select the criteria based on objective measures.

Table 13.4 Example of structure, process, and outcome criteria

	Structure	Process	Outcome
Criteria	Staffing in the NICU	Door to balloon insertion time	Surgical site infection rate
Target	1:1 nursing staff for ventilated patient	<30 min	<1%

- Define and design the data collection tool and decide on data collection methodology and sample size.
- Multidisciplinary team conducts the audit and collects the data.
- Data analysis, interpretation, and identification of improvement, and develop an action plan to address deficiencies.

The clinical audit cycle cannot be completed until there is evidence that changes are made on identified areas of improvement and have been effective. Typically, clinical audits are often carried out retrospectively; however, growing digital technology also enables the team to record ongoing real-time data collection. The clinical audit findings identified areas of improvement, and the action required should be shared with all concerned clinical care team members to facilitate learning.

Plan-Do-Study-Act

This process is also referred to as the Shewhart cycle or PDSA method. It is the quality improvement model that is a combination of building and applying knowledge to make a continuous improvement. PDSA (Plan, Do, Study, Act) iteratively helps to evaluate the impact of test changes and ensures that new ideas improve quality before they are rolled out on a large scale. Since process changes can lead to unexpected results, it is safer and more efficient to test quality improvements on a small scale prior to large-scale implementations, and a sample of relevant stakeholders has been suggested. You can evaluate the execution of changes. With the introduction of these small changes, it is also possible to test the interaction with other systems without having a significant impact on the quality of service; for example, pilot a new fall risk assessment tool in one unit with a limited patient group before using the new tool across the facility patients.

Used for?

Use for potential quality improvements, test them, and make small improvements before implementing them on a large scale.

When to Use It?

If you need to change a process or system, or if you want to introduce a new procedure, process, or system.

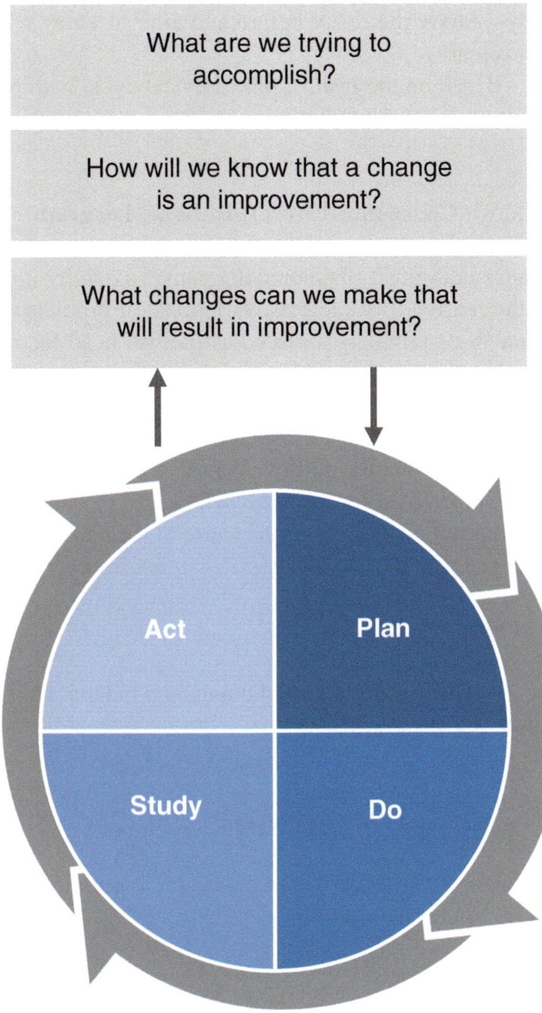

Fig. 13.3 Reference—key topics in healthcare management: understanding the big picture. (By Robert Jones, Radcliffe Publishing, 2007)

How to Use PDSA Effectively?

Processes or systems that require change, or new processes or systems that are planned and implemented on a small scale for a specified period of time with a minimum cohort of stakeholders (do), evaluated (study) and adjusted (act), with repeated PDSA cycles, until it is fit for purpose and wholesale implementation. Engaging all concerned stakeholders in all four phases of the PDSA cycle facilitates involvement in proposed changes and provides input for adaptation when potential users are aware of barriers to change. Please refer to the PDSA cycle (Fig. 13.3) [12]:

Plan—the implementation you are going to do.
Do—Carry out the test or changes preferably on a small scale to start with.

Study—Study the result before and after to know whether a plan works and what was learned.
Act—Based on the results, plan the next cycle with required changes and/or go for full-scale implementation.

Ishikawa Cause-and-Effect (Fishbone) Diagram

A cause-and-effect (fishbone) diagram is a quality improvement tool that helps find out the reason(s) for defects, variations, or problems within a process. The defect, variation, or problem is placed as the fish head facing on the right and the causes extend to the left as the bones of the skeleton; the ribs branch off the back, branch reflects the major cause, and sub-branches denote root causes. The fishbone diagram enables the source of a defect, variation, or problem to be identified so that resources for quality improvement can be appropriately directed towards the true cause, rather than towards the symptoms. A fishbone diagram is often used as a reactive method to identify the cause of the defect, variation, or problem.

Used for?

Use to identify the physical, human, and hidden and real causes of events affecting the service or product.

When to Use a Fishbone Diagram?

To identify the root causes of events for quality improvement which is affecting the service or product.

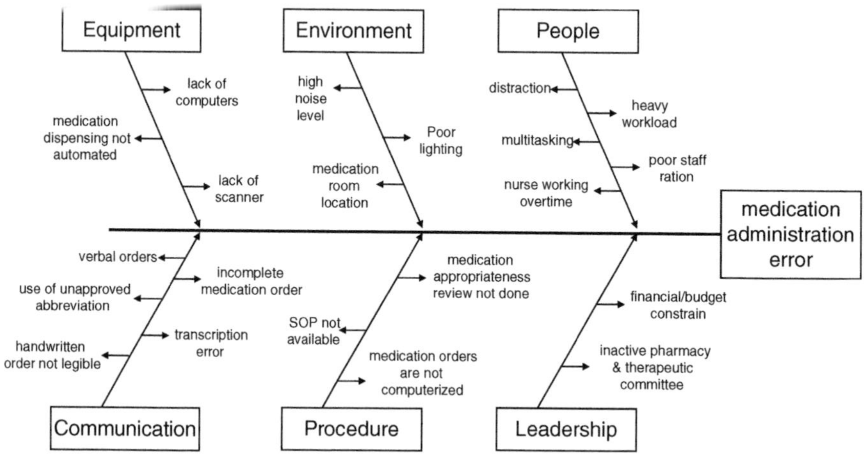

Fig. 13.4 Sample medication administration error in fishbone diagram

How to Use It Effectively?

The fishbone diagram helps identify a wide range of all possible causes behind the defect, variation, or problem and the associated effects. The defect, variation, or problem is placed as the fish head facing on the right, e.g., medication administration error; the causes extend to the left as the bones of the skeleton; the ribs branch off the back; the branch reflects the major cause such as process, environment, manpower, and material; and sub-branches denote root causes. All direct and indirect concerns of stakeholders such as physicians, nurses, and pharmacists should be involved in conducting the root-cause analysis using a fishbone diagram to identify the cause of the defect, variation, or problem. In an event when the patient is affected, then whenever appropriate the patient or family member should be involved to add their valuable perspective and insight during a root-cause analysis process. The fishbone diagram allows identifying the cause of a defect, variation, or problem so that efforts and resources for quality improvement can be appropriately navigated towards the real cause of the deviation, variation, or problem, rather than towards the symptoms (Fig. 13.4).

Statistical Control Chart

The process typically has two types of variation, abnormal variation that arises under unusual circumstances and normal variation that occurs under normal conditions, and often can be traced to a source or cause. The control chart is a graph used to investigate how a process changes over time. The data is plotted in a chronological order. The control chart always has a central line for the average, an upper line for the upper control limit, and a lower line for the lower control limit, and these lines are derived from historical data. By comparing the present data with these lines, we conclude whether process variability is consistent (controlled) or unpredictable or uncontrolled, affected by a particular source of variation. The statistical control chart has been widely used in many other industries to control quality in the management process. It is known as one of the seven basic quality tools.

Used for?

Often it is used to measure and control processes against predefined parameters.

When to Use Statistical Control Chart?

When determining whether a process is stable or requires monitoring and control to maximize its full potential. Also, to analyze patterns of process variation from unusual causes or common causes and to determine whether quality improvement

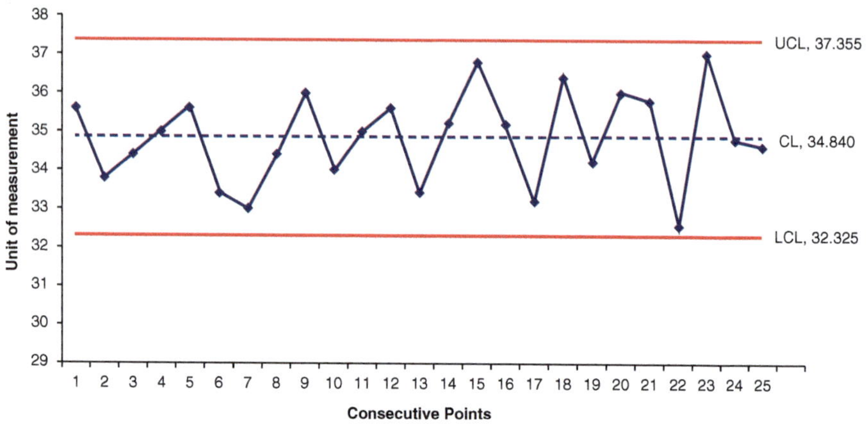

Fig. 13.5 Sample statistical process control chart

should aim to prevent specific problems or to make an essential change to the process.

How to Use It Effectively?

A lower control limit and an upper control limit are set using standard deviations from past or baseline data, and outputs are plotted for variation in quality (Fig. 13.5). Data must be collected for charting and for statistical rigor, and the number and frequency of measurements are important; the more measurements that are charted, the graph will give a more robust overview of variation in output. Analysis of variation makes it possible to identify shortfalls in the baseline and highlights opportunities for improvement. Such gaps require targeted investigation, process modification, and ongoing monitoring to know that the changes made have reduced variation or led to further variation, which may appear at a different point within the process. Control charts can be used throughout the life cycle of a process improvement project, during project identification, setting baselines, checking progress, reviewing the project impact, and knowing whether the changes made are sustainable.

Healthcare Failure Modes and Effects Analysis (HFMEA)

Healthcare failure modes and effects analysis (HFMEA) is a systematic, proactive quality improvement method for process evaluation, used to identify where and how a process might fail and to assess the relative impact of different failures, for identification of the process elements in most need of change. HFMEA includes a review of the following [13]:

- Steps in the process

- Failure modes (what could go wrong)
- Failure causes (why would the failure happen)
- Failure effects (what would be the consequences of each failure)

Used for?

It is used to systematically and proactively evaluate the processes to identify improvement opportunities.

When to Use HFMEA?

When a process needs a meticulous and systematic review and further improvement to avoid failure.

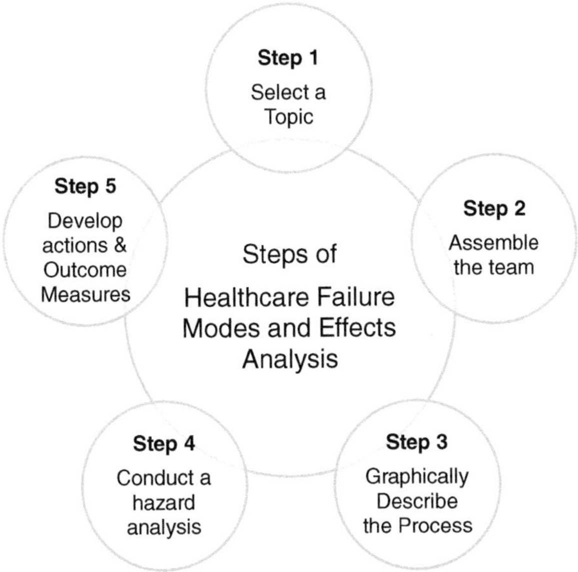

Fig. 13.6 HFMEA steps (source: Cohen, M. R., & American Pharmacists Association. (2006). *Medication errors*. Washington, DC: American Pharmacists Association)

How to Use It Effectively?

The multidisciplinary team collaborates to conduct HFMEA to prevent errors by proactively reviewing and modifying the process, rather than responding to post-error adverse events. Focusing on prevention reduces the risk of harm to patients, visitors, and staff. HFMEA is especially useful for assessing new critical processes prior to implementation or for evaluating the impact of proposed changes on current critical processes.

Failure mode contains any issue or process that could go wrong and that can prevent the execution of process steps. There are multiple possible causes for each failure mode. The causes are prioritized, eliminated, controlled, or accepted by systematic risk classification.

Control measures should be included in the process as early as possible. You can manage a single hazard with multiple controls, and each control can be used multiple times in a process. To seek feedback from the process owner or representative, each recommended process change requires simulation for testing before it is implemented across the facility. Please refer to the HFMEA steps (Fig. 13.6) [14].

Pareto Chart

A Pareto chart is a bar graph; it helps to show the relative contribution of the different causes of the problem. The Pareto principle states that 80% of the results are determined by 20% of the causes. So, one should try to find 20% of the types of issues and defects that cause 80% of all problems. Pareto chart bar lengths represent frequency and are arranged with the longest bars on the left and the shortest bars on the right. Thus, the diagram clearly shows which situations are more significant. Without analyzing or inspecting the data, the leaders may assume that all causes contribute equally to poor quality or that one or more causes are the leading ones.

Used for?

To identify the most common causes resulting or leading to poor quality.

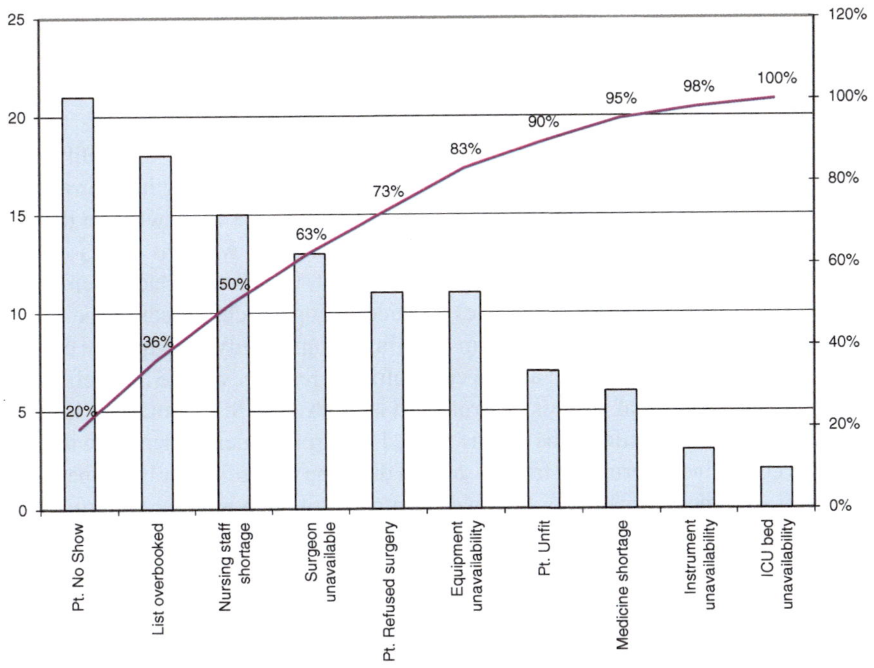

Fig. 13.7 Sample surgery OT cancellation—Pareto chart

When to Use Pareto Chart?

When analyzing data about the frequency of problems or causes in a process. There may be many problems or causes, but only a significant one or more causes needs focus for quality improvement.

How to Use It Effectively?

The multidisciplinary team collaborates to identify the causes resulting in poor quality using the Pareto chart. A multidisciplinary team should group the causes into specific categories and choose appropriate measurements. The team shall define the period of the time chart, which will cover and use the data collected and compute the subtotal for defined categories. Then adjust the scale of the left axis to accommodate the largest subtotal from the different defined categories. Based on those constructed bars, the tallest bar is at the far left, and the shortest bar is at the far right. The percentages for each subtotal category are then calculated, dividing them by the total of all categories that represent 100%, as indicated by the right vertical axis. The cumulative sum is calculated, starting from the far left to the right, and a line graph represents the percentage of the sum relative to the right vertical axis. Please refer to the sample Pareto chart (Fig. 13.7).

Six Sigma

Six Sigma is a data-driven methodology that provides tools and techniques to define and evaluate each step of a process and seeks to improve flow in the value stream and eliminate waste. The aim of Six Sigma is to achieve a level of quality that resides in the 6-standard deviation of average performance, resulting in an error rate of 3.4 defects per million opportunities. Six Sigma uses the framework to define, measure, analyze, improve, and control (DIMAC) process, which is a data-driven quality strategy used to understand root causes of variation, reduce them, and improve processes. Six Sigma provides a structured approach, to reduce the variation in medical services; it also helps in ensuring a consistently high-quality patient experience, reduces waste, and aids in concentrating resources in the most effective locations. The statistical process control chart is a subset of Six Sigma, and it helps in monitoring the variation. The data is plotted in chronological order, showing the average centerline determined from historical data, the upper line for the upper control limit, and the lower line for the lower control limit bounds. After the process is set up, it helps in concluding the variability of the process by comparing the current data with these lines.

Used for?

To evaluate the systems to study the cause of variation, to eliminate waste, and for continuous improvement.

When to Use Six Sigma?

When the systems are unproductive, inefficient, and varying.

How to Use It Effectively?

Six Sigma uses process mapping, and it should be done by involving all concerned stakeholders to identify inefficient or non-value-added steps, which are affecting the service and aiding action planning for quality improvement.

- Define the problem, specify the target group, identify goals, and plan the target process.
- Measure: decide the criteria or indicators to be quantified and find a way to measure them. Then collect the required baseline data and measure again after changes have been applied.
- Analyze: identify the gaps between actual performance and defined goals, find the causes of those gaps, determine how process inputs affect output, and aim for further improvement.

- Improve: formulate potential solutions, identify the most feasible solutions for implementation, trial hypothetical solutions, and implement the improvement solutions.
- Control: develop a detailed solution monitoring strategy, observe implemented solutions for success, and update on a periodical basis.

13.2 Continue Development in Healthcare Quality

The credible reports from the Institute of Medicine and other organizations have raised significant awareness of medical errors, patient safety, and quality concerns in the medical system. Patient safety remains the top priority as healthcare professionals are becoming more and more aware, and quality improvement will be the focus for many coming years. Also, medical schools, regulatory bodies, and healthcare accreditation bodies around the world have adopted various initiatives to bridge the gap and improve patient safety and quality. It is essential that healthcare providers make every possible effort to instill knowledge of quality improvement in their healthcare workers to improve patient safety and quality of care.

References

1. Codman EA. The product of a hospital. Surg Gynecol Obstet. 1914;18:491-496
2. Donabedian, A. (1988). "The quality of care: how can it be assessed?". JAMA. 260 (12): 1743–8. https://doi.org/10.1001/jama.1988.03410120089033.
3. Shewhart W. Economic Control of Quality of Management Product. New York: D. Van Nostrand Co.; 1931
4. Deming, W. Edwards. Out of the Crisis (MIT Press) (1986:pp. 23-24)
5. Crosby PB. Quality is Free: The Art of Making Quality Certain. New York: McGraw-Hill: 1979.
6. Juran JM. Juran on Leadership for Quality. New York: Free Press; 1989.
7. Chassin MR, Galvin RW. The urgent need to improve healthcare quality. Institute of Medicine National Roundtable on Healthcare Quality. JAMA. 1998;280(11): 1000-1005
8. Committee on Quality of Healthcare in America, Institute of Medicine. Kohn LT, Corrigan JM, Donaldson MS, eds. To Err is Human: Building a Safer Healthcare System. Washington DC: National Academies Press; 2000.
9. Improving the safety and quality of nursing care through standardized operating procedures in Bosnia and Herzegovina - PubMed (nih.gov)
10. Batalden P, Davidoff F. Teaching quality improvement: the devil is in the details. JAMA 2007;298:1059–61.
11. NHS Institute for Innovation and improvement, 2008 A conventional model of process mapping.
12. Key Topics in Healthcare Management: Understanding the Big Picture By Robert Jones, Radcliffe Publishing, 2007
13. Institute for Healthcare Improvement, 2004. Failure modes and effects analysis
14. HFMEA Steps reference - Cohen, M. R., & American Pharmacists Association. (2006). Medication errors. Washington, DC: American Pharmacists Association.

Chapter 14
Barrier-Free Healthcare Design for Patients with Disabilities

Moonis Mirza, Tarun Goyal, and Lata Goyal

14.1 Introduction

The terms "access to healthcare" and "barriers to access" have been metaphorically used to define the overall appropriateness of the healthcare system to satisfy the needs of an individual or a region timely and effectively. Accessibility may refer to the utilization of services in terms of availability of the right technology, supplies, cultural barriers, affordability, acceptability, relevance, or equity. An essential part of accessibility refers to the ability of a person with special needs to navigate the existing healthcare building to avail the services being provided. Any facility that cannot meet the physical needs of a disabled patient by overcoming its architectural barriers cannot deliver barrier-free healthcare.

Hospitals are places that see a proportionately much larger number of temporarily or permanently disabled persons than any other public buildings. Denying this vulnerable population their right to equal accessibility fails our commitment to social justice and human rights. The World Report on Disability transcribes that 60% of physically challenged individuals fail to fully utilize health facilities due to architectural barriers [1]. Disabled-friendly hospital design has been identified as a universal concern. The Global Burden of Disease 2004 projected that 15.3% of the

M. Mirza
Department of Hospital Administration, All India Institute of Medical Sciences, Bathinda, India

T. Goyal (✉)
Department of Orthopaedics, All India Institute of Medical Sciences, Bathinda, India

L. Goyal
Department of Dentistry, All India Institute of Medical Sciences, Bathinda, India

D. Bhatia et al. (eds.), *A Guide to Hospital Administration and Planning*,
https://doi.org/10.1007/978-981-19-6692-7_14

population are facing "moderate or severe disability" and 2.9% of the population have "severe disability" [2]. The female gender, old age, and people belonging to low socioeconomic status are more likely to have a disability [3]. In India, 2.21% of the total population lives with disability [4], with the prevalence of mild, moderate, and severe disability estimated at 17%, 35%, and 16%, respectively [5].

Barrier-free healthcare building design should be viewed from the eye of a disabled patient that expects and has a right to access healthcare with ease and comfort. The patient pathway is one of the best guides that can be considered to cover the complete journey of any patient, right from entry to exit of that patient. Based on various national guidelines for barrier-free healthcare, multiple sections have been discussed.

14.2 Need for Barrier-Free Healthcare

2030 Agenda for Sustainable Development by the United Nations explicitly mentions people with disabilities 11 times in the document, including the 4th, 8th, 10th, 11th, and 17th Sustainable Development Goals (SDGs) [6]. "Disabled-inclusive development across the world" is one of the main priority areas of the 2030 Agenda for Sustainable Development Goals. Human Rights, Disability, and Sustainable Development Goals had established a strong link in-between that can be undoubtedly anticipated. A study from Ethiopia presented that 74.6% of its disabled population faced problems, with at least one access barrier to healthcare services [7]. Another study from South Africa highlighted the correlation between health outcomes and access to health services for people with disabilities [8]. It has been documented that access-related problems, particularly in low-income countries, may compromise the targets set by the United Nations in the Millennium Development Goals [9]. Alkawai et al. [10] showed that 88% of disabled patients needed somebody to accompany them to a healthcare facility. Mean ratings for satisfaction with hospital services were significantly lower in disabled populations. Parking for the disabled was reported as non-satisfactory in 52% of the patients, 49.8% were dissatisfied with the lounge, 51.3% were dissatisfied with wheelchair services, and 45% were unhappy with toilets for the physically disabled [9]. Out of 67 primary health centers included in a study in India, only 25 (36%) had accessible doors for the disabled [11]. No PHCs had height-adjustable examination tables or disabled-friendly toilets. Even the best healthcare facilities are behind in the design plan suitable for differently abled patients [11].

14.3 Design Considerations in Barrier-Free Healthcare

14.3.1 Anthropometric Requirements for Accessible Inbuilt Environment for Patients with Disability

Space Required for Mobility Devices

Walkways, patient examination areas, toilets, etc. should have sufficient space to provide unhindered mobility for the disabled patients using assistive devices for walking or a wheelchair.

Wheelchair

Overall length, width, lap height, etc. of a standard wheelchair should be known to a hospital architect/planner while designing/planning the pathway and user controls in a building for patients with disability.

A reach zone for wheelchair users can be defined as the area around the wheelchair that a user can access while sitting on a wheelchair. All the amenities in a disabled-friendly building should be planned considering the forward, side, and standard reach zone, touch, and grasp reach forwards and sideways. In any case, amenities to be contacted by a wheelchair user should not be more than its maximum reach zone in a sitting position (Fig. 14.1).

Crutch Users and White Cane Users

A minimum of 900 mm of clear vast pathway space without any obstruction on the ground, at least 300 mm, is required for movement (Fig. 14.2).

Vision Zone

Placement of signages should be based on the vision zone of a wheelchair holder and should be placed between 900 and 1800 mm, with the smallest letters of signage being not less than 15 mm.

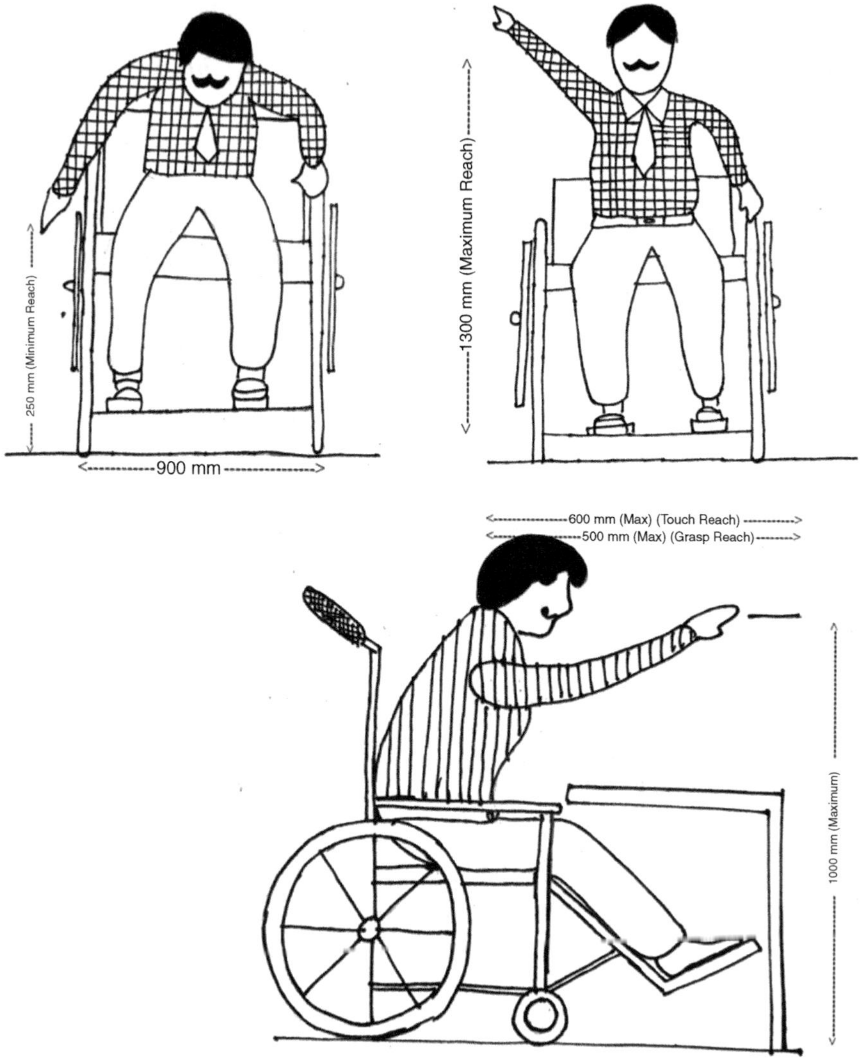

Fig. 14.1 Reach zones of a wheelchair use

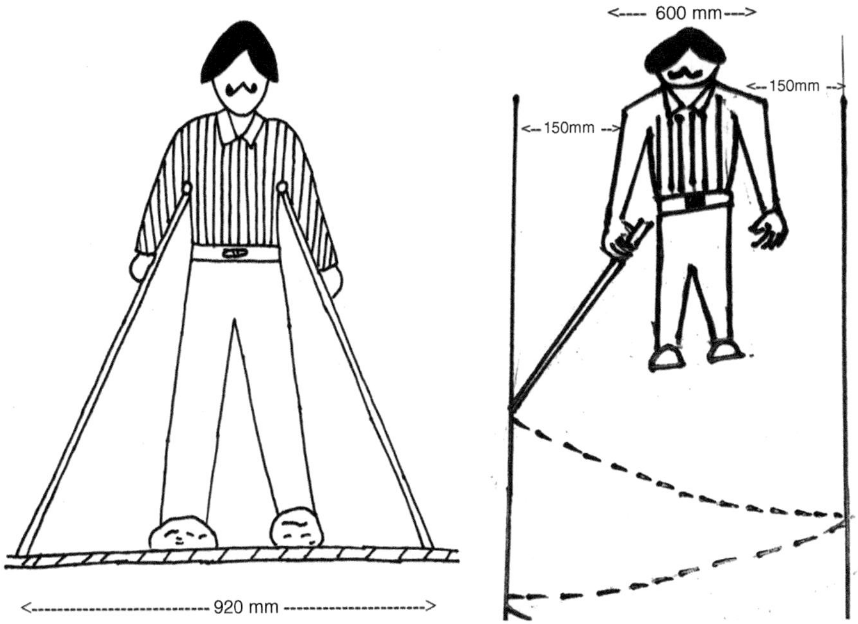

Fig. 14.2 Crutch users and white cane users

Height of Controls

Reach zones for persons with a disability need to be well versed by any hospital planner. A person sitting in a wheelchair cannot reach the same controls as an average person without a disability. A specific range of height from the ground is thus essential to understand and implement for creating a barrier-free environment.

Height of controls from floor level	400–1200 mm
Height for switches (power)	400–500 mm
Height for switches (light)	800–1200 mm
Height of door handles	800–1100 mm
Opening controls for windows	800–1100 mm
Space required under the counter for wheelchair footrest	350 mm deep

Entrance/Exit Door

- Minimum width of entrance/exit door: 900 mm
  Minimum front-approach doorway space: 600 mm
- Minimum latch side-approach doorway space: 1250 mm

14.3.2 External Area

Walkways

Smooth, non-slip, complex, and leveled surface suitable for walking and wheeling with curbs for level change should be provided. Walkways exceeding 60 m approx. in length should be provided with a rest area adjacent to the walk in the form of benches/resting seats. A ramp should accompany the stepped path and stair along with handrails. The landings of steps, as well as ramps, should not have any waterlogging. It shall be drained correctly to avoid water flowing down steps and ramps.

Barriers and Obstacles

Obstacles, gratings, maintenance holes, signs mounted on walls, columns, or freestanding supports along the walking path shall be avoided. Special care should be taken to leave proper headroom, a clear walkway, and protruding objects.

Tactile Ground Surface Indicators (TGSI)

Tactile guiding and warning tiles/blocks should be placed along the entire length of the route and in open spaces to guide blind and vision-impaired patients.

Width of the Walkways

For two-way and one-way traffic, the width of pathways should be at least 1.8 m and 1.2 m, respectively, with a passing and turning space at convenient intervals (25 m approx.).

Lighting for Walkways

Proper illumination focusing on walkways should be planned.

14.3.3 Designated Accessible Parking Space

Location

It should be planned near the building entrance, with curbs connecting the pathway. Curb is a small ramp built to accommodate level changes between footpaths and pavement towards vehicular area/road (Fig. 14.3).

Several dedicated disabled parking per number of standard parking spaces:

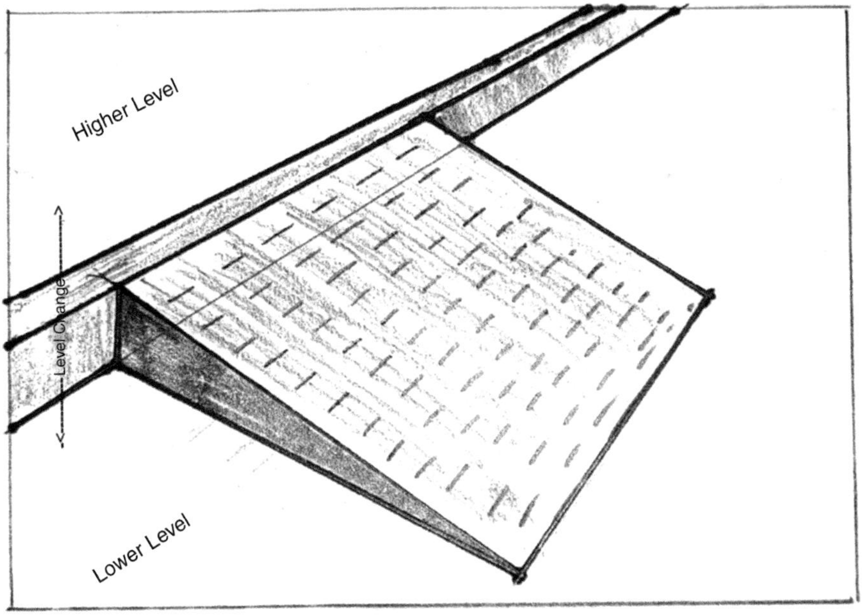

Fig. 14.3 Curb connecting the pathway accommodating level changes

Parking space	No. of accessible designated parking spaces for disabled
10	01
25	02
50	03
100	04
200	06
Above 200	One for each additional 100 parking spaces shall be provided

Signage for Parking

International symbol of accessibility should be displayed at the entrances to a car parking area.

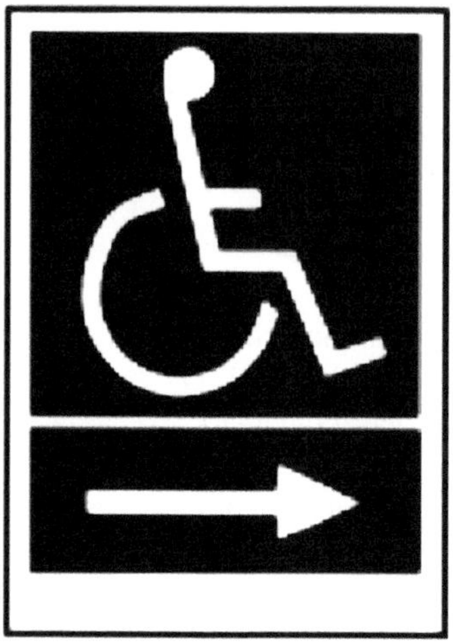

Space Dimensions and Surface Requirements

Planning the space for disabled parking should accommodate a large car with a wheelchair transfer area. The area should be marked in yellow or white. The level surface for disabled parking should be without an aeration slab. Also, parking should be covered with a shelter to protect from rain and sunlight.

14.3.4 Approach to the Building

Approach to any building, particularly a healthcare building, is a combination of various elements that work in sync and give overall accessibility to disabled patients. There should be proper signages to locate accessible entrances. Marked drop-off points for vehicles should be near the accessible entrance. A tactile ground surface indicator (TGSI) should be provided on the pathway. Curbs should be installed in case of any level change.

14.3.5 Access at Entrance and Within the Building

A leveled and firm pathway for one-way or two-way traffic of persons with disability should be planned. An accessible route to lifts should be available. A tactile floor plan should be provided at the entrance for visually compromised patients. In addition to the tactile pavers (TGSI), beepers may be placed at entrances to help visually compromised patients locate accessible entrances. Evenly diffused and glare-free lighting in the corridor should be planned. The door opening in the gallery should not open outwards except for accessible toilets and service ducts.

Doors

Easily visible doors for visually impaired patients that should be easy to manure, with visual contrast to the leading edges and frame, should be placed, and at least 900 mm clear space for wheelchair and crutch users with wheelchair maneuvering space should be planned. Location of latch and handles should be consistent throughout the building. Glass doors should be glazed at hand and eye level for easy identification for visually compromised patients.

Handrails and Grab Bars

Materials used should be able to withstand the weight of a heavy man. Tactile marking should be provided at the beginning and the end of handrails. A continuous both-sided handrail should be provided at a height between 700 and 900 mm.

14.3.6 Level Changes

Ramps, staircases, lifts, and escalators should be practically planned and designed for vertical circulation and level changes so that it is easily identifiable and usable for persons with disability. Ramps should be planned with stairs with a leveled platform at the end. Tactile warning blocks are placed at the ramps' beginning and end. Ramps should be provided with regular landings for rest. The number of steps in a stair riser should not be more than 12 per flight, with a maximum riser of 150 mm. Stairs should be provided with handrails, tactile floor indicators, and color contrast between landing and steps for visibility.

At least one lift accessible to disabled patients should be planned in a multistorey building, with an international symbol of accessibility placed on the lift and its accessible route. Lift should have a space to maneuver a wheelchair. Braille/tactile operating buttons inside and outside lifts should be placed according to the height of a wheelchair user. Emergency communication and alarm system should be installed in the accessible lifts.

14.3.7 Operating Controls and Devices

Operating controls for fire alarm call points, fire extinguishers, meter indicators, socket outlets, horizontal pull bars, toilet room doors, vertical handles, and lever-type handles should be installed at an accessible height. All-important controls should have a braille/tactile raised surface. Drinking water facilities should be wall mounted with clear floor space for wheelchair users.

14.3.8 Seating Spaces

Seating facilities at a regular interval should be provided for waiting and rest. Seating space should be planned not to obstruct the common circulation area.

14.3.9 Toilet Rooms and Sanitary Rooms

Toilets for persons with disability should be located in a way that the traveling distance should not exceed more than 30 m. Proper tactile signage to indicate male and female toilets should be placed at an accessible height for wheelchair users. International symbols of accessibility should be marked at the most visible location near the toilet entrance. Space inside the toilets should have a clear maneuvering space for wheelchair users. Urinals for wheelchair users should be placed in male toilets. Doors for accessible toilets should have a two-way opening. Operating controls for emergency assistance alarm, water tank, soap dispensers, waste bins, etc. should be placed at an accessible height for wheelchair users.

14.3.10 Reception Areas, Counters, Desks, and Ticket Offices

While planning reception counters for wheelchair users, special consideration should be taken for accessible height and approach for both receptionist and the visitor. At least one counter should be fitted with a hearing enhancement system with appropriate signage. Approaches to the counters should be marked with a tactile ground surface for easy identification. Proper illumination should be provided to facilitate lip-reading.

14.3.11 Lighting

Glare-free lights illuminating accessible routes should be uniformly planned to coordinate with the natural lighting and facilitate patients for easy moments during the day or nighttime.

14.3.12 Emergency Evacuation in Buildings

Planning an emergency evacuation route at the time of internal disasters like fire and earthquakes should be by fire safety norms, particularly in a high-rise building. Fire signage, emergency lighting, and evacuation plans should be statistically placed.

14.3.13 Signage

Signages for persons with disabilities should focus on the format of two senses, i.e., audio and visual indicators. For patients with visual impairment, audible and tactile wayfinding solutions should be planned. Public address systems, auditable warning signals, and lift voice announcement systems should be meticulously designed in an acoustically ambient environment. For the visually disabled, tactile signage including braille signages, and tactile floor plan should be placed at key locations. Visual information needs to be correctly displayed with adequate contrast between letters and background for patients with hearing impairment. A specific size by the viewing distance should be used. Signages are mainly divided into orientation signs (floor directories, plans, models, etc.), directional signs (information related to route plans and arrows between two points), functional signs (explanatory information), informative signs (name of departments, doctors, etc.), and emergency exit signages (evacuation plans, exit signs in accordance to "fire safety" guidelines). The use of universal pictograms and letters helps better orient wayfinding for persons with disabilities and all. Placing of signages at specific heights and locations with proper size and font with a minimum of 70 points light reflection value should be planned. Avoid using excess information that can confuse a person rather than guiding them.

14.3.14 Accessible Medical Equipment

All people have a right to receive equal medical service, whether standard or disabled. Planning of equipment and examination rooms keeping in view the patients with disabilities is essential. Poorly planned medical equipment can be a barrier to individuals with disabilities. Height-adjustable exam tables and chairs, height-flexible radiologic equipment, weighing scales for wheelchair users, and examination room patient lifts should be planned.

14.4 International Guidelines Related to Disabled-Friendly Infrastructure

Internationally, "disability considerations for infrastructure programs" [12] summarize evidence about the effect of non-accessible infrastructure on the disabled. The United Nations Convention on the Rights of Persons with Disabilities (CRPD) [13] defines disability as "... an evolving concept that results from the interaction between persons with impairments and attitudinal and environmental barriers that hinders their full and effective participation in society on an equal basis with others."

The following national guidelines have discussed what is required to make a building barrier free:

1. "Guidelines and space standards for barrier-free building environment for disabled and elderly persons" (1998) [14] published by the Central Public Works Department
2. "Design Manual for a Barrier-Free Built Environment" (2004) [15] published by the UNNATI-Organisation for Development Education and Handicap International (HI)
3. "Handbook on Barrier-Free and Accessibility" (2014) [16] issued by the Central Public Works Department
4. "Harmonized Guidelines and Space Standards for Barrier-Free Built Environment for Persons with Disability and Elderly Persons" (2016) [17] issued by the Minister of Urban Development, Government of India
5. "Model Building Bye-Laws—2016" [18], issued by the Ministry of Urban Development, Government of India, 2016
6. "National Building code 2016" [19]

   Despite existing guidelines, emphasis on norms of building design for barrier-free access to public buildings is lacking in India.

14.5 National Guidelines and Laws Related to Disabled Persons

Laws have been formulated worldwide [20–22] to support the disabled population. In India, Chapter V, clause no. 25, (1) (b) of the Rights of Persons with Disabilities Act, 2016 [23], clearly mentions "barrier-free access in all parts of Government and private hospitals and other healthcare institutions and centers." Also, Chapter VIII, clause 45, (1) writes, "All existing public buildings shall be made accessible by the rules formulated by the Central Government within a period not exceeding five years from the date of notification of such rules: Provided that the Central Government may grant an extension of time to the States on a case-to-case basis for adherence to this provision depending on their state of preparedness and other related parameters." Clause 45 (2) says, "The appropriate Government and the local authorities shall formulate and publish an action plan based on prioritization, for providing accessibility in all their buildings and spaces providing essential services such as all primary health centers, civil hospitals, schools, railway stations, and bus stops."

14.6 Gap Analysis

Most of the guidelines focus mainly on general buildings, not particularly on special healthcare infrastructure needs. Also, most people involved in architectural planning have experience in designing a general public building rather than a hospital. During the initial planning of any healthcare facility, the end users, like hospital administrators and doctors, are involved only in the broad medical needs of the building, like equipment and operation theaters; micro-planning of the building design that mainly focuses on the needs of a disabled population is often ignored. Engineers and architects are not the final users of the healthcare building, nor do they converse about the unique needs of a disabled population. Thus, they have a limited vision for casting the needs of a disabled population using the structure in the future. Also, the existing guidelines are so complexly written that it is practically impossible for the user organizations to assess the current building or include barrier-free design in a greenfield project. Lack of knowledge and lack of user-friendly tools that can be used to evaluate the building design to be barrier free are possibly two factors for the omission of disabled-friendly methods in most hospital buildings. Thus, the disabled population is left with no choice but to accept what is offered to them.

14.7 Limitations in the Implementation of Laws

The Persons with Disabilities Act does not clarify the gaps in a building design for disabled-friendly healthcare. It further does not explain the financial commitment of local governments to include the changes required in new and existing buildings. The National Human Rights Commission, in its reports, writes that due to a lack of clarity in the funding resources, organizations find an easy way out to escape from the implementation of disabled-friendly building design. Many of the recommendations made in the Act come with the condition "within the limits of their [the states'] economic capacity" [24]. Hence, many authorities argue that they do not have the assets to provide proper facilities for disabled people. Another unsung challenge is the lack of knowledge regarding the need for a disabled-friendly design.

14.8 Recommendations

This chapter concludes with a few recommendations to achieve the goal of barrier-free healthcare design:

- Gap analysis: Large-scale studies need to be planned to evaluate the gaps in barrier-free healthcare design in the existing buildings and the newly constructed field projects in healthcare.
- **Multidimensional and intersectoral participation**: There is a need to bring different stakeholders on the same platform during the planning of a hospital design. The center of attention should be the end users, i.e., disabled persons, doctors, and other healthcare providers. Engineering and architectural experts to be involved in planning hospital buildings should know the essential components of an accessible building design and incorporate them into the plan.
- The components of a disabled-friendly building design should be categorized into **vital, essential, and desirable** (VED) categories. At least **vital gaps** should be rectified in all existing buildings. For new healthcare buildings, all three parts, i.e., **vital, essential, and desirable** (VED) categories, should be included in the building design.
- Like other building byelaws and essential clearances (e.g., air, water, and fire clearance) for a new building design, barrier-free healthcare design should be included as the essential minimum requirement for all the latest healthcare buildings. Building plans should be approved only after scrutinizing the building designs against the **vital, essential, and desirable criteria**.

14.9 Conclusion

It appears that this struggle for the rights of the disabled for accessible healthcare shall continue for some more time. Academicians from the medical sciences, engineering, and architecture seem to have filled their roles by creating an awareness and laying down guidelines for a barrier-free healthcare design. The onus of responsibility to look after these people now lies in the hands of statutory authorities. Executive and judicial commitment to the cause can bring a new ray of hope to our differently abled people in need to approach their hospitals.

References

1. World Health Organization (WHO). World Report on Disability 2011. Geneva: World Health Organization; 2011. ISBN-13: 978-92-4-156418-2.
2. World Health Organization (WHO). The Global Burden of Disease. Update 2004. Available on:https://www.who.int/healthinfo/global_burden_disease/GBD_report_2004update_full.pdf.
3. World Health Organization (WHO) – Western Pacific Region. Disability-Inclusive Health Services Toolkit. A Resource for Health Facilities in the Western Pacific Region. 2020. Available on: https://iris.wpro.who.int/bitstream/handle/10665.1/14639/9789290618928-eng.pdf.
4. Census of India 2011 Report on Post Enumeration Survey. Available on: https://censusindia.gov.in/2011Census/pes/Pesreport.pdf
5. World Health Organization. (WHO). Brief model disability survey: result for India, Lao People's Democratic Republic, and Tajikistan: executive summary, 2019. Available on: https://apps.who.int/iris/handle/10665/330013. License: CC BY-NC-SA 3.0 IGO
6. International Disability and Development Consortium (IDDC), International Disability Alliance (IDA). The 2030 Agenda the Inclusion of Persons with Disabilities. Comprehensive Guide. Available on: https://www.cbm.org/fileadmin/user_upload/Publications/2030_Agenda_Comprehensive_Guide_for_persons_with_disabilities.pdf
7. Tesfaye T, Woldesemayat EM, Chea N, Wachamo D. Accessing healthcare services for people with physical disabilities in Hawassa city administration, Ethiopia: A cross-sectional study. Risk Manag Healthc Policy. 2021 Sep 24; 14: 3993-4002.
8. Moodley J, Ross E. Inequities in health outcomes and access to health care in South Africa: a comparison between persons with and without disabilities. Disabil Soc 2015; 30(4): 630-44.
9. Eide AH, Mannan H, Khogali M, et al. Perceived barriers for accessing health services among individuals with disability in four African countries. PLoS One. 2015 May 20; 10(5): e0125915.
10. Alkawai FM, Alowayyed AS. Barriers in accessing care services for physically disabled in a hospital setting in Riyadh, Saudi Arabia, cross-sectional study. J Commun Hosp Intern Med Perspect 2017 Jun 6; 7(2): 82-6.
11. Nischith KR, Bhargava M, Akshaya KM. Physical accessibility audit of primary health centers for people with disabilities: an on-site assessment from Dakshina Kannada district in Southern India. J Family Med Prim Care 2018 Nov-Dec; 7(6): 1300-3.
12. Agarwal A, Steele A. Disability considerations for infrastructure programmes. 2016 Mar 8. https://doi.org/10.12774/eod_hd.march2016.agarwaletal. Available on: https://assets.publishing.service.gov.uk/media/57a08954ed915d3cfd0001c4/EoD_HDYr3_21_40_March_2016_Disability_Infrastructure.pdf

13. United Nations. Convention on the Rights of Persons with Disabilities and Optional Protocol, 2007, preamble (e). Available on: https://www.un.org/disabilities/documents/convention/convoptprot-e.pdf. [Last accessed: 2021 Dec 16].
14. Government of India – Central Public Works Department (CPWD). Guidelines and Space Standards for Barrier-Free Environment. CPWD; 1998. Available on: https://cpwd.gov.in/publication/aged&disabled.PDF
15. UNNATI-Organisation for Development Education and Handicap International (HI). Design Manual for Barrier. Free Built Environment. India, Reprint 2006 Nov. Available on: http://www.unnati.org/pdfs/manuals/barrier-free-built-environment.pdf
16. Government of India - Central Public Works Department (CPWD). Handbook of Barrier-Free and Accessibility. CPWD; 2014. Available on: https://cpwd.gov.in/Publication/HandbookonBarrier.pdf
17. Government of India - Central Public Works Department. Harmonised Guidelines and Space Standards for Barrier-Free Built Environment for persons with Disability and Elderly Persons'. CPWD; 2016. Available on: https://cpwd.gov.in/publication/harmonisedguidelinesdreleasedon23rdmarch2016.pdf. [Last accessed: 2021 Dec 16].
18. Government of India – Ministry of Urban Development. Model Building Bye-Laws- 2016. http://mohua.gov.in/upload/uploadfiles/files/MBBL.pdf
19. National Building Code of India (NBC) (2016). Available on: http://www.bis.org.in/sf/nbc.htm.
20. Waddington L, Lawson A. Disability and non-discrimination law in the European Union. Publications Office of the European Union; 2009. Available: https://tandis.odihr.pl/bitstream/20.500.12389/20813/1/06267.pdf
21. International Disability Laws Index [Internet]. [Last accessed: 2022 Feb 9]. Available from: https://dredf.org/legal-advocacy/international-disability-rights/international-laws/.
22. United Nations Enable - Disability Laws and Acts by Country/Area [Internet]. [Last accessed: 2022 Mar 1]. Available from: https://www.un.org/development/desa/disabilities/disability-laws-and-acts-by-country-area.html
23. Ministry of Law and Justice (Legislative Department). The Rights of Persons with Disabilities Act, Dec 27 2016, No. 49. India Code Digital Repository of All Central and State Acts. Available on: https://www.indiacode.nic.in/handle/123456789/2155?locale=en
24. Mohit A, Pillai M, Rungta P. Rights of the Disabled. New Dheli, India: National Human Rights Commission; 2006. Available on: https://nhrc.nic.in/sites/default/files/DisabledRights_1.pdf

Chapter 15
Technological Advancements and Challenges in the Management of Hospital Functions and Public Health

Sohini Paul and Josephine Princey

15.1 Introduction

Hospital settings form an essential part of a societal and medical institution, the function of which is to provide for the population's complete healthcare, both curative and preventive, and whose outpatient services reach out to the family and its home environment; the hospital is also a center for the training of health worker and for biosocial research.

According to hospital definition, any district hospital is usually said to be the region's primary health care facility with a greater number of intensive care beds and extra beds for patients who need long term care. Trauma centres, children's hospitals, rehabilitation hospitals, and seniors'(geriatric) hospitals for coping with particular medical conditions such as psychiatric care are also examples of specialised hospitals and several other disease categories.

At few hospitals, there are outpatient departments separately and a chronic care center separately, wherein specialty units and common support units like radiology, pharmacy, and pathology are available. A drastic and a striking progress has taken place in the hospital consciousness and healthcare in the last few decades. The well-said needed services by a hospital that is required for the society can be met at low cost only with necessary thinking given to planning, design, construction, and operation of healthcare facilities. Any expert usually says that when we need to look into future changes, one should plan for a smart hospital necessarily meeting the current needs of the people.

S. Paul (✉)
Exercise Physiology and Ergonomics Laboratory, Faculty of Health and Wellness, Sri Sri University, Cuttack, India
e-mail: sohini.p@srisriuniversity.edu.in

J. Princey
KG College of Health Sciences, Coimbatore, Tamil Nadu, India

D. Bhatia et al. (eds.), *A Guide to Hospital Administration and Planning*,
https://doi.org/10.1007/978-981-19-6692-7_15

Anytime availability, anytime accessibility, and highly qualified healthcare to patients are ensured by the start of better hospital management. Without any genuine clinical procedures and systems in place, it is hard to achieve the abovementioned needs and excellent care of hospitals and clinics. Hospitals and clinics consist of manifold settings that have various departments, specialties, teams, schedules, data collection, and so many other aspects to manage. Almost all types of organizations have a similar management function that revolves around planning, objectives of the individual, objectives of the institution, policy and strategy of the hospital, rules and procedures of a hospital, various health programs of the hospital, priorities of the hospital, and patient experience. In any field when one has to achieve the desired goals, the required activity is organizing and forecasting planning. Without planning, nothing can be achieved in a well-defined manner. Any successful hospital is built on the best planning methods, good design, and construction with excellent administration. A hospital must be staffed with a competent and adequate number of efficient doctors, nurses, and other professionals. The main aim of creating this hospital need with advance learning and planning must be useful to serve people in a right way.

In planning for a new hospital, a complete functioning of all requirements needed for the people must be implemented in the study management. All the other types of construction and building totally differ in the complex functional relationship that prevails among various parts of the hospital. Planning also involves the process of currently appearing issues and existing trends required for the growth of hospitals. It is not enough in contributing the necessary environment for patients and caregivers, but one should look into the want of the visitors. It is very crucial to scrutinize the upcoming issues, study the challenges, appreciate the spotlight trends, and learn the various important options available for planning, designing, and constructing a hospital.

The present development in technology collides with leading processes for design, construction, and operations, imparting a superior environment that strengthens the occupant comforts and productivity while decreasing the energy consumption and operations staffing. There is a new concept of Go Green that is used sparingly and which means different for everyone. To preserve energy, decrease pollution, and save money are the steps involved in going green. The principle of hospital designing includes shaping of the building or object that must be initially based on its intended purposes or function.

The sequences and the important aspects of planning a hospital indulge more with the society interest over single-person interest, preventive care over curative care, care provided to the weaker sections of the people, and city over village to mention a few. Planning of regionalization in healthcare is about to bring necessary and appropriate allocation and togetherness of resources according to the common population needs in health and community engagement in order to improve the quality and optimize delivery.

When we need to serve patients adequately, hospitals must meet the two fundamental requirements: definitely, it should be in size and proportion where the owners or promoters should be able to construct and operate. A sound structural planning, economic viability, effective society orientation, and high-quality patient care are the requirements for the guiding principles for a hospital planning. For a smooth undergoing of hospitals, ancillary care planning, plan towards revenue generation, recurrent cost, and financial planning are very important. The rest of the planning includes data collection, feasibility study, land acquisition project and implementation, building planning, and strategic planning.

Hospital commissioning is the process that ensures that every building system in a facility is completed with predetermined criteria. It is defined by the ASHRAE Standards and Guidelines as "a quality-focused process for improving project delivery as the process ensures that all commissioned systems and assemblies are planned, designed, installed, tested, operated, and maintained in accordance with the Owner's Project Requirements." To attain the proprietor's requirements as expected by the owner of the building and as designed by the architects and engineers, the process of verifying an emerging building construction involves subsystems for plumbing, electrical, and fire safety; building envelops; interior systems; co-generation; utility plants; sustainable systems; lighting; wastewater; controls; and building security. This is the procedure by which an equipment, facility, or plant (already installed, yet to install) is checked to confirm if the functions are according to its design objectives or specifications.

To culminate with the planning of hospital management, telecommunications must be fulfilled. Safety is one of the vital factors which have to be noted while planning for a hospital, and all the clinical needs should be taken into account. Henceforth, the importance of the role of hospital staffs in building and design must also be considered.

15.2 Management in Terms of Technology

To enhance care and prevent inadvertent outcomes, new measures can be brought into health information technology (IT) with a multiplex adaptive healthcare system.

The vital challenging aspect in a clinical setting is the use and safety of health IT. The technical society is making an attempt to clearly understand the multiplex connections between people, environment, conditions, processes, and technologies as they try to safely grow, implement, and sustain the present new digital infrastructure. The current proof reveals that in patient settings care can be made safer with health IT and can also bring in new safety measures and ideas after implementing new technologies [1]. We spot out and connect nine key, short-term challenges to help healthcare institutions, health-related IT developer researchers, policy makers, and funders focus their achievement on health information technology and patient-related safety. As per the stages and life cycle of the health information technology, the challenges are related to (a) enlarging models, methods, and tools to enable risk assessment; (b) enhancing regular user of interface design features and functions; (c) establishing the security of software in an interfaced network—enabled clinical environment; (d) executing a technique for unambiguous patient identification; (e) improving safety by promoting and implementing decision support; (f) finding out the action to safely control information technology system transitions; (g) progressive real-time methods to permit automated surveillance and monitoring of system performance and security; (h) beginning the cultural and legal framework to allow sharing of information about hazards and adverse events; and (i) growing models and methods for patients to improve health information technology.

Telehealth or digital healthcare is a comprehensive, multifaceted conception that comprises models from a connection between healthcare and technology. Telehealth or digital health applies digital transformation to the healthcare field, installing software, hardware, and services. Digital health is a regulation that adds in digital care programs and technologies with health, healthcare, living, and society to enhance the efficiency of healthcare delivery and to make medicines highly personalized and precise.

Technology with healthcare-coalesced digital health aspires to offer advanced and economical medical-related facilities. By employing innovative technology such as apps related to health, real-time data, ingestible sensors, and wearables, patients can now remain fit enough in an easy way. The application of information and communications technology to give away digital health interventions to prevent disease and improve quality of life is not a present concept. The related technology continues to grow in importance and advances in the face of world concerns linked to aging, child illness and mortality, epidemics and pandemics, high costs, and effects of poverty and racial discrimination on access to healthcare—digital health platforms and health systems. Additionally igniting the fire of change, the COVID-19 pandemic has helped to fuel the ongoing digital transformation in healthcare. According to Forrester Research, the highly influenced pandemic technologies include patient-facing tools, such as tethered online personal health records, symptom checkers, patient portals, telehealth, and remote patient-monitoring tools.

According to many insights, digital health allows more than just technologies and tools; it also views "radically compatible data, artificial intelligence (AI), and open, secure platforms as central to the promise of more consumer-focused, prevention-oriented care." By using smartphone, mobile app that is connected to pacemaker devices can be designed to securely and wirelessly transmit data to a patient's network, giving patients better insight into the health data from the pacemakers and transmitting the health information to their physicians.

mHealth, including wearables, apps, and mobile technology that provide access to healthcare support and monitoring, is experiencing growth, particularly for helping manage long-term, chronic conditions. The COVID-19 pandemic has led to a rise in demand for personal health monitoring via wearables, which straddles the line between consumers and medical devices [2]. Vendors of wearable devices have added features for heart rate variability, pulse oximeters, electrocardiography, and continuous glucose monitoring. Another significant application is blockchain-based electronic medical records (EMRs), which aim to reduce the time needed to access patient information while improving data quality and interoperability. Blockchain's benefits—access security, data privacy, and scalability—are attractive in digital healthcare. Using AI in the healthcare applications can augment human decision-making by automating and speeding up previously labor-intensive tasks. Many hospitals, for example, use AI-based patient monitoring tools to collect data and treat a patient based on real-time reports. In medical imaging, the use of AI can reduce the number of clicks needed to perform a task and determine the next steps based on context. Another AI application, digital twins, can be used to model medical devices and patients and show how devices would work under actual conditions. Augmented reality, which integrates digital information with the user's environment in real time, is applicable in patient and doctor education, surgical visualization, and disease simulation. Big data draws information from all these health systems and applications and poses both benefits and challenges. The amount of data is massive and continues to proliferate.

15.3 Critical Challenges in Digital Health

15.3.1 Factors Related to the Society

Even with technology being the heart of any digital health system, the necessary transformations cannot be seen purely through a technological lens. Technologies offered through digital systems have to deliver affordable, easy-to-use healthcare solution to an extending and aging mass in which current technologies are often slow to be adopted and accepted by the general populace. Components that influence the lack of acceptance include regulatory factors, such as unreliability focusing on digital health policies and legislation as well as perceived lack of accountability within the commercial sector. Fewer levels of digital and health literacy seen in common population, mostly in the elderly, seem to be a major contributing factor. Constant efforts are therefore required to normalize the use of digital health at a societal level. Through a far-reaching educational initiative, all the efforts taken must include both health professionals and the common public. The COVID-19 pandemic has spotlighted the necessity to accustom and update the clinical care delivery systems. Concerns have been made to increase the efforts and move away from traditional one-to-one medicine and against remote, digital, solutions that have highlighted as earlier existing socioeconomic gaps between groups of people who can very well get along and use such services or cannot use [2].

Social media in fact plays a major role in encouraging communication between social and family groups during lockdowns, and it has deliberately made it wider and easier to spread medical misinformation across community. The government and societal efforts are urgently necessary to help counter this negative phenomenon. Using remote apps, contact tracing has enabled mass data collection to aid public health and research actions. However, this raises concerns relating to data ownership and other ethical concerns.

15.3.2 Ethical Challenges in Digital Healthcare

According to the researchers, there are six key indicators of ethical challenges in digital healthcare: procedure importance, accountability, confidentiality, autonomy, protection, and integrity. The chief ethical concerns, as observed, were "patients' rights, equity of resources, confidentiality of the patients, patient safety, conflict of interests, ethics of privatization, informed consent, dealing with the opposite sex, beginning and end of life, and healthcare team ethics." The foremost challenging situation in designing, developing, and deploying digital health technologies and its purposes will be to ascertain the constitution of ethics and the criteria for adherence of the codes of ethics. There are numerous structures and directives instituted for dealing with the effect of digital technologies on communities. The mounting healthcare digitization and the augmentation of mobile and IoT tools as devices for data collection may hoist many ethical concerns. In fact, particular tech companies as Amazon, Apple, Google, and Facebook offer apparent resolutions for assembling, accumulating, and examining "health data, which raises issues relating to privacy, data protection, and informed consent."

15.3.3 Solutions Related to Connected Health

"Connected health is a socio-technical model for healthcare management and delivery by using technology to provide healthcare services remotely." It utilizes already accessible end-user expertise for delivering patient care without visiting the hospital or the clinician. Top connected health devices comprise telehealth, distant scrutinizing devices for patients, wearables, protected communication devices for sending messages, applications of mobiles, and automated devices, which assist in connecting patients to their caregivers. "Connected health" is a handy tool since it provides a link among the patient, doctors, and health of a patient. However, more of highly "connected health solution" approaches require higher levels of security as there might be some safety concerns also.

Internet of Things (IOT) which represents a network for communicating comprises devices, software, and admittance services. Therapeutic care and healthiness care in relation to IoT symbolize one of the major alluring implementation domains; thus, IoT and connected health are extremely essential. IoT tools suggest many innovative prospects for clinicians and caregivers to scrutinize not only the patients, but also monitoring of the patients by oneself.

15.3.4 Healthcare Scrutinizing Devices

Distant monitoring of patients is the major purpose of IoT tools of healthcare. In addition to the above monitoring of glucose concentration, heart rate, hygiene of the hands, depression and mood, and Parkinson's disease, connected inhalers and ingestible sensors can also be helpful for the basic treatment of patients. The utilization of IoT tools in bonded health means a larger assistance for anytime anywhere resolutions as well as real-time examination.

15.3.5 Role of Artificial Intelligence (AI)

AI augments the capability of clinicians and caregivers to comprehend the daily routine and requirements of the people; thereby, with the help of the obtained knowledge, they might give a preferable advice, management, and aids for continuing to lead a healthy life [3]. One of the major instances of artificial intelligence in healthcare is thought to be precision medicine. Its institution depends on the huge quantity of records collected from various automation novelties, such as inexpensive genome sequencing, progressive biotechnology, and health sensors employed by patients at home.

It has been suggested that "the ten common applications of AI in healthcare are in the domain of managing medical records and other data, doing repetitive jobs, treatment design, digital consultation, virtual nurses, medication management, drug creation, precision medicine, health monitoring, and healthcare system analysis." The utilization of AI will diminish the hindrances in recognizing and evaluating abnormal medical images. This aspect is particularly very essential in chest and brain imaging where time duration plays a very important role. Based on the reports of GE Healthcare, "over 90% of healthcare data comes from medical imaging and more than 97% of medical images are not analyzed." It is further suggested that "the comprehensive subject of digital health and medicine in the use of AI in orchestrating, storing, and interpreting the huge amounts of data derived from the devices facilitates acute and chronic disease diagnosis and management via AI-enabled acquisition and interpretation of data." This approach will not only help in augmenting the capability to dynamically arbitrate when required but also at the same time diminish the load of both the patient and the healthcare providers when the assessments and results are comparatively uncomplicated. The incidence of AI-based resolutions in digital health strengthens confrontations related to security, accountability, and equitableness. The previous decade has observed the advancement of AI constantly, having a significant role in diverse domains of information such as medicine and robotics. The next decade will witness AI transforming the field of biomedical sciences globally. Deep learning (DL) programs could assist in evolving novel drugs, inferring images, etc.

15.3.6 The Potential of Genomics

Genomic medicine is the learning of the genetic constitution and their interlinkage with human healthiness. The field of genomics explores an individual's genetic particulars that can be utilized to ameliorate the patient's medical care and health-related effects by the help of effectual evaluation and treatment [4].

Genetic profiling is being increasingly accepted by people due to the technological progression, growing demand, and a decline in cost. Genomic medicine has the potentialities of providing evaluation related to genetics for a diseased condition more proficiently and economically. The genetic makeup and variability of an individual enlighten the threat of an ailment and can also be used as a screening tool in various stages of human life for accurately characterizing healthiness states, improving medicine choices that include treatment which might be planned to aim the fundamental illness. Progressions in the domain of genomics are interconnected with health-related challenges. It has been suggested that "for truly personalized medical care, genomics information should be combined with environmental, behavioral, and medical history information."

15.3.7 Technology and the Prospect of Progression of Healthcare

The prospect of healthcare comprises programs that impeccably coalesce information of a patient's medical history; present health status of a patient, insurance, and other financial related information that will assist health professionals in the decision-making process; ameliorate a patient's physical condition; and lessen the expenditure. There is a drastic change in healthcare due to technological developments, from anesthetics and antibiotics to magnetic resonance imaging scanners and radiotherapy. Technology is altering all phases of our lives, and it is creating remarkable alterations in the healthcare industry as well. Innovative progression in the areas of robotics, analytics, and systems for scanning is aiding in making surgeries more specific and precise. Robotic help is lowering the expenditure of patients in hospitals also.

An improvement of day-to-day technology leading to the novel advancement is persistently penetrating our lives. The six ways by which technology is improving healthcare are mentioned below:

1. The internet has turned into a chief foundation of therapeutic database.
2. Healthcare services are being extended to the patients by the use of social network.
3. An enhanced treatment and reduced agony.
4. Advanced care for patient and worker efficiency.
5. Clinicians may be approached effortlessly, and the database may provide assistance to the doctor.
6. Online record databases may precisely speculate the therapeutic trends.

Clinicians can also utilize online databases for easily observing case studies and verify case history of a patient in a detailed manner. An expertise with technology has also facilitated the medical professional to utilize e-mails, videos, and conferencing amenities to discuss with contemporaries globally. The ten ways technology is changing healthcare by the help of AI are "virtual reality, augmented reality, healthcare trackers, wearables and sensors, medical tricorder, genome sequencing, revolutionizing of drug development, nanotechnology, robotics, and 3D printing." Therefore, our duty at this instance is to combat the frights of the future with valor and to embrace the role of technologies in an unbiased manner and also simultaneously organize ourselves for the altering world with likely most of the available information. The field of public health has been sluggish in taking up digital innovations when compared with other segments. In this context, the World Health Organization has issued its primary strategic plan on digital health interventions for supporting healthcare system in 2019. The exceptional humane and financial requirements necessitated by the pandemic are propelling the advancement and implementation of novel digital technologies at a rapid rate.

15.3.8 Implementation of Digital Technologies and Its Effectiveness

Digital technologies may not function in segregation and require to be amalgamated into subsisting community healthcare systems. Digital information resources are required to be amalgamated and made compatible in several platforms, for example with computerized patient documentations. Investigation and utilization of these records will be dependent on the programmed framework and promptness of the public health networks. The harmonization of evaluations is also a confrontation with several symptom description sites in a particular nation, thus risking disintegration. In future times to come, there is urgency for a network-level process for the idea of the perfectly befitting computerized public health structure that bonds "symptom-tracking apps, rapid testing and case isolation, contact tracing and monitoring of aggregated population-mobility levels, access to care, and long-term follow-up and monitoring, with public communication."

Substantiation of the effectuality of any novel tool is required for broader implementation, but as the existing pandemic of COVID-19 is in progress, several digital tools have not yet been critically reviewed, nor been incorporated into public health structures, nor have undergone thorough assessments or been assessed by standardized digital health verification frameworks. "Contact-tracing apps" have been initiated in different countries, but there is presently no confirmation of the efficiency of these applications. Even though it is difficult, owing to the necessity of the pandemic, assessment of the efficacy of the interventions is crucial. The World Health Organization has sketched a draft of its universal approach on digital health for the period of 2020–2024 on 22nd March 2020 [5].

15.4 Conclusion

The COVID-19 pandemic is still continuing, and it is too soon to completely enumerate the additional worth of digital automation in this scenario. Although they provide tools for sustaining a pandemic situation, it cannot be considered as an elixir. The budding concurrence is that digital technologies have a significant task to play in response to the widespread pandemic, harmonizing traditional public health issues and thus in this manner contributing to plummeting the effect of the pandemic in terms of human health and economy. Cost-effectiveness and sustainability will have the need of systems-level techniques in constructing online care pathways digitally, and this will connect the swift and extensive investigation with digital indicator assessors, epidemiological intelligence follow-up studies, etc. The present pandemic situation has substantiated the requirement of not only data sharing but also the necessity of scrupulous evaluation and principled structures with a population involvement to develop together with the budding domain of mobile and digital healthcare [6]. The future of the public health domain is possibly rising digitally, and identifying the significance of digital technology in this domain and in pandemic vigilance planning has turned out to be very vital. There is an essential requirement for the configuration of global policies for the guideline, assessment, and utilization of digital technologies to reinforce the pandemic management and potential readiness for infectious diseases.

References

1. Sittig DF, Wright A, Coiera E, Magrabi F, Ratwani R, Bates DW, Singh H. Current challenges in health information technology-related patient safety. *Health Inform. J.* 2020; 26:181–189. https://doi.org/10.1177/1460458218814893
2. Budd J, Miller BS, Manning EM, Lampos V, Zhuang M, Edelstein M, Rees G, Emery VC, Stevens MM, Keegan N, Short MJ, Pillay D, Manley E, Cox IJ, Heymann D, Johnson AM, McKendry RA. Digital technologies in the public-health response to COVID-19. Nature Medicine 2020; 26: 1183–1192.
3. Cummins N and Schuller BW. Five Crucial Challenges in Digital Health. Front. Digit. Health, 2020 https://doi.org/10.3389/fdgth.2020.536203
4. Moore J. From personalised nutrition to precision medicine: the rise of consumer genomics and digital health. Proc Nutr Soc. 2020; 79:300–10. https://doi.org/10.1017/S0029665120006977
5. World Health Organization. Draft Global Strategy on Digital Health 2020–2024. https://www.who.int/docs/default-source/documents/gs4dhdaa2a9f352b0445bafc79ca799dce4d.pdf?sfvrsn=f112ede5_42 (2020).
6. The Academy of Medical Sciences. Interdisciplinary research in epidemic preparedness and response. https://acmedsci.ac.uk/policy/policy-projects/multidisciplinary-research-in-epidemic-preparedness-and-response (2019).

GPSR Compliance

The European Union's (EU) General Product Safety Regulation (GPSR) is a set of rules that requires consumer products to be safe and our obligations to ensure this.

If you have any concerns about our products, you can contact us on ProductSafety@springernature.com

In case Publisher is established outside the EU, the EU authorized representative is:

Springer Nature Customer Service Center GmbH
Europaplatz 3
69115 Heidelberg, Germany

Batch number: 10732090

Printed by Printforce, the Netherlands